Neurology
Pearls

Neurology Pearls

ANDREW J. WACLAWIK, MD
Associate Professor
Department of Neurology
University of Wisconsin–Madison Medical School
Madison, Wisconsin

THOMAS P. SUTULA, MD, PhD
Detling Professor and Chairman
Department of Neurology
University of Wisconsin–Madison Medical School
Madison, Wisconsin

Series Editors

STEVEN A. SAHN, MD
Professor of Medicine and Director
Division of Pulmonary and
  Critical Care Medicine
Medical University of South Carolina
Charleston, South Carolina

JOHN E. HEFFNER, MD
Professor and Vice Chairman
Department of Medicine
Medical University of South Carolina
Charleston, South Carolina

HANLEY & BELFUS, INC. / Philadelphia

Publisher: HANLEY & BELFUS, INC.
                Medical Publishers
                210 S. 13th Street
                Philadelphia, PA 19107
                (215) 546-7293, 800-962-1892
                FAX (215) 790-9330
                Website: http://www.hanleyandbelfus.com

Library of Congress Cataloging-in-Publication Data

Neurology Pearls / edited by Andrew J. Waclawik, Thomas P. Sutula.
        p.   cm.—(The Pearls Series®)
    Includes bibliographical references and index.
    ISBN 1-56053-261-0 (alk. paper)
    1. Nervous system—Diseases—Case studies.   2. Neurology—Case studies.
I. Series.   II. Waclawik, Andrew J., 1958–   III. Sutula, Thomas.
    [DNLM: 1. Nervous System Diseases—diagnosis—Case Report.
2. Nervous System Diseases—diagnosis—Problems and Exercises.
WL 141 N485 2000]
RC359.N48 2000
616.8'049 21—dc21

                                                        99-040818

NEUROLOGY PEARLS   ISBN 1-56053-261-0

Last digit is the print number: 9 8 7 6 5 4 3 2 1

CONTENTS

Patient **Page**

Patient	**Page**

MUSCLE STRENGTH AND REFLEX GRADING SCALES

Throughout this book we used the following modified British Medical Research Council muscle strength grading scale:

0 = no movement or muscle contraction
1 = a trace of contraction or barely discernible movement
2 = movement with gravity eliminated
3 = movement against gravity
4 = movement against gravity and mild resistance
+ 4 = moderate resistance needed to overcome the limb
– 5 = slight but definite weakness
5 = normal strength

We used the following muscle stretch reflex grading scale:

0 = absent (even with reinforcement, if applicable)
1 = present but diminished
2 = normal
3 = hyperactive but not necessarily pathologic
4 = pathologically hyperactive, often with sustained clonus

FOREWORD

In all ages, physicians have delighted in solving challenging clinical problems. Not only do patients benefit from a well-directed diagnostic approach, but clinicians experience a unique sense of professional satisfaction when years of experience pry open a diagnostic dilemma.

The Pearls Series® is directed toward this aspect of the physician's nature. In editing these books, we have attempted to develop a consistent format and style that challenge the reader with the salient features of a clinical problem and direct attention to an important question in management. The discussion that follows presents a review of the patient's general disorder as well as a focus on the unique aspects of the presented patient's condition. Throughout the discussion, aspects of diagnosis and care that are especially important, "cutting edge," or not widely recognized are captured and listed at the end of the text as "Clinical Pearls." Finally, so as not to lose sight of our interest in the individual patient, the discussion closes with the clinical outcome of the patient at hand. In the process, we hope that the student readers beginning their medical careers, residents in training, and experienced clinicians honing their skills will find something of value in each of the patient presentations.

We compliment Drs. Waclawik and Sutula for presenting a challenging array of neurologic case studies in the Pearls format. We believe that *Neurology Pearls* will serve as a valuable resource and trustworthy guide to assist physicians in the diagnosis and care of patients with neurologic disorders.

John E. Heffner, MD
Steven A. Sahn, MD
SERIES EDITORS

Acknowledgment

The authors acknowledge the following physicians from the Department of Neurology, University of Wisconsin Medical School, and gratefully appreciate their contributions and assistance in preparation of this book:

Staff
Drs. Ross L. Levine, Barend P. Lotz, John O. Fleming, Douglas A. Dulli, Christopher C. Luzzio, William W. Lytton, Miroslav Backonja, Paul A. Rutecki, Raj D. Sheth, Catherine Gallagher, Brad R. Beinlich, John C. Jones, Henry A. Peters, Henry S. Schutta, Benjamin R. Brooks, Shahriar Salamat (Neuropathology), Richard E. Appen (Neuro-ophthalmology), Bruce P. Hermann (Neuropsychology)

Residents and Fellows
Drs. Shanker Dixit, Ivo Tremont, Katalin Juhasz-Pocsine, Sankar Bandyopadhyay, Dominic Fee, Opas Nawasiripong, Faizan Hafeez, Mohammad Ghouse, Xiang-Yan Yi, Carlos Rosario, Michael Vesali, Nihal Herath, Allauddin Khan

We also thank Ms. Anna Dresang, Ms. Cheryl Miller, and Mr. Daryn Belden for their technical assistance.

PREFACE

This book is a collection of some interesting cases encountered at the Neurology Service of the University of Wisconsin Hospital and Clinics and the William S. Middleton Memorial Veterans Hospital in Madison, Wisconsin during the last several years. The cases include a diverse range of both common and rare neurologic disorders, but the main intent is to provide an opportunity to develop an appreciation of the process of clinical decision making in the evaluation and management of patients with diseases of the nervous system.

The reader should first analyze the symptoms, signs, and other available information in the case presentation. At this point, one should "Stop and Consider" the neuroanatomic localization of the process, think about a differential diagnosis, and formulate a plan for diagnostic studies before a final diagnosis is considered and discussed. We hope that the book will be an interesting and useful educational tool for medical students, residents, neurologists preparing for board examinations, and practicing physicians who seek to understand the clinical approach to patients who suffer from neurologic disorders.

The diagnosis and care of patients who are afflicted with diseases of the nervous system has been immeasurably improved by the introduction of the diagnostic tools such as EEG and EMG, and the remarkable ability to detect structural lesions through MR and CT imaging. Despite these powerful tools, diagnosis and management of patients with acute and chronic neurologic deficits, cognitive and developmental problems, and alterations in consciousness still rely primarily on the clinical skills of eliciting a history of symptoms and bedside examination. We hope that this volume captures the dynamic and logical interplay between bedside history and examination, laboratory studies, and thoughtful initiation of a treatment approach from the increasing range of medical and surgical options for diseases of the nervous system.

Andrew J. Waclawik, MD
Thomas P. Sutula, MD, PhD

Dedication

To our wives

Bożena Waclawik
Eileen Sutula

for their love and support

PATIENT 1

A 42-year-old man with a 7-year history of progressive disequilibrium, slurred speech, jerking extremities, and cognitive decline

A 42-year-old man presented with deteriorating cognitive skills, frequent falls, and abnormal movements of arms and legs. His parents reported a 3-year history of progressive disequilibrium, clumsiness, choking on food, and slurred speech. For the last 5 years he was unable to "sit still." He had difficulty holding or manipulating objects and was unable to tie his shoes. The patient had an MS degree in English but had never held a steady job. He had 3 children, but gradually lost any interest in family life and got divorced. His family history was negative for neurologic conditions.

Physical Examination: Vital signs: normal. General: normal. HEENT: normocephalic head, nontender skull, supple neck, no bruits. Mental status: alert, oriented to place, person, and time; marked difficulty with calculations and 10-minute recall. Neuropsychological testing: IQ 87, premorbid cognitive ability estimated at > 105. Speech: dysarthric, no aphasia. Cranial nerves: mild limitation of upward gaze, delay in initiation of saccadic eye movements, dyskinetic, grimacing, intermittent jerking movements of tongue, lips, face, and neck. Motor examination: muscle bulk normal, tone mildly increased (rigid), strength grade +4 throughout, prominent choreiform movements of upper and lower extremities. Sensory examination: normal. Muscle stretch reflexes: grade 3 and symmetric throughout. Plantar reflexes: flexor. Coordination: severe dysmetria with some intention tremor in both upper extremities. Gait: broad-based, ataxic.

Stop and Consider: How would you classify the abnormal movements experienced by this patient, and what neural systems/structures are likely to be involved? What is the differential diagnosis?

Laboratory Findings: CBC, ESR, liver function tests, electrolytes, antinuclear antibody, serum ceruloplasmin, urine copper: normal. Slit-lamp examination: no Kayser-Fleischer ring. Head MRI: see figures. DNA analysis: increased number of CAG repeats (46, normal 11–35) in one allele of the *IT15* gene located on chromosome 4p16.3.

Question: What abnormalities does the brain MRI show? What is the significance of the DNA testing result?

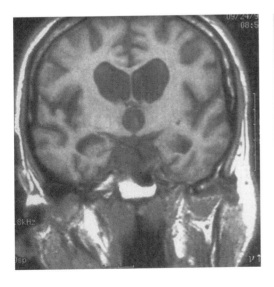 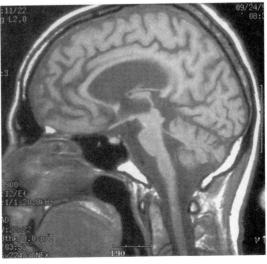

1

Diagnosis: Huntington's chorea

Discussion: The clinical presentation of this patient, with gradual development of dementia, dysarthria, dysphagia, prominent chorea with limb and gait ataxia, and dystonia, is suggestive of Huntington's disease (HD), even with lack of positive family history. Metabolic, systemic, drug-induced, toxic, infectious, inflammatory/autoimmune (vasculitis), and other neurodegenerative conditions should be considered. Wilson's disease should be specifically excluded.

The brain MRI showed prominent atrophy of both cerebral hemispheres, corpus callosum, and brain stem. There was ventriculomegaly with flattening of the caudate. The DNA analysis provided an unequivocal confirmation of the suspected clinical diagnosis. It showed an abnormal expansion of the CAG trinucleotide repeats in the coding region of the *IT15* gene (HD gene) on chromosome 4.

HD is a relentlessly progressive, hereditary condition with an autosomal dominant inheritance. In some patients there are behavioral problems, depression, personality changes, or frank psychotic behavior preceding chorea by up to 10–15 years. However, the movement disorder may occur first or present together with cognitive decline and personality changes. The onset is usually in mid-adult life, but symptoms may develop in early childhood or as late as 8th decade of life. The motor impairment with chorea usually develops insidiously. Patients become fidgety, clumsy, and with progression of chorea they have increasing difficulty with activities of daily living such as dressing or eating. Speech becomes slurred and eventually is unintelligible. Dysphagia is probably the major source of morbidity and mortality (risk of aspiration pneumonia). Intellectual decline progresses to severe dementia, usually when the movement disorder is advanced. From the time of diagnosis patients may survive up to 15–30 years.

The putative protein product of the HD gene ("huntingtin") has not been well characterized and its function is unknown. The CAG repeats code for glutamine, and toxic "gain of function" mechanism, leading to degenerative changes in the central nervous system, has been postulated. The brain abnormalities are diffuse, but most characteristic is severe neuronal loss in the caudate nucleus and putamen.

About 10% of HD cases have an early (childhood) onset. In this group it is inherited usually from the father. This form of HD is frequently associated with muscle rigidity, minimal or no chorea, and seizures. Late-onset cases may be associated with a wide spectrum of cognitive and psychiatric presentations and may be misdiagnosed as Alzheimer's disease. There is usually inverse correlation between the number of CAG repeats and age of onset. New cases appear to be very rare (approximately 3%). In those patients the possibility of late-onset, unrecognized HD in the parents and critical evaluation of paternity should be considered. The possible mechanism of new mutations is the potential meiotic instability of so-called intermediate alleles in unaffected individuals. Such persons usually have between 27–35 CAG repeats in the HD gene (normal < 36) and their offspring may have expansion of the length of repeats and develop HD.

The diagnosis is usually relatively easy in patients with positive family history, progressive dementia, and movement disorder. When the family history is negative or difficult to obtain, especially in early stages of the disease, the diagnosis may be difficult to make. The DNA analysis is most helpful. Genetic testing should be offered to all potentially affected family members with appropriate pre- and post-testing counseling.

There is no effective treatment that can alter the relentlessly progressive course of this condition. Neuroleptics (e.g., haloperidol) may transiently improve chorea. Most patients eventually have to be institutionalized.

The present patient underscores possible diagnostic difficulty in patients with HD who have negative family history. The available DNA testing was most helpful in confirming the diagnosis of HD. His chorea initially responded to haloperidol and he was also treated with antidepressants; however, his dementia and movement disorder were relentlessly progressive and he had to be placed in a nursing home.

Clinical Pearls

1. "Premorbid" behavioral and personality changes may precede the development of the movement disorder by more than a decade.

2. Consider late-onset Huntington's disease in the differential diagnosis of elderly patients with dementia.

3. DNA testing can be helpful to confirm the diagnosis of Huntington's disease.

4. Pre- and post–DNA testing counseling should be offered to asymptomatic family members.

REFERENCES

1. Goldberg YP, Kremer B, Andrew SE, et al: Molecular analysis of new mutations for Huntington's disease: Intermediate alleles and sex of origin effects. Nat Genet 1993; 5:174–179.
2. Myers RH, Vonsattel JP, Stevens TJ, et al: Clinical and neuropathologic assessment of severity in Huntington's disease. Neurology 1988; 38:341–347.
3. Shulman KI, Lenox A, Karlinsky H: Late-onset Huntington's disease: A geriatric psychiatry perspective. J Geriatr Psychiatry Neurol 1996; 9:26–29.
4. Snell RG, Mac Millan JC, Cheadle JP, et al: Relationship between trinucleotide repeat expansion and phenotypic variation in Huntington's disease. Nat Genet 1993; 4:393–397.

PATIENT 2

A 32-year-old woman with progressive headache, somnolence, and seizures

A 32-year-old previously healthy woman experienced progressive bilateral frontal headaches during the previous 3 weeks that were unresponsive to acetaminophen and codeine. She became increasingly drowsy and required up to 12 hours of sleep per day. On the day of admission she was found in her apartment in an unresponsive state. During evaluation in the emergency department of a local hospital, a generalized tonic-clonic seizure occurred. A cranial CT scan showed a relatively small left posterior frontal hemorrhagic infarct. During transfer to the hospital she was given an infusion of 20 mg/kg of phenytoin. Her medical history was significant for morbid obesity, use of oral contraceptives, and recent amoxicillin therapy for sinusitis. She smoked one pack of cigarettes a day and drank alcohol regularly in social settings. There was no history of a previous seizure disorder, illicit drug use, head injury, or other chronic illness.

Physical Examination: Temperature 37.4°; pulse 116; respirations 18; blood pressure 145/88. General: normal. Mental status: obtunded, localizing only deep pain stimuli. Cranial nerves: pupils equal, reactive to light, marked papilledema, roving, conjugate eye movements, right lower facial paresis evident with elicited grimace. Motor function: right hemiparesis. Muscle stretch reflexes: diffusely suppressed (grade 1). Plantar reflexes: extensor bilaterally.

Stop and Consider: Can the left hemispheric lesion producing the right hemiparesis account for the patient's abnormal mental status? What is the differential diagnosis of this clinical presentation?

Laboratory Findings: Cranial CT scan: see figure, *left*. Brain MRI: similar findings to cranial CT scan. MR angiogram with venous phase: see figure, *right*. CBC, glucose, renal and liver function tests, electrolytes: normal. ESR: 38 mm/hr (normal 0–25). Thyroid-stimulating hormone (TSH): 0.03 μIU/ml (normal: 3–4.3), T_3 by radioimmunoassay: 388 ng/dl (normal 80–160). Protein S, protein C, activated protein C resistance, anticardiolipin antibody, lupus anticoagulant: normal or negative.

Question: What therapy should be initiated?

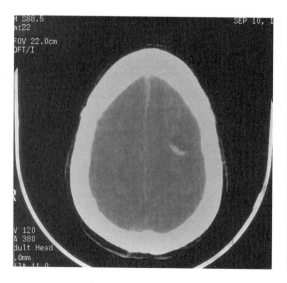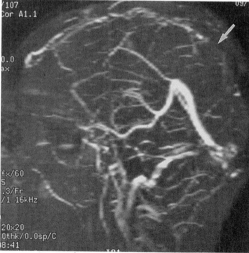

Diagnosis: Cerebral venous (sinus) thrombosis with intracranial hypertension

Discussion: The differential diagnosis of severe, progressive headaches when associated with fever, abnormal mental status, seizures and abnormal vital signs includes important and life-threatening entities such as subarachnoid hemorrhage, diencephalic tumor, subdural hematoma, brain abscess, extradural infections such as mucormycosis, herpes encephalitis, cerebral vasculitis, chronic meningitis, and cerebral venous thrombosis (CVT). In this patient, cranial CT and brain MRI scans showed a left parietal hemorrhagic infarct. In addition, there was evidence of generalized cerebral edema. MR venogram demonstrated absence of flow within the posterior sagittal sinus (arrow), left transverse sinus, and left sigmoid sinus, compatible with venous sinus thrombosis. Flow was visualized in the basal vein of Rosenthal, vein of Galen, straight sinus, and internal cerebral veins. Multiple small medullary and superficial cortical veins were visualized due to collateral venous flow. Laboratory studies revealed hyperthyroidism.

Cerebral venous (sinus) thrombosis (CVT) is an important cause of headaches that can progress to altered mental status, seizures, and death. The lateral sinuses and superior sagittal sinus are most commonly involved in noninfective (primary) symptomatic CVT. This condition typically presents with a triad of progressive headache, somnolence, and papilledema. Focal deficits and seizures often accompany an associated venous cortical infarction, which is frequently hemorrhagic. Unfortunately, the venous thrombosis itself is often missed until the patient presents in the more dire condition. The diagnosis can be established by noninvasive tests such as MRI or MR venography.

Multiple risk factors are present in most patients with CVT. Patients who are particularly susceptible to cerebral venous thrombosis include newborns and the elderly, particularly with dehydration, infections, and malignancies, young women in the puerperium or in association with recent use of birth control pills, cigarette smoking, or other risk factors for coagulopathy. Less common associated conditions include hemolytic anemia, sickle cell trait, thrombocytosis, ulcerative colitis, hyperthyroidism, and inherited coagulopathies, including protein C and protein S deficiency and anticardiolipin syndrome.

Another more recently demonstrated CVT risk factor is activated protein C resistance. This condition is in most cases due to modification of factor V. The modified factor V is called "factor V Leiden." In this condition, the abnormal factor V is resistant to cleavage by activated protein C. This condition probably represents the most common cause of inherited thrombophilia.

Anticoagulation as a treatment for cerebral venous thrombosis, particularly sagittal sinus thrombosis, has been controversial in the past. There has been concern about the danger of anticoagulation in the presence of hemorrhagic infarcts, which are commonly associated with venous thrombosis. Anticoagulation actually reduces the risk of hemorrhage by lowering the increased venous pressure, which is the cause of venous infarction. Because CVT is a progressive and frequently fatal condition, anticoagulation is recommended since it improves the outcome. Other therapeutic approaches have included intrasinus thrombolysis.

The present patient was intubated, hyperventilated, and received intravenous mannitol to reduce intracranial pressure. She was anticoagulated with heparin. There was no increase in the size of her parenchymal hemorrhage with anticoagulation but she remained obtunded for the next 3 days and then recovered consciousness rapidly. She had a residual, mild dysphasia and right hemiparesis, which improved markedly over the next 2 weeks with rehabilitation. Her headaches rapidly resolved, and she had no further seizures. Cranial MR angiogram obtained 1 year after presentation demonstrated interval recanalization of all sinuses as well the development of a collateral drainage vessel in the posterior neck. Her thyroid status was normalized and birth control pills were discontinued. Warfarin was continued for 1 year following her hospitalization.

Clinical Pearls

1. Progressive headaches with somnolence or delirium indicate the possibility of several life-threatening intracranial conditions.

2. Cerebral venous thrombosis is underdiagnosed; its prompt recognition requires a heightened awareness of the patient at risk and the typical presenting clinical manifestations.

3. MR venography is a noninvasive test, which enables prompt and accurate diagnosis in most patients with cerebral venous thrombosis.

4. Anticoagulation for cerebral venous thrombosis, despite the apparent risk when associated with parenchymal venous hemorrhage, can often be life-saving.

REFERENCES

1. Ameri A, Bousser MG: Cerebral venous thrombosis. Neurol Clin 1992; 10:87–111.
2. Dahlback B: Inherited resistance of activated protein C, a major cause of venous thrombosis, is due to a mutation of factor V gene. Haemostasis 1994; 24:139–151.
3. Einhaupl KM, Villringer A, Meister W, et al: Heparin treatment in sinus venous thrombosis. Lancet 1991; 338:597–600.

PATIENT 3

A 4-year-old boy with large calves and difficulty running

A 4-year-old boy presented with progressive difficulty walking, climbing stairs, and clumsiness. He was delivered by cesarean section after a normal pregnancy. His early developmental milestones were normal. He was able to walk independently at the age of 14 months. A 20-year-old uncle has a severe muscle disease with onset at the age 5.

Physical Examination: Vital signs: normal. General: normal. Spine: slightly exaggerated lumbar lordosis. Mental status, speech, cranial nerves: normal. Motor examination: marked enlargement of both calves, muscle tone slightly decreased, mild, grade +4 proximal weakness in upper and lower extremities; positive Gowers' sign. Sensory examination: normal. Muscle stretch reflexes: decreased (grade 1 throughout). Plantar reflexes: flexor. Coordination: normal. Gait: mildly waddling.

Stop and Consider: What is the differential diagnosis of this boy's weakness?

Laboratory Findings: CBC, electrolytes: normal. Creatine kinase (CK): 13,938 IU/L (normal 0–250). Nerve conduction studies: normal. Needle electromyography (EMG): fibrillation potentials and short-duration, low-amplitude, rapidly recruiting motor unit potentials. DNA testing: no deletion or duplication in the dystrophin gene on chromosome Xp21. Muscle biopsy with immunocytochemical studies for dystrophin: see figure *(right)*, with normal control *(left)*; arrows indicate normal immunocytochemical staining for dystrophin. Western blot: only residual amount of dystrophin (5%) of abnormally small size (380 kDa, normal 427 kDa).

Question: What is the significance of the muscle biopsy findings?

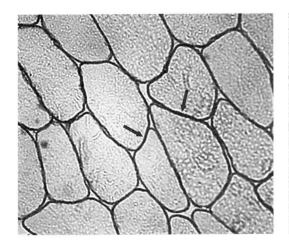 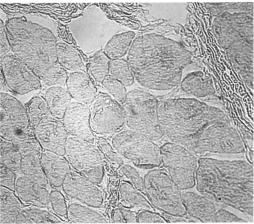

Diagnosis: Duchenne muscular dystrophy (dystrophinopathy)

Discussion: Normal mental status and normal cranial nerves with diffuse weakness, decreased reflexes and muscle tone, and normal sensation suggested a peripheral lesion within a motor unit. Normal nerve conduction study pointed away from a condition affecting peripheral nerves. Needle EMG was consistent with a myopathic process and the very high CK level indicated severe muscle fiber breakdown. Muscle biopsy unequivocally demonstrated abnormalities in the muscle as the cause of weakness. It showed clusters of necrotic and regenerating muscle fibers and severe proliferation of fibrous and fatty connective tissue. Immunocytochemical staining against the C-terminal, N-terminal, and rod portion of the dystrophin molecule showed absent or markedly diminished reactivity in subsarcolemmal regions.

Duchenne muscular dystrophy (DMD) is an X-linked recessive condition caused by a mutation in the dystrophin gene on chromosome Xp21. About two thirds of cases are inherited and one third are caused by *de novo* mutations. The dystrophin gene is one of the largest in humans, therefore it is prone to spontaneous mutations. The dystrophin protein is important for the function of the muscle membrane (sarcolemma). Defects in the muscle membrane lead to muscle fiber necrosis.

There is marked clinical heterogeneity in DMD with differences in age of onset and rate of progression. The onset of weakness is usually in early childhood; however, affected children typically have marked CK elevation at birth. Girls are unaffected but up to 8% of DMD carriers may manifest mild to moderate myopathy that can resemble limb-girdle muscular dystrophy. Girls with Turner's syndrome (46 X0) or patients with X-autosomal translocation may exhibit a typical Duchenne phenotype.

A milder form of X-linked muscular dystrophy, also caused by mutation of the dystrophin gene, is called Becker muscular dystrophy (BMD). These patients usually have milder disease course and may be able to ambulate independently until the third or fourth decade of life. Intermediate phenotypes are sometimes referred to as "outliers." Since the time of identification of the dystrophin gene, the clinical spectrum of dystrophinopathies has been evolving and includes patients that may present with a cramp and myalgia syndrome or dilated cardiomyopathy without muscle weakness.

DMD is a progressive disorder. Most boys lose the ability to ambulate independently before or by the age of 12. Weakness of respiratory muscles leads to respiratory failure and death before the age of 20, usually due to associated respiratory infections. In many patients there is involvement of the heart muscle and cardiac failure or arrhythmias can be causes of death. Approximately one third of patients may have some degree of cognitive impairment.

In about 60% of patients diagnosis can be made by DNA analysis (patients with DNA deletions or duplications), in the remaining 30–40% (point mutations) diagnosis is made by muscle biopsy and by immunocytochemical staining or Western blotting using dystrophin-specific antibodies. In some patients the phenotype may be predicted from the nature of the mutation. Deletions with preservation of the reading frame ("in-frame" mutations) usually lead to a relatively benign phenotype (Becker), whereas mutations causing a shift of the reading frame ("out-of-frame" mutations) lead to premature termination of translation and produce truncated dystrophin that is associated with a severe phenotype. There are, however, exceptions from this general rule. Some rare forms of muscular dystrophy caused by mutations in different genes and presenting with a phenotype similar to DMD have been identified (defects in the dystrophin-glycoprotein complex or merosin deficiency).

Because of the devastating nature of this condition, genetic counseling is of paramount importance. It should be offered to all families with affected children and their relatives. In families with identified mutations (deletions or duplications) carriers can be identified and prenatal diagnosis is possible by a DNA analysis. When the DNA study is negative (point mutations), some carriers may be identified by CK measurements or by a linkage study.

Currently there is no effective curative treatment for DMD. Supportive treatment includes management of contractures, scoliosis, and cardiorespiratory complications and psychosocial support. Corticosteroids may transiently improve muscle strength and slow down progression of the disease, but have significant side effects. Gene therapy may bring some progress in the future.

In the present patient, the molecular findings and quantitation of the dystrophin expression by Western blotting or immunocytochemistry present a very interesting dilemma about prognosis and prediction of the rate of progression. In typical DMD cases there is no detectable dystrophin in the skeletal muscle. In this patient, despite very early onset of weakness, there was residual amount of dystrophin of lower molecular weight expressed in the skeletal muscle. These observations suggest that progression of weakness in his case may be relatively slower than in typical DMD. Interestingly, his uncle, who was subsequently examined, had early onset of weakness (at age 5); however, at age 20 he was still able to ambulate independently for short distances.

Clinical Pearls

1. In patients with Duchenne or Becker phenotypes and high serum CK levels, the diagnostic evaluation should be initiated with a DNA analysis for a deletion or duplication in the dystrophin gene.

2. Patients with suspected dystrophinopathy and negative DNA analysis (most likely point mutations or undetectable deletions) should have a muscle biopsy with immunocytochemistry or Western blot testing for dystrophin abnormalities.

3. Consider dystrophinopathy in patients with idiopathic cardiomyopathy.

4. Genetic counseling should be offered to all families with children affected by Duchenne/Becker muscular dystrophy. Carriers can be identified and prenatal diagnosis is possible.

REFERENCES

1. Koenig M, Beggs AH, Moyer M, et al: The molecular basis for Duchenne versus Becker muscular dystrophy: Correlation of severity with type of mutation. Am J Hum Genet 1989; 45:498–506.
2. Mendell JR, Moxley RT, Griggs RC, et al: Randomized, double-blind 6-month trial of prednisone in Duchenne's muscular dystrophy. N Engl J Med 1989; 320:1592–1597.
3. Mirabella M, Servidei S, Manfredi G, et al: Cardiomyopathy may be the only clinical manifestation in female carriers of Duchenne muscular dystrophy. Neurology 1993; 43:2342–2345.

PATIENT 4

A 62-year-old woman with sudden onset of right hemiparesis, diplopia, and dysarthria

A 62-year-old woman arrived at the emergency department 45 minutes after the onset of severe weakness of the right extremities accompanied by double vision and slurring of speech. She denied difficulty finding words, loss of consciousness, headache, numbness, or recent head injury. There was no history of stroke, seizure, head injury, diabetes, hypertension, or other risk factors for stroke. She took no medications.

Physical Examination: Afebrile; pulse 82 and regular; respirations 18; blood pressure 150/80. Mental status: alert, no acute distress other than severe anxiety. Speech: severely dysarthric, but could name, repeat, read, and follow instructions with her left hand. Cranial nerves: pupills and visual fields intact, no papilledema, left gaze paresis, facial sensation normal, mild left facial paresis involving upper and lower facial muscles. Motor examination: severe right hemiplegia in the right upper and lower extremity. Sensory examination: mildly decreased to light touch and pain on the right, normal vibration sense. Muscle stretch reflexes: grade 2, symmetric throughout. Plantar reflexes: right extensor, left flexor. Coordination of left extremities intact.

Stop and Consider: What is the time course and localization of the neurologic dysfunction?

Laboratory Findings: Noncontrast head CT: negative except for an abnormality in the basilar artery (see figure). CBC, chemistry panel, electrolytes, PT, PTT, platelet count: normal. EKG: normal.

Question: What disorder is suggested by the basilar artery abnormality on the CT scan?

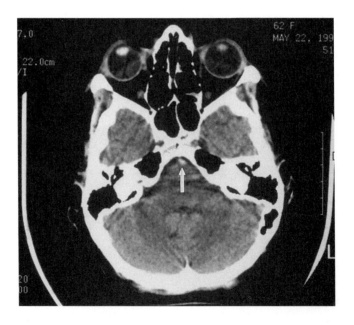

Diagnosis: Left pontine infarction

Discussion: The neurologic examination indicated an acute pontine lesion affecting the paramedian pontine reticular formation, pyramidal tract, and the ipsilateral facial nucleus (Foville's syndrome). It typically results from a lesion involving the pontine paramedian artery, or, as in this case, the basilar artery itself. An initial noncontrast head CT scan demonstrated a hyperdense basilar artery (arrow), which may be seen as an early sign of basilar artery thrombosis.

Approximately 15–30% of ischemic strokes are cardioembolic, caused most frequently by atrial fibrillation and valvular disease. Most cardioembolic strokes affect the territory of the middle cerebral artery, but posterior circulation embolism is also relatively common. A typical clinical feature of a cardioembolic stroke is an abrupt onset of maximal neurologic deficit.

Transesophageal echocardiogram (TEE) has been increasingly used in evaluation of patients with suspected cardioembolic stroke. However, the TEE and transthoracic echocardiogram (TTE) should be considered as complementary procedures and the decision whether a patient should be studied directly with TEE without prior TTE should be made on a case-by-case basis. The TEE provides better visualization of the thoracic aorta, atrial septal defects, patent foramen ovale, and cardiac valves. The TTE is superior in visualization of the left ventricle, especially its apex. The data about possible association of some cardiac anomalies (e.g., atrial septal aneurysm or patent foramen ovale) with embolic stroke are still controversial and more studies are needed to optimally guide the selection of the most appropriate diagnostic tests. To perform a TEE, patients need both light anesthesia and the ability to swallow safely. A careful dysphagia evaluation should precede a TEE since many cerebral deficits caused by stroke may impair swallowing.

Cautious anticoagulation can be started early in cardioembolic strokes with mild to moderate deficits. With large infarctions, repeat CT scan should be done in 3–5 days, and if there is no evidence for hemorrhagic transformation, heparinization can be started if useful recovery is expected. Warfarin is usually recommended for long-term preventive therapy. Thrombolytic therapy with intravenous recombinant tissue plasminogen activator (rt-PA) may be considered in selected cases within 3 hours from the onset. In the multicenter clinical trial of rt-PA conducted by the National Institute of Neurologic Disorders and Stroke, no difference between patients treated with rt-PA or placebo were noted within the first 24 hours. Improvement was observed after 3 months in patients treated with rt-PA, who were at least 30% more likely to have minimal or no disability on graded assessment scales. The intravenous thrombolytic therapy significantly increases the risk of intracranial as well as extracranial bleeding; therefore, the risks and potential benefits should be carefully weighed in each patient who may be a candidate for thrombolytic therapy. It should never be used by physicians who do not have sufficient experience with evaluation of patients with stroke. Rapid clinical improvement may be attributable to either thrombolysis or flow-related migration of the clot.

In the present patient, the neurologic exam and neuroimaging findings indicated an acute ischemic pontine stroke caused by an embolic event within the basilar artery circulation. After careful consideration of possible risks and benefits of thrombolytic therapy, rt-PA was infused intravenously at 0.9 mg/kg, with 5.4-mg initial bolus, and the remainder of the 54-mg dose administered over 1 hour. While awaiting transfer to the intensive care unit, she had a sudden and dramatic reversal of her deficit preceded by a sensation of an "electric shock" affecting the right side of her body. Her exam 24 hours after admission was abnormal only for very mild clumsiness limited to the right upper extremity and mild tandem-gait ataxia. On further diagnostic evaluation, cranial MRI and MR angiography were entirely normal. A TEE, however, revealed a significant atrial septal defect estimated at greater than 1 cm in size. Twenty four hours after rt-PA infusion the patient was placed on heparin anticoagulation followed by long-term warfarin therapy. She remains well and without recurrent stroke 1 year later.

Clinical Pearls

1. Acute stroke is a medical emergency. Specific therapy for the hyperacute ischemic stroke is now available and is both effective and safe in properly selected patients.

2. Thrombolytic therapy should always be considered in acute ischemic stroke in appropriately selected patients for whom its potential benefits best outweigh its risks.

3. The transesophageal echocardiogram has played an increasingly important role in the diagnosis of previously unrecognized cardioembolic stroke risk factors, such as atrial septal defect and patent foramen ovale. Embolic strokes associated with such lesions are best treated with long-term anticoagulation therapy and surgical repair in selected patients.

REFERENCES

1. Bogousslavsky J, Regli F, Maeder P, et al: The etiology of posterior circulation infarcts: A prospective study using magnetic resonance imaging and magnetic resonance angiography. Neurology 1993; 43:1528–1533.
2. Ehsan T, Hayat G, Malkoff MD, et al: Hyperdense basilar artery: An early computed tomography sign of thrombosis. J Neuroimag 1994; 4:200–205.
3. Leung DY, Black IW, Cranney GB, et al: Selection of patients for transesophageal echocardiography after stroke and systemic embolic events: Role of transthoracic echocardiography. Stroke 1995; 26:1820–1824.
4. Minematsu K, Yamaguchi T, Omae T: "Spectacular shrinking deficit": Rapid recovery from a major hemispheric syndrome by migration of an embolus. Neurology 1992; 42:157–162.
5. National Institute of Neurologic Disorders and Stroke rt-PA Stroke Study Group: Tissue plasminogen activator for acute ischemic stroke. New Engl J Med 1995; 333:1581–1587.
6. Wijdicks EFM, Nichols DA, Thielen KR, et al: Intra-arterial thrombolysis in acute basilar artery thromboembolism: The initial Mayo Clinic Experience. Mayo Clin Proc 1997; 72:1005–1013.

PATIENT 5

A 63-year-old man with a 1-week history of rapidly progressing weakness and numbness of all extremities

A 63-year-old man presented with a 1-week history of weakness with tingling and numbness that started in both legs and eventually spread to his upper extremities. He was unable to walk or feed himself. He denied shortness of breath, difficulty swallowing, or problems with bowel or bladder function. There was no preceding illness, trauma, or toxic exposure. His medical history was positive for hypertension and asthma.

Physical Examination: Temperature 36.5°; pulse 70; respirations 20; blood pressure 150/80. General: normal. Extremities: no edema, good peripheral pulses. Mental status, speech, cranial nerves: normal. Motor examination: muscle bulk normal, muscle tone diminished in all four extremities, severe weakness (grade 1–2) in distal muscles of both upper and lower extremities with proximal muscles strength grade 4. Sensory examination: diminished to vibration in lower extremities. Muscle stretch reflexes: absent, except for bilaterally markedly diminished biceps reflexes. Coordination: impaired in proportion to weakness. Gait: unable to walk independently but no ataxia.

Stop and Consider: What is the most likely neuroanatomic localization of this patient's progressive weakness, paresthesias, and numbness?

Laboratory Findings: CBC, liver function tests, electrolytes, urinalysis, porphyria screen: normal. Pulmonary function tests: vital capacity 2.9 L, negative inspiratory force: – 60 cmH$_2$O, ABGs (room air): normal. Lumbar puncture/CSF examination: opening pressure normal, nucleated cell count 1/µl, protein 42 mg/dl (15–45), glucose 83 mg/dl (serum glucose 143), cultures negative. Needle EMG: rare fibrillation potentials in the right gastrocnemius muscle; markedly decreased motor unit recruitment in all muscles tested in both upper and lower extremities. Nerve conduction studies: see tables (normal values in parentheses).

Question: What is the likely interpretation of the electrodiagnostic findings?

Motor	Latency (ms)	CMAP (mV)	F-waves	CV (m/s)
Ulnar$_{wrist/ADQ}$	5.1 (< 3.6)	3 (> 4) dispersed	NR	37 (> 51)
Median$_{wrist/APB}$	7.1 (< 4.5)	0.5 (> 6) dispersed	NR	29 (> 48)
Peroneal$_{ankle/EDB}$	7.1 (< 6.0)	1.1 (> 2) dispersed	NR	34 (> 41)

Sensory	Latency (ms)	SNAP (mV)
Sural$_{calf/ankle}$		NR
Median$_{wrist/2nd digit}$	4.9 (< 3.6)	0.003 (> 0.015)
		NR with proximal stimulation

CMAP, Compound muscle action potential; SNAP, sensory nerve action potential; ADQ, abductor digiti quinti; APB, abductor pollicis brevis; EDB, extensor digitorum brevis; NR, no response.

Diagnosis: Acute inflammatory demyelinating polyneuropathy (Guillain-Barré syndrome)

Discussion: Diffuse weakness and sensory symptoms (paresthesia) with absent stretch reflexes and decreased muscle tone are all suggestive of a condition affecting the peripheral nervous system. Nerve conduction studies (NCSs) showing prolongation of distal latencies, small motor and sensory action potentials with temporal dispersion, absent F-waves, and slowing of conduction velocities unequivocally point to dysfunction of the peripheral nerves as the cause of the patient's weakness and sensory findings. The pattern of electrodiagnostic abnormalities on NCS/EMG is consistent with an acquired, primarily demyelinating process.

Guillain-Barré syndrome, also known as acute inflammatory demyelinating polyneuropathy (AIDP), is an acquired, immune-mediated disorder affecting the peripheral nervous system. The pathologic hallmark of this condition is demyelination of peripheral nerves. Although known as primarily motor polyneuropathy, many patients have evidence of mild or more severe sensory nerve involvement as well. In most cases, the demyelinating process also affects the nerve roots; therefore, this condition is frequently referred to as acute polyradiculoneuritis.

About one half of patients have a history of preceding acute, usually viral, infection. Guillain-Barré syndrome may also be associated with recent immunizations, surgery or trauma, pregnancy, and systemic conditions such as connective tissue diseases, malignancies, and medications (e.g., D-penicillamine). In typical cases the weakness is symmetric, progresses in an ascending fashion, and in approximately one third of patients leads to respiratory failure necessitating ventilatory support. In almost all patients there is early loss of tendon reflexes. In many instances there are signs of autonomic fiber involvement. These patients may have severe fluctuations in blood pressure (hypotension and/or hypertension), severe irregularities of heart rate, loss of sweating, gastrointestinal dismotility and sphincter dysfunction.

Cerebrospinal fluid (CSF) analysis is most helpful in the diagnostic evaluation. It typically shows very high protein content (in some cases as high as 1–2 gm/dl) with usually normal or only slightly elevated cell count. The CSF protein content is typically highest between the first and third week after the onset of symptoms but within the first few days it may be normal. It may be necessary to repeat the lumbar puncture 7–10 days after the initial examination, especially if the clinical or electrodiagnostic findings are atypical. The CSF cell count may be much higher in Guillain-Barré syndrome associated with HIV infection.

The most important diagnostic test to confirm the diagnosis is NCS/EMG, which shows slowing of conduction velocities as well as other changes indicative of peripheral nerve demyelination. In some patients there may be evidence of coexisting axonal injury. Guillain-Barré syndrome should be differentiated from other neurologic conditions, such as acute spinal cord compression (usually brisk reflexes, sensory level, increased muscle tone), transverse myelitis, myasthenia gravis, acute porphyria, poliomyelitis, toxic neuropathies, botulinum intoxication, and diphtheric neuropathy.

There are several variants of Guillain-Barré syndrome. In Miller Fisher syndrome patients typically develop ataxia, ophthalmoplegia, and areflexia with rather mild to moderate weakness. This form of Guillain-Barré syndrome is frequently associated with high titers of anti-GQ_{1b} antibodies. "Pure" motor, sensory, or primarily dysautonomic forms have been described. The primarily axonal form of Guillain-Barré syndrome is associated with severe disability, relatively high mortality, and very slow and frequently incomplete recovery. In many cases it follows infection with *Campylobacter jejuni.*

Most patients have full recovery provided they receive diligent supportive care. All patients with a suspicion of Guillain-Barré syndrome should be hospitalized since the progression from the onset of symptoms to respiratory failure may be dramatic in some cases (over 24 hours.) Adequate management of respiratory condition is crucial. Prevention of secondary complications (deep vein thrombosis, decubiti, pneumonia, etc.) frequently determines successful outcome. Neuropathic pain is common in the acute stage and may require narcotics. Physical and occupational therapy should be initiated as soon as possible. Severe reactive depression is common and there is a need for psychological support and reassurance about the generally favorable prognosis. Because the immune mechanisms play a role in pathogenesis, immunomodulatory treatments such as plasmapheresis (plasma exchange) and high-dose intravenous immunoglobulin (IVIG) have significantly improved the outcome if initiated early, within the first week of illness. At the present time there is no convincing evidence about which treatment is superior. Most clinicians currently initiate the treatment with IVIG, because of the ease of administration and relative safety.

Prognosis is good in most cases. Approximately 75–80% of patients have complete recovery, 10% have mild residual disability, and only about 5–10% of patients have severe disability. Mortality rate is usually less than 3–5% and can be reduced by aggressive treatment of complications.

The present patient received IVIG treatment of 0.4 gm/kg/day for 5 consecutive days. However, his weakness became profound and he subsequently underwent plasmapheresis (total of 5 exchanges). Despite profound weakness of all extremities, his respiratory function remained satisfactory and endotracheal intubation with ventilatory support was not necessary. Despite typical precautions, he developed deep vein thrombosis and was treated with heparin and later warfarin. His condition stabilized but recovery was slow. After 6 months on intensive physical therapy he regained ability to walk independently, but had mild, residual distal leg and hand weakness and paresthesias.

Clinical Pearls

1. Evidence of significant early axonal injury in the course of Guillain-Barré syndrome is associated with slow and frequently incomplete recovery.

2. Acute polyneuropathy resembling Guillain-Barré syndrome may develop in the early stages of HIV infection or may precede HIV seroconversion. In HIV-negative patients with risk factors for HIV infection, repeat HIV testing is recommended for up to 6 months.

3. Declining mental status may be related to increased intracranial pressure caused by very high protein concentration in the CSF with impairment of spinal fluid absorption.

4. Diligent supportive care with monitoring of all vital functions is still the cornerstone of successful management.

5. If initiated within the first week of illness, immunotherapy (IVIG or plasmapheresis) may arrest progression and accelerate recovery.

REFERENCES
1. Cornblath DR: Electrophysiology in Guillain-Barré syndrome. Ann Neurol 1990; 27(Suppl):S17–S20.
2. Ropper AH: The Guillain-Barré syndrome. N Engl J Med 1992; 326:1130–1136.
3. van der Meché FGA, Schmitz PIM, and the Dutch Guillain-Barré study group: A randomized trial comparing intravenous immune globulin and plasma exchange in Guillain-Barré syndrome. N Engl J Med 1992; 326:1123–1129.

PATIENT 6

A 50-year-old woman with sudden onset of severe orthostatic headache

A 50-year-old previously healthy woman developed sudden, severe headache while boating during stormy weather. The headache transiently improved when she returned to land, but worsened while driving home later that day. During the next 10 days she complained of almost constant, severe headache that was most intense in the occipital region and improved in the recumbent position. Occasionally there was some throbbing quality of the headache, with mild nausea and right upper neck pain radiating to her occiput. A head CT scan and cervical spine x-ray obtained by her family physician were negative. She had no prior history of migraine or significant injuries or illnesses. She denied any visual symptoms, weakness, numbness, or vertigo.

Physical Examination: Vital signs: normal. General: normal. Mental status, speech: normal. Cranial nerves: normal, no papilledema. Motor and sensory examination: normal. Muscle stretch reflexes: grade 2 and symmetric. Plantar reflexes: flexor. Coordination: normal. Gait: complains of excruciating headache immediately after standing up, otherwise unremarkable.

Stop and Consider: How would you classify this type of a headache? What are the possible mechanisms of headache that worsens with postural changes?

Laboratory Findings: CBC, glucose, renal and hepatic tests, electrolytes, ESR: normal. Cervical spine MRI: mild degenerative joint disease. Brain MRI: mild scattered white matter changes most likely related to small-vessel ischemia, prominent, diffuse enhancement of meninges (see figure, arrow). Lumbar puncture (lateral decubitus position): CSF opening pressure 40 mmH$_2$O (normal 60–200), no xantochromia or white cells; protein level: 98 mg/dl (normal 15–45).

Question: What is the likely cause of low CSF pressure?

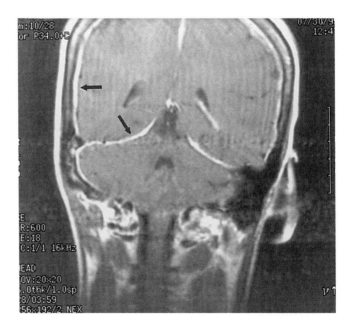

Diagnosis: Intracranial hypotension syndrome, most likely caused by a CSF leak

Discussion: The differential diagnosis of a patient presenting with sudden, severe headache includes several conditions. Subarachnoid hemorrhage (SH) was ruled out by negative noncontrast cranial CT and lumbar puncture that showed no red cells or xantochromia. This patient's clinical course and symptoms were most suggestive of a postural headache related to intracranial hypotension, but other headache types, including intracranial lesions, especially within the posterior fossa, may also have a significant postural component. The finding of very low CSF opening pressure on lumbar puncture strongly supported the notion that her headache was caused by low intracranial pressure.

Intracranial hypotension syndrome (IHS) typically presents as a postural headache in a patient with low CSF pressure (usually < 60 mmH$_2$O). The diagnosis of IHS is based on a combination of clinical evaluation, neuroimaging studies, and measurment of the CSF opening pressure. The diagnosis of this type of headache may be very difficult in a patient with preexisting migraines. The headache is typically postural, in erect position, and resolves or markedly improves with recumbency. It is typically most severe in the occipital region and may have a throbbing quality. In some patients there may be co-existing neck pain, nausea or emesis, blurred vision or intermittent diplopia, or imbalance. The IHS may develop insidiously, but a proportion of patients present with a sudden excruciating headache and in those cases it is necessary to rule out a subarachnoid hemorrhage. The headache is most likely caused by traction forces on pain-sensitive intracranial structures (blood vessels, meninges) after standing or postural change that alters the CSF pressure.

Lumbar puncture with CSF examination and measurement of the opening pressure is the most important diagnostic test. The CSF pressure in lateral decubitus position in cases of IHS is usually less than 60 mmH$_2$O (normal 60–200). The CSF protein content elevation and mild lymphocytic pleocytosis may be present. In some patients this syndrome may persist for years, leading to erroneous alternative diagnoses (e.g., migraine).

The IHS is typically divided into spontaneous and symptomatic. The most frequent cause is the CSF leak related to lumbar puncture. However, many surgical, cranial, spinal, or thoracic procedures, injuries, and some metabolic conditions (e.g., diabetic coma, uremia, dehydration) may lead to the development of IHS. Sometimes it may follow relatively benign trauma or coughing or sneezing spells.

Brain MRI frequently shows prominent enhancement of meninges, which is most likely related to the increased blood flow through the meningeal vessels secondary to decreased intracranial pressure. However, before these MRI findings were recognized as typical of low intracranial pressure, many patients were thought to have either infectious or even a malignant process and menigeal biopsy was not infrequently performed. In some cases there is evidence of downward displacement of cerebellar tonsils and small subdural fluid collections. In some patients the site of the leak can be localized by a radionuclide cysternography or CT/myelography scan. However, in many typical cases the precise site of the leak cannot be localized.

Management of IHS is similar to treatment of post–lumbar puncture headache. In many patients symptoms resolve spontaneously with bed rest, oral hydration, caffeine, and analgesics. If the headache persists, intravenous normal saline or caffeine infusions may be helpful. However, in intractable cases the epidural blood patch might be the most effective treatment. The mechanism of this treatment is unclear, but it may be due to the closure of the CSF leak site in the dura or vasoconstriction induced by deactivation of the adenosine receptor by sudden increase in the CSF pressure. The latter mechanism, like caffeine treatment, may be responsible for the near-immediate headache resolution in some cases, possibly by inducing blood vessel constriction with subsequent decrease of blood flow.

In a majority of cases the CSF leak is within the spinal dura. Therefore, in cases with typical clinical, MRI, and lumbar puncture findings it may not be necessary to perform radioisotope cisternography or other studies to document the site of the leak. Most patients respond to an epidural blood patch performed in the lumbar region (even if not done in close proximity of the CSF leak site). There is evidence from several studies that after epidural injection of approximately 15 ml of blood in the lumbar region there is a caudal and rostral blood migration spanning up to 7–14 spinal levels. If the epidural blood patch is not successful, a careful search for the site of the leak should be undertaken since neurosurgical treatment to close the leak may be necessary.

The present patient was treated with an epidural blood patch with compete resolution of symptoms within a few hours.

Clinical Pearls

1. Consider CSF leak in a patient with a sudden onset of postural headache.
2. MRI is a helpful diagnostic tool in evaluating patients with intracranial hypotension headache and frequently shows prominent dural enhancement.
3. In most patients, visualization of the CSF leak site with different radiographic techniques is not necessary.
4. Epidural blood patch is an effective treatment of headache caused by spinal CSF leak.
5. Some patients may need neurosurgical intervention to close a CSF leak.

REFERENCES

1. Fernández E: Headaches associated with low spinal fluid pressure. Headache 1990; 30:122–128.
2. Khurana RK: Intracranial hypotension. Semin Neurol 1996; 16:5–10.
3. Marcelis J, Silberstein SD: Spontaneous low cerebrospinal fluid pressure headache. Headache 1990; 30:192–196.
4. Mokri B, Piepgras DG, Miller GM: Syndrome of orthostatic headaches and diffuse pachymeningeal gadolinium enhancement. Mayo Clin Proc 1997; 72:400–413.
5. Pannullo SC, Reich JB, Krol G, et al: MRI changes in intracranial hypotension. Neurology 1993; 43:919–926.

PATIENT 7

A 29-year-old man with severe neck pain and diffuse skin abnormalities

A 29-year-old man presented with severe, progressive left-sided neck pain for the last several months. The pain was nonradiating and there was no recent trauma. He reported multiple focal areas of numbness on his limbs and chest. Since childhood he has developed diffuse, multiple hyperpigmented skin lesions and nodules over his entire body. There was no weakness, bowel or bladder involvement, or loss of hearing or vision. He denied any headaches or memory problems.

Physical Examination: Vital signs: normal. General: normocephalic, numerous cutaneous/subcutaneous tender nodules over the forehead and other areas of the skull, some tender; supple neck, good range of motion, numerous subcutaneous tumors of different sizes, tender to palpation, the largest felt over the left sternocleidomastoid muscle. Skin: diffuse hyperpigmented areas, numerous cutaneous or subcutaneous soft nodules of various sizes in diffuse distribution (see figure, *left*). Spine: no deformity, spinal processes nontender, good range of motion. Mental status, speech, cranial nerves, motor examination: normal. Sensory examination: numbness to pain stimuli over both thumbs, anterolateral left thigh, and right lower leg. Muscle stretch reflexes: normal. Plantar reflexes: flexor. Coordination, gait: normal.

Stop and Consider: What is the significance of the skin lesions and development of neurologic symptoms in this patient?

Laboratory Findings: CBC, chemistry, electrolytes, ESR: normal. Nerve conduction studies and needle electromyography (NCS/EMG): multiple focal neuropathies in upper extremities and multiple, bilateral cervical radiculopathies. Cervical spine MRI: see figure, *right*.

Question: What potential complication is indicated by the MRI findings?

Discussion: The hyperpigmented skin lesions are typical café-au-lait lesions and the nodular

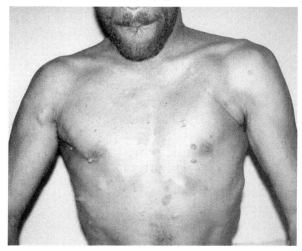
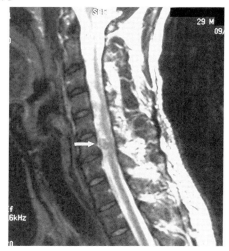

Diagnosis: Neurofibromatosis type 1 (von Recklinghausen's disease)

changes are cutaneous and subcutaneous neuro-fibromas. The MRI showed multiple, bilateral "dumbbell" tumors typical of neurofibromas involving spinal nerve roots from C1 through T1 (depicted by an arrow in the cervical spine MRI). The NCS/EMG studies showed features of mononeuropathy multiplex and cervical polyradiculopathy, presumably caused by neurofibromas compressing peripheral nerves and nerve roots. However, his neck tenderness was caused by the palpable subcutaneous tumors and not radiculopathies.

Neurofibromatosis is a hereditary neurocutaneous disorder that may present in a few clinical forms. The most typical and most frequent is neurofibromatosis type 1 (NF-1), also known as von Recklinghausen's disease or "peripheral" neurofibromatosis. The disease is characterized by multiple hyperpigmented skin lesions known as café-au-lait spots, cutaneous or subcutaneous neurofibromas, plexiform neurofibromas, smaller hyperpigmented lesions resembling freckles in the axillary and inguinal regions, and iris hamartomas (Lisch nodules). Other associated abnormalities may include optic gliomas, macrocephaly (with or without hydrocephalus), musculoskeletal abnormalities, vascular disease, hypertension (due to neurofibromatosis of renal artery or pheochromocytoma), rhabdomyosarcoma, or Wilms' tumor.

The clinical spectrum and the distribution of lesions in NF-1 are highly variable. Most patients have a relatively benign form of the disease manifesting as cosmetic problems without functional impairment. About 30% of patients with NF-1 may have some degree of mild cognitive impairment.

The most common CNS tumor in NF-1 is optic glioma, but meningiomas, astrocytomas, and shwan-nomas may also be observed. Large plexiform neurofibromas, such as those observed on the cervical MRI of the present patient may cause cord compression or radiculopathies.

The hallmark of neurofibromatosis type 2 (NF-2), also known as central neurofibromatosis, is the presence of acoustic neuromas (usually bilateral), meningiomas, schwannomas, gliomas, spinal cord ependymomas, cutaneous or plexiform neurofibromas, and subcapsular cataracts.

Both NF-1 and NF-2 are autosomal dominant disorders. The NF-1 gene is on the proximal long arm of chromosome 17 (locus q11.2). The NF-2 gene is located on the long arm of chromosome 22. There is significant overlap between different types of neurofibromatoses. The major difference is the bilateral presence of acoustic neuromas in NF-2.

Skin tumors associated with neurofibromatosis should be removed when they cause significant pain, compromise function, or produce significant cosmetic disfiguration. Some neurofibromas may degenerate into sarcomas; therefore, all surgically removed lesions should be examined pathologically. MRI is the best diagnostic test to identify lesions affecting the central nervous system. Spinal tumors causing cord compression need surgical treatment. Surgery, radiation, and chemotherapy should be considered in treatment of associated malignant and nonmalignant tumors in individual cases.

The present patient underwent removal of subcutaneous neck tumors with resolution of neck tenderness. Histopathologic examination was typical of a neurofibroma.

Clinical Pearls

1. Neurofibromas affecting the spinal roots may reach very large size and result in myelopathy due to cord compression.

2. MRI of the brain and spine should be considered in all patients with neurofibromatosis who present with signs or symptoms of the peripheral or central nervous system dysfunction.

3. Changing skin lesions should be surgically removed since they may indicate development of a sarcoma.

4. There is significant clinical overlap between the different forms of neurofibromatosis. The DNA analysis is helpful in diagnostically difficult cases.

5. Genetic counseling should be offered to families of patients with neurofibromatosis. Prenatal diagnosis is possible for NF-1.

REFERENCES

1. Mackool BT, Fitzpatrick TB: Diagnosis of neurofibromatosis by skin examination. Semin Neurol 1992; 12:358–363.
2. National Institute of Health Consensus Development Conference: Neurofibromatosis: Consensus statement. Arch Neurol 1988; 45:575–578.
3. Riccardi VM: Neurofibromatosis: Clinical heterogeneity. Curr Probl Cancer 1982; 7:1–34.

PATIENT 8

A 48-year-old man with a 1-week history of unilateral headache, anisocoria, and ptosis

A 48-year-old man with a history of migraines and hypertension was awakened by severe right hemicrania and neck pain unlike the usual headaches he experienced occasionally. His right eyesight was blurred but there was no double vision. His wife observed that his left pupil was larger than the right and that his right eyelid was drooping. After waiting 5 days, the patient presented to an outpatient clinic for neurologic consultation. His headache and visual symptoms had partially resolved. He denied recent head or neck trauma, limb weakness, or numbness. He suffered facial trauma in a motor vehicle accident 20 years earlier that required facial reconstructive surgery.

Physical Examination: Temperature, pulse, respirations: normal; blood pressure 140/90. General: normal, except mild right-sided neck tenderness. Mental status, speech: normal. Cranial nerves: normal fundi, visual fields and visual acuity normal; right and left pupils 3 mm and 4.5 mm in diameter, respectively; pupillary reflexes, ocular movements: intact; mild right ptosis; right side of forehead felt dryer than left side; facial muscles: normal and symmetric; oral and pharyngeal structures: midline. Motor and sensory examination: normal. Muscle stretch reflexes: grade 2 and symmetric. Plantar reflexes: flexor. Coordination, gait: normal.

Stop and Consider: What is the localization of the neurologic dysfunction in this patient?

Laboratory Findings: CBC, serum chemistries, ESR: normal. Head MRI: see figure.

Question: What diagnosis is confirmed by the MRI?

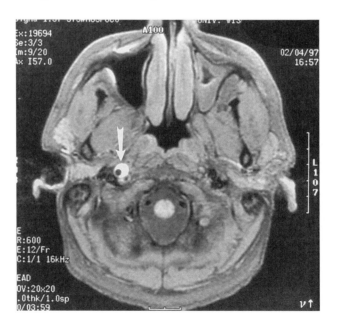

Diagnosis: Acute right internal carotid artery dissection

Discussion: The clinical presentation of acute right ptosis, miosis, and forehead anhidrosis (partial or incomplete Horner's syndrome or oculosympathetic palsy) indicates interruption of the right-sided oculosympathetic pathways. The differential diagnosis includes any process that can interrupt the sympathetic pathway, including the 1st-order neuron (hypothalamus to upper thoracic cord), 2nd-order neuron (intermediolateral column in upper cord to superior cervical ganglion) or 3rd-order neuron (superior cervical ganglion with branches that ascend the carotid vessels to the orbit). Typical pathologies at these sites include brain stem infarction (e.g., lateral medullary syndrome affecting 1st-order neuron), apical lung or neck masses (affecting 2nd-order neuron), and carotid trauma or dissection (affecting 3rd-order neuron).

The presence of a unilateral headache is an important clue that carotid dissection has occurred. The head MRI confirmed the diagnosis by showing increased signal on T1 and T2 weighted images surrounding the right carotid lumen, which is consistent with the presence of a mural thrombus (see figure, arrow). MR angiogram (MRA), which was subsequently obtained in this patient, also showed a corresponding narrowed carotid lumen.

Internal carotid artery (ICA) dissections can occur spontaneously, after major or even relatively insignificant neck trauma, or in patients with diseases that cause structural weakness in arterial vessels. Blood enters a defect in the endothelium and splits layers of media to form a false lumen that propagates distally and causes narrowing of the vessel's true lumen. The term dissecting aneurysm is reserved for carotid dissections that balloon out within the media because of an expanding hematoma that remains directly connected to the true lumen. These structures can form thrombi prone to distal embolization.

The overall incidence of spontaneous ICA dissection in the U.S. is about 3/100,000. Most patients are younger than 50 years. Common presenting findings in ICA dissection are unilateral headache or face pain, transient ischemic attacks and stroke, Horner's syndrome, carotid bruit, and neck pain. Cranial nerve palsies, amaurosis fugax, and syncope are less frequently observed. ICA dissection can compromise brain tissue because of hemodynamically altered blood flow through a stenotic lumen, which occasionally completely occludes from thrombosis or because of thrombi that embolize distally into tributaries of intracranial vessels. ICA dissection is an important diagnosis to consider in the work-up of ischemic strokes occurring in young to middle-aged patients. Currently,

MRI and MRA technologies are the most efficient means of detecting ICA dissection. MRI will show cross-sections of a narrowed arterial lumen surrounded by crescents of thrombosed blood within the vessel wall. MRA may show a string sign, narrowed lumen, no flow, or large aneurysms. Some patients may require contrast angiography to verify or supplement MRA studies.

Because thromboemboli can propagate within the narrowed true lumen or within the false space of dissection, recommended treatment for acute ICA dissection is intravenous heparin followed by at least 3 months of oral anticoagulation with warfarin. In dissections that extend intracranially there is a risk for subarachnoid hemorrhage, and in such cases anticoagulation may not be indicated.

Surgery may be indicated for patients with dissecting aneurysms that are a source of embolization or for those with critically stenosed true lumens causing clinically evident cerebral ischemia. Superficial temporal artery to middle cerebral artery bypass is used to provide an alternative blood supply to intracranial vessels in patients with ischemic symptoms caused by hemodynamically significant ICA stenosis. When the ICA recanalizes or its narrowed lumen expands, the bypass usually becomes nonfunctional. Also, surgery may be considered in cases of a subarachnoid hemorrage resulting from leaking intracranial dissection or aneurysm. Overall, most patients with spontaneous ICA dissection have an excellent long-term prognosis, with less than 10% suffering from significant neurologic injury.

Horner's syndrome in this case is partial in that the patient had only forehead anhidrosis. The sympathetic fibers supplying sweat glands to the most of the face travel along the external carotid artery, while those carried by the ICA innervate only those in part of the forehead via the supraorbital nerve. Complete Horner's syndrome includes ipsilateral miosis, enophthalmos (paralysis of the muscle of Müller), upper and lower tarsal muscle weakness causing pseudoptosis with some elevation of the lower lid, ocular hypotonia, anhidrosis of the entire ipsilateral face, and dilatation of blood vessels to the ipsilateral face, head, and neck. Pain fibers from the trigeminal nerve ascend along the ICA and branch along the anterior and middle cerebral arteries to innervate pain-sensitive structures within the anterior and middle cranial fossae, causing referred pain to the head or hemicrania in ICA dissection (Raeder's syndrome).

Frequently, in patients with evidence of Horner's syndrome, the exact location (1st-, 2nd-, or 3rd-order neuron) or nature of the lesion in the sympathetic pathways is not obvious and application of pharmacologic agents to the affected eye may be helpful. Hydroxyamphetamine (1%) releases norepinephrine from sympathetic nerve terminals causing dilatation of a normal pupil. Pupillary dilatation in response to hydroxyamphetamine requires an intact 3rd-order postganglionic neuron. The pupil will dilate normally if the lesion causing Horner's syndrome is located within the 1st- or 2nd-order neurons but will not dilate if the lesion involves the 3rd-order neuron.

About one fifth of arterial dissections in the neck occur within the vertebral vessels and may cause symptoms and signs of ischemia in posterior fossa structures. Principles behind etiology, pathophysiology, imaging, and treatment are similar to those for ICA dissection.

The present patient was placed on 6-month anticoagulation therapy with warfarin and the INR was maintained between 2–2.5. His neurologic exam normalized and pain gradually resolved. Repeat MRI and MRA showed resolution of the mural thrombus, minimal narrowing of the right internal carotid artery, and no evidence for significantly diminished flow or aneurysm formation.

Clinical Pearls

1. Patients presenting with Horner's syndrome and ipsilateral neck pain or headache may have carotid dissection and require immediate evaluation.

2. Carotid dissection may also present with severe unilateral headache without Horner's syndrome or any other neurologic signs.

3. Carotid dissection may be visualized on MRI as a crescent of increased signal intensity surrounding the vessel and on MRA as a tapering narrowed lumen.

4. Treatment for carotid or vertebral dissection is anticoagulation; however, when dissection extends intracranially, there is an increased risk of subarrachnoid hemorrhage.

5. Surgical treatment consisting of ECA-ICA bypass may be indicated in selected cases.

REFERENCES

1. Humphrey PW, Keller MP, Spadone DP, Silver D: Spontaneous common carotid artery dissection. J Vasc Surg 1993; 18:95–99.
2. Karacagil S, Hardemark HG, Bergqvist D: Spontaneous internal carotid dissection. Int Angiol 1996; 15:291–294.
3. Leys D, Lucas C, Gobert M, et al: Cervical artery dissections. Eur Neurol 1997; 37:3–12.
4. Mokri B: Spontaneous dissections of internal carotid arteries. The Neurologist 1997; 3:104–119.
5. Provenzale JM: Dissection of the internal carotid and vertebral arteries: Imaging features. Am J Roentgenol 1995; 165: 1099–1104.
6. Russo CP, Smoker WRK: Nonatheromatous carotid artery disease. Neuroimaging Clin North Am 1996; 6:811–830.

PATIENT 9

A 39-year-old man with a whiplash injury

A 39-year-old man was in his car at a stop sign when his car was suddenly struck from behind by another vehicle. His head was rapidly jerked backward. Initially he did not have pain or other symptoms, but a few hours later he noticed numbness of the tip of his left index finger. He also developed left-sided neck pain radiating to the upper trapezius region, which was markedly aggravated by neck motion. Within a few days he was experiencing numbness involving the whole left index finger and radial aspect of the left forearm as well as weakness of the left elbow extension. He reported no difficulty with bowel or bladder function. There was no numbness or weakness in his legs.

Physical Examination: Vital signs: normal. HEENT: normocephalic head, nontender skull; neck tenderness and some muscle spasm on palpation of the left cervical paraspinal muscles and the trapezius; neck flexion or rotation aggravate the pain. Mental status, speech, cranial nerves: normal. Motor examination: normal except for mild weakness (grade +4) of left elbow extension. Sensory examination: decreased to pin prick over the left index finger and part of the extensor surface of the left forearm. Muscle stretch reflexes: mildly depressed left triceps reflex compared to the opposite side. Plantar reflexes: flexor. Coordination, gait: normal.

Stop and Consider: What nerve or nerve root could account for the pain, weakness, and sensory deficit in this patient?

Laboratory Findings: Cervical spine MRI: see figures. Nerve conduction studies: normal. Needle electromyography (performed 4 weeks after the accident): fibrillation potentials in the left triceps, pronator teres, and cervical paraspinal muscles; motor unit potentials in the same muscles characterized by very large amplitude and long duration, abundant polyphasic units present, motor unit recruitment markedly decreased in the left triceps.

Question: What is your interpretation of the MRI and electrodiagnostic findings?

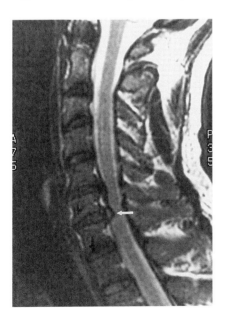 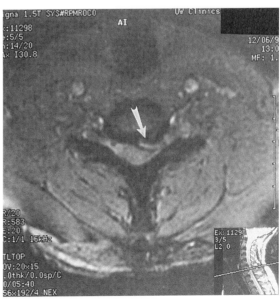

Diagnosis: Left C7 radiculopathy

Discussion: The pattern of sensory deficit, pain radiation, weakness of the left triceps muscle, and depressed left triceps reflex indicate the presence of an acute left C7 nerve root compression. The clinical diagnosis was confirmed by the MRI and electrodiagnostic findings. The MRI of the cervical spine showed a very large herniated disc at the C6–7 level compressing the left C7 root (arrows). There is also a smaller disc at the C5–6 level. At both C6–7 and C5–6 levels there is some degree of spinal stenosis with compression of the anterior aspect of the spinal cord. The EMG showed evidence of acute and chronic changes in the C7-innervated muscles on the left as well as cervical paraspinal muscles. The marked decrease in motor unit recruitment and spontaneous activity is consistent with an acute or recent event; however, the prominent reinnervation changes observed within 4 weeks from the accident suggest that although the acute symptoms and signs of the radiculopathy were directly related to the accident, this patient very likely had some preexisting, most likely asymptomatic C7 radiculopathy.

Ninety percent of cervical disc herniations occur at the C5–6 and C6–7 spine levels. The C6–7 herniated discs, causing C7 nerve root compression, are the most common. In typical C7 radiculopathies, paresthesias and pain radiate to the index and middle fingers. Sensory loss may be found within the C7 dermatome. Weakness and atrophy involve the triceps muscle, pectoral muscles, and wrist extensors. Triceps reflex is diminished or absent.

MRI is the best diagnostic study to evaluate patients with radiculopathy. It may visualize the herniated disc or demonstrate spinal canal or foraminal stenosis ("spondylotic" radiculopathy) and exclude spinal cord compression. In some cases EMG may help to confirm the diagnosis and localize specific level of root dysfunction and is especially useful when the clinical or MRI findings are equivocal. In some patients, when surgical treatment is considered, a myelogram with a follow-up CT may be necessary. MRI and EMG are not necessary in most patients who do not show signs of focal neurologic dysfunction.

Most patients with cervical radiculopathy can be treated successfully with a conservative approach.

In a majority of patients the symptoms, especially the radicular pain, resolve within a few weeks or months. Neck immobilization with a neck collar, muscle relaxants, analgesics, and physical therapy are the mainstay of treatment. Some patients may require mild narcotics, usually for short periods of time. Once the acute pain subsides (usually within 1–3 weeks), some stretching and strengthening exercises are beneficial. Neck "manipulations" are contraindicated with disc herniations. The benefit of epidural steroids is questionable.

Surgical treatment is indicated in patients who have acute cervical disc herniation and signs of myelopathy. In patients who present with purely radicular signs, a conservative approach should be attempted first, but in some cases of herniation with severe loss of function, early surgical intervention may be necessary.

It should be emphasized that the vast majority of neck injuries of a "whiplash" type cause only injuries to soft tissues (muscles, ligaments, tendons) that are not associated with focal neurologic signs but may be accompanied by symptoms that mimic a radicular pattern. Symptomatic management with physical therapy is the cornerstone of treatment. Some relatively "benign" whiplash injuries may be associated with prolonged recovery with persisting neck pain or headache for many months and some of those patients develop a chronic syndrome commonly referred to as whiplash syndrome. Careful neurologic examination and evaluation for potential cervical spine instability, including cervical x-rays with flexion/extension films, if necessary, should be done in all patients.

The present patient was initially scheduled for surgical treatment; however, his pain resolved before the surgery and, without signs of myelopathy, a conservative approach was pursued. This included physical therapy, muscle relaxants, and nonsteroidal anti-inflammatory medications. Three months later he showed markedly improved strength in his left triceps. The EMG at that time showed only minimal spontaneous activity with prominent reinnervation changes and significantly improved recruitment. After 5 months his strength was back to normal and he was asymptomatic.

Clinical Pearls

1. A detailed neurologic examination is of paramount importance in patients presenting with a whiplash-type injury to exclude radiculopathy and myelopathy.

2. MRI is the imaging modality of choice in the evaluation of patients with radiculopathy.

3. Electromyography (EMG) may help to confirm the diagnosis, localize the process to a specific nerve root, evaluate the severity and duration of the radiculopathy, and provide useful information in the evaluation of recovery in some patients.

4. EMG should not be used routinely in all cases presenting with neck or arm pain, especially in patients with no focal neurologic deficits.

5. In most instances surgical treatment of radiculopathies is not necessary and the outcome is good with medical treatment.

REFERENCES

1. Dubuisson A, Lenelle J, Stevenaert A: Soft cervical disc herniation: A retrospective study of 100 cases. Acta Neurochirur 1993; 125:115–119.
2. Tan JC, Nordin M: Role of physical therapy in the treatment of cervical disc disease. Orhtop Clin North Am 1992; 23:435–449.

PATIENT 10

A 48-year-old woman with a 20-year history of recurrent unilateral headache, visual scotomata, and hemibody numbness

A 48-year-old woman with history of hypertension and cigarette smoking presented for evaluation of recurrent episodes of neurologic symptoms, which started at age 21. She described approximately 50 events, from age 21 through age 45, that consisted of visual scotomata, lasting from 5–20 minutes, associated with right retro-orbital headache, lasting hours to days, and left-sided numbness of the face, tongue, arm, and leg, lasting 25 minutes or less. Typical spells would progress from visual changes to numbness to headache, with headache lingering for hours to days. At age 45 she was placed on aspirin therapy and her spells significantly decreased, only to increase in frequency after she started estrogen replacement therapy at age 47. She denied having any other recent neurologic symptoms or events of any kind. Her family history was significant for females with onset of arterial hypertension in their twenties and two family members who died from ruptured intracranial aneurysms.

Physical Examination: Temperature: normal; pulse 68 and regular; respirations: normal; blood pressure 132/86. General: loud carotid artery bruits on the neck, right greater than left. Mental status, speech, language: normal. Cranial nerves: eye fundi normal, pupils equal and reactive to light and accommodation, visual acuity, visual fields and extraocular eye movements normal, facial muscles symmetric and normal, oral and pharyngeal structures midline. Motor and sensory examination: normal. Muscle stretch reflexes: grade 3 and symmetric. Plantar reflexes: flexor. Coordination, gait: normal.

Stop and Consider: How would you classify the headache? What feature of the headache pattern is of concern?

Laboratory Findings: CBC, chemistry panel, coagulopathic profile, ESR: normal. Head CT: normal. Intra-arterial angiography of the right internal carotid artery: see figure. Similar, but less severe findings were present in the left internal carotid artery.

Question: What abnormality is shown on the angiogram?

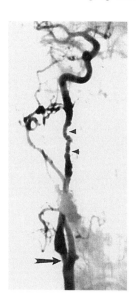

Diagnosis: Symptomatic fibromuscular dysplasia of the right internal carotid artery

Discussion: The clinical presentation of this patient with transient and self-limited episodes of visual scotomata, right retro-orbital headache, and left hemibody numbness suggests a pathophysiologic process affecting the right internal carotid artery. The "positive" phenomena, including presence of headache, visual obscurations, and paresthesias, suggest that these transient attacks may not necessarily be ischemic in nature. Ischemic transient neurologic events typically have "negative" phenomena, such as loss of sight, loss of feeling, loss of power, or loss of speech. Positive phenomena are more suggestive of either migrainous, epileptic, or demyelinating processes. This patient's family history, combined with her history of arterial hypertension and the long-standing nature of these transient events, suggests an underlying arterial vasculopathy. The differential diagnosis for this patient's problems should also include fibromuscular dysplasia, excessive tortuosity of extracranial vessels (Ehlers-Danlos syndrome, Marfan syndrome), and moyamoya disease. However, the images of her right internal carotid artery showed a classic presentation of both tubular stenosis at the origin of the right internal carotid artery (arrow) and the typical luminal irregularities (arrowheads) seen in fibromuscular dysplasia. This patient was also found to have renal artery stenosis.

Fibromuscular dysplasia of extracranial vasculature was first described in 1965. In typical series of patients with this disorder, women predominate and their mean age is around 50. Dysplastic vessels in the carotid circulation are found in 90–95% of all patients with extracranial fibromuscular dysplasia, while only 20% of the patients have vertebral artery dysplasia. The major neurologic presentations of fibromuscular dysplasia include: (1) temporary or permanent cerebral ischemia in 40–50%; (2) cerebral hemorrhagic phenomena in 20–30%; and (3) symptoms and neurologic signs associated with cerebral aneurysms in 20–25%. The typical symptomatologies include: (1) headache in 70–75%; (2) "mental distress" in 40–50%; (3) pulsatile tinnitus in 30–40%; (4) vertigo in 30–40%; (5) transient ischemic attacks (TIAs) in 30–40%; (6) syncope in 25–30%; and (7) throbbing or pounding lateral neck pain in 15–20% of patients. Angiographic features include: (1) classic "string of beads," as in this patient; (2) tubular stenosis, as in this patient; (3) tubular stenosis plus poststenotic dilation or aneurysmal formation; and (4) semicircumferential arterial wall changes distal to the carotid bifurcation. Diseases often associated with fibromuscular dysplasia include intracranial aneurysms, arteriovenous malformations in the brain, aberrant renal arteries, and renal dysplasia.

Patients with fibromuscular dysplasia are typically treated with risk factor modification, surveillance for the associated diseases as listed above, treatment with antiplatelet agents, and, on rare occasions, surgical reconstructive procedures to try to reestablish a more normal intravascular lumen. Surgery is quite controversial in patients with fibromuscular dysplasia and has included intraoperative dilation of dysplastic vessels as well as a number of different bypass procedures. On rare occasions, warfarin anticoagulation is used in patients whose transient ischemic attacks or other ischemic symptoms continue in spite of adequate antiplatelet therapy. Obviously, in these patients exquisite control of arterial hypertension is necessary before warfarin can be used safely.

The present patient was treated with risk factor modification, angioplasty to repair the bilateral renal artery stenosis, discontinuation of estrogen therapy, and continued administration of aspirin. Her medication regimen was also modified in that her residual hypertension was treated with propranolol. She remained well with no further neurologic events. Her most recent neurologic events were believed to be related to complicated migraine and control of her symptoms was probably related to treatment with a combination of propranolol and an antiplatelet agent (aspirin), both of which have antimigraine properties.

Clinical Pearls

1. Suspect fibromuscular dysplasia of extracranial arteries in young patients (especially female) with transient neurologic events, vascular headaches, carotid bruits, and associated arterial hypertension.

2. Appropriate and specific therapy for transient ischemic attacks (TIAs) can only be offered when a precise diagnosis of both anatomic and pathophysiologic factors is made.

3. Risk factor modification and aggressive treatment of associated diseases can minimize neurologic and cerebrovascular events.

REFERENCES

1. Luscher TF, Lie JT, Stanson AW, et al: Arterial fibromuscular dysplasia. Mayo Clin Proc 1987; 62:931–952.
2. Mettinger KL: Fibromuscular dysplasia and the brain. II. Current concept of the disease. Stroke 1982; 13:53–58.
3. Mettinger KL, Erickson K: Fibromuscular dysplasia and the brain. I. Observations on angiographic, clinical, and genetic characteristics. Stroke 1982; 13:46–52.

PATIENT 11

A 40-year-old woman with a 1-year history of episodic visual blurring

A 40-year-old woman was referred to the neurology clinic after two attacks of visual blurring. The first occurred 1 year prior to her evaluation and involved the right eye. She saw an ophthalmologist after her vision had gradually deteriorated over 6 weeks and reported mild pain in the right eye. She was given prednisone and her sight returned to virtually normal in about a week. However, later that year she had similar symptoms in the left eye. On this occasion prednisone treatment also was followed by improvement, but during periods of heat or stress she experienced deterioration of central vision in the right eye. On further questioning it became apparent that she had a history of paresthesias 5 years earlier, which had spontaneously remitted after 3 months. There was no family history of neurologic or ophthalmologic disorders.

Physical Examination: Vital signs: normal. HEENT, cardiac, chest, abdomen, spine: normal. Mental status: normal, except for mild depression thought to be due to concern about her disease. Speech: normal. Cranial nerves: mild but definite diminution of the corrected visual acuity to 20/30 OU, peripheral fields full to confrontation; central scotoma in the left eye on testing of the central fields with a 2-mm red pin target; formal field testing with the Amsler's grid: marked diminution of color vision in both eyes as judged by Ishihara plates; funduscopic examination: equivocal disc pallor in the left eye and definite disc pallor in the right eye; extraocular movements: full, but "jerky" and irregular on pursuing a target. Motor examination: normal bulk, tone, and strength. Muscle stretch reflexes: brisk throughout (grade 3). Sensory examination: diminution in the subjective intensity of perceived pin prick and light touch at all segments below the T11 dermatome bilaterally. Plantar reflexes: extensor bilaterally. Coordination/gait: slight clumsiness on finger-to-nose testing, gait slightly hesitant, support required during tandem walking, falling backward during the Romberg maneuver.

Stop and Consider: What CNS structures are most likely affected in this patient? What disease process most likely accounts for her symptoms?

Laboratory Findings: CBC, chemistry, ESR, ANA: normal. Visual evoked responses: marked conduction delay in both optic nerves, particularly on the left. Brain MRI: see figure.

Question: Are the MRI findings consistent with this patient's symptoms?

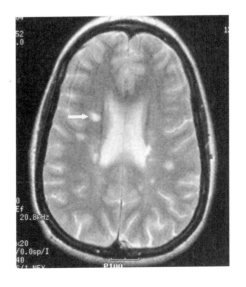

Diagnosis: Optic neuritis and multiple sclerosis

Discussion: Transient disturbance of visual acuity lead to the suspicion of optic neuritis in this patient. It was confirmed by careful ophthalmologic evaluation that failed to show a hereditary, compressive, or primary rheumatologic, infectious, or dysimmune disease that would account for her symptoms. A central scotoma is characteristic of optic nerve dysfunction, and the pale appearance of her optic discs as well as the diminished visual acuity indicate some degree of permanent fiber loss in the optic nerves. Bilateral Babinski signs and brisk muscle stretch reflexes indicate involvement of the corticospinal tracts. The sensory symptoms and findings also suggest a more diffuse CNS involvement. The MRI scan of the brain showed multiple areas of increased signal in the periventricular white matter on T2 weighted images (arrow), most consistent with a diffuse demyelinating process. The MRI of the cervical and thoracic spinal cord also showed several demyelinating lesions.

Optic neuritis can be defined as an idiopathic inflammation of one or both optic nerves. The pathology of this disorder is demyelinating, and many authors feel that optic neuritis is simply one manifestation of multiple sclerosis. In fact, on follow-ups of 10–20 years as many as 80% of patients initially diagnosed with optic neuritis subsequently develop disseminated white matter disease that can be clinically recognized as multiple sclerosis. This patient had a history of paresthesias prior to the onset of optic neuritis, suggesting that her disease was disseminated. Also, after the initial evaluation she continued to have episodes of paresthesias, ambulatory difficulty, and transient visual disturbance. Her initial evaluation showed evidence of corticospinal tract and sensory pathway disturbance in addition to optic neuritis.

The differential diagnosis of optic neuritis includes all conditions that result in progressive visual failure, especially those that preferentially affect the optic nerve. Optic nerve swelling in the setting of relatively preserved visual acuity may indicate papilledema secondary to increased intracranial pressure. Also, ischemic optic neuropathy should be considered, particularly when visual failure is associated with sudden onset or stepwise progression in a patient with known cerebrovascular risk factors. In some cases, infectious conditions such as syphilis or tuberculosis or primary inflammatory diseases such as sarcoid or systemic lupus erythematosus will produce ocular and central nervous system inflammation. A family history of progressive visual failure suggests a genetic cause for the patient's deficits, such as Leber's optic neuropathy. Rarely, optic neuropathy is caused by toxic exposures, as in methanol poisoning, ethambutol toxicity, and tobacco-alcohol amblyopia. Relentless visual failure associated with pain and focal neurologic signs suggests a compressive cause, such as tumor or giant aneurysm. Carcinoma may affect optic nerves by means of metastatic tumors or malignant infiltration of the meninges. Optic nerve failure may also follow nutritional deficiencies, e.g., vitamin B_{12} deficiency.

If the pattern of visual loss is typical of optic neuritis, the diagnosis may be established reliably on the basis of the history and physical examination without recourse to expensive laboratory testing, which is of very low yield in this setting and may be of some risk to the patient. Findings typical of optic neuritis include ocular pain, relative involvement of central or paracentral visual fields, and unilaterality. Often, the course of optic neuritis will consist of an insidious onset, progressive loss of vision in approximately a week, and substantial improvement over subsequent weeks. If visual failure is relentlessly progressive and associated with focal neurologic findings, a positive family history of similar disorder, or an evident systemic disease, further testing, including neuroimaging, immunologic assessment, genetic counseling, and other investigations may be appropriate.

Although the etiology and pathogenesis of multiple sclerosis remain areas of intense controversy and research, there is a general consensus that abnormalities of the immune system underlie this disease. The triggering event for the immune dysfunction is uncertain, but viral or other infectious processes or reactions to other antigens have received attention. On the basis of such theories, clinical trials with immunomodulating treatments, such as beta interferon and copolymer-1, have been initiated. This has led to the development of medications that significantly influence the frequency of relapses in active multiple sclerosis.

The present patient was treated for 3 years with interferon beta-1b. Initially she had a period of stability during which her relapses became less frequent. However, after 3 years she developed fatigue, malaise, and elevated liver function tests, indicative of the development of neutralizing antibodies to the beta interferon. This medication was stopped and the patient improved dramatically. Her occasional flares of the disease have been managed with intravenous corticosteroids. This class of medications has been shown to hasten recovery from acute flares of multiple sclerosis or optic neuritis, although their effect on the ultimate disability has not been established. Although this patient remains in a relapsing, remitting phase of the disease, many patients unfortunately develop a secondarily progressive course after the first decade of the disease. Presently there are many experimental trials of treatment in progressive multiple sclerosis; however, to date there is no proven effective treatment for this phase of the disease.

Clinical Pearls

1. Patients with optic neuritis are at considerable risk for subsequent development of multiple sclerosis.

2. Immunomodulating agents show a favorable but incomplete reduction of the relapse rate. These treatments should be considered in patients with active disease that causes substantial recurrent disability.

3. Treatment of acute relapses with intravenous corticosteroids may accelerate short-term recovery but does not appear to change the long-term outcome of the disease.

REFERENCES

1. Lucchinetti CF, Rodriguez M: The controversy surrounding the pathogenesis of the multiple sclerosis lesion. Mayo Clin Proc 1997; 72:665–678.
2. Lynch SG, Rose JW: Multiple sclerosis. Dis Mon 1996; 42:1–55.
3. Rizzo JF, Lessell S: Risk of developing multiple sclerosis after uncomplicated optic neuritis: A long-term prospective study. Neurology 1988; 38:185–190.

PATIENT 12

A 62-year-old man with abrupt onset of left-sided weakness and numbness

A 62-year-old man with a history of excessive alcohol use awoke one morning with profound weakness and numbness of his left face, arm, and leg. He was seen in the emergency department and was admitted for further evaluation. He denied any prior episodes of transient weakness, numbness, or other symptoms suggestive of possible transient ischemic attacks. There was no history of hypertension, cardiac disease, diabetes, or any other cerebrovascular or cardiovascular risk factors.

Physical Examination: Temperature 36.5°; pulse 88 and irregular; respirations 18; blood pressure 120/78. Skin, neck, chest, abdomen: normal. Rectal exam: stool mildly positive for blood. Mental status: alert, awake, follows commands. Speech: mild dysarthria but no evidence of aphasia. Cranial nerves: pupils equal and reactive to light; fundi and vision normal; left homonymous hemianopia on visual field testing; gaze preference to the right; moderate facial weakness involving the left lower face; tongue and palatal movements normal. Motor examination: muscle tone flaccid on the left; muscle bulk normal; muscle strength grade 0 throughout the left arm and left leg musculature. Sensory examination: significant decrease in light touch, pinprick, pain, and vibratory sensation of the left face, arm, and leg; diminished joint position sensation in left upper and lower extremities. Muscle stretch reflexes: absent on the left, grade 2 on the right. Coordination: unable to be tested on the left; normal on the right. Plantar reflexes: flexor on the right, extensor on the left. Gait: unable to be tested.

Stop and Consider: What CNS lesions can account for the neurologic signs described above? What is the differential diagnosis in a patient presenting with these symptoms and neurologic findings?

Laboratory Findings: CBC, chemistry, electrolytes, coagulation profiles: normal. Head CT scan 1 hour after presentation: normal. Follow-up head CT scan on day 3 after admission: see figure. Carotid Doppler ultrasound: normal. Electrocardiogram: atrial fibrillation with a rate of 110 bpm.

Question: What is the likely cause of the brain lesion shown on the CT?

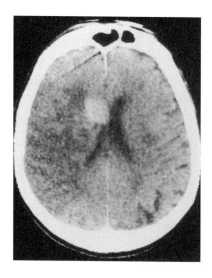

Diagnosis: Hemorrhagic infarction caused by a cardioembolic trunk occlusion of the right middle cerebral artery

Discussion: The clinical presentation of this patient with acute onset of left-sided weakness, sensory loss, and hemianopia indicates an acute lesion affecting the descending right corticospinal tract, the ascending sensory tracts from the left side of his body, and visual pathway in the right hemisphere. Localization of this lesion is in the arterial territory of either the right internal carotid artery or the right middle cerebral artery, and the presenting physical signs did not allow further differentiation based on clinical examination alone. Strokes in the distribution of an acutely occluded carotid artery and those with a middle cerebral artery trunk occlusion are often clinically indistinguishable. The first CT scan was normal and excluded primary intracerebral hemorrhage and traumatic brain hemorrhage, and made a tumor diagnosis highly unlikely. The follow-up head CT scan confirmed the presence of a hemorrhagic infarction consistent with the trunk occlusion of the right middle cerebral artery. This appearance of the lesion is rather typical of cerebral infarction with secondary conversion to a partially hemorrhagic infarction. The finding of atrial fibrillation on the EKG indicated the possibility of a cardioembolic occlusion of the right middle cerebral artery, which was supported by the normal carotid Doppler study.

Autopsy studies reveal that hemorrhagic infarctions occur in 51–71% of embolic strokes compared to 2–21% of nonembolic strokes. Hemorrhagic transformation visible on CT is delayed for variable intervals following stroke; early hemorrhagic transformation, within 48 hours of stroke onset, appears particularly frequent with cardioembolic strokes. Fragmentation and migration of the embolus from its initial site of arterial occlusion to more distal sites appears to be a key factor in reperfusion injury and secondary hemorrhagic conversion of a "bland" infarct to a transformed hemorrhagic infarct.

Atrial fibrillation is a marker of increased risk for ischemic stroke, with a fivefold increased risk as compared to patients in normal sinus rhythm. At least 20% of all ischemic strokes and more than one third of ischemic strokes in the elderly are associated with atrial fibrillation. Atrial fibrillation patients who appear to be at highest risk for subsequent development of stroke include those with mitral stenosis, congestive heart failure, previous stroke, and prosthetic mitral valves. Intermittent atrial fibrillation is also associated with increased risk for stroke, especially in the elderly. Stroke recurrence in patients with nonvalvular atrial fibrillation is reported to be as high as 1% per day in the first 2 weeks following the first cardioembolic stroke. The high risk of recurrent stroke has been regarded as a reason for acute and chronic anticoagulation in patients with cardioembolic stroke. Typically, anticoagulation is delayed in cases of moderate-to-large cardioembolic strokes, severe neurologic deficit, associated uncontrolled hypertension, or any other systemic conditions that would make anticoagulation unsafe and unwarranted. Secondary stroke prevention research studies show that aspirin and warfarin significantly decrease the rate of recurrent stroke in patients with nonvalvular atrial fibrillation. These studies favor warfarin as more effective anticoagulant than aspirin in secondary stroke prevention in patients with atrial fibrillation. Warfarin treatment was associated with slightly higher risk of bleeding as compared to aspirin.

This patient was not anticoagulated because of his heme-positive stool. The gastrointestinal evaluation did not reveal any significant abnormalities, and on repeat testing the stool was negative for blood. In addition, he developed gross hematuria during his rehabilitation stay and was found to have invasive cancer of the urinary bladder wall. His neurologic deficits remained severe during a protracted hospitalization for rehabilitation and treatment of bladder cancer. At 6 months following stroke onset, he had made no substantial neurologic recovery. He died from metastatic bladder cancer in the seventh post-stroke month.

Clinical Pearls

1. Cardioembolic strokes are initially "bland" infarctions, but in up to 40% of cases transform to hemorrhagic infarctions within hours to days of the initial presentation.

2. Cardiac emboli arising from the left atrium and its appendage underlie many of the devastating and unheralded strokes in patients with atrial fibrillation, but these patients also may have large-vessel arterial occlusive disease, making a specific stroke etiology determination difficult.

3. Small-to-moderate cardioembolic strokes in nonhypertensive patients who have no evident risk of hemorrhagic complications are typically treated with acute and chronic anticoagulation to prevent recurrent stroke.

4. Transformation from a bland infarction to a hemorrhagic infarction does not necessarily correspond to clinical worsening, but the presence of a hemorrhagic infarction typically delays the start of chronic anticoagulation.

REFERENCES

1. Caplan LR: Brain embolism, revisited. Neurology 1993; 43:1281–1287.
2. Halperin JL, Hart RG: Atrial fibrillation and stroke: New ideas, persisting dilemmas. Stroke 1988; 19:937–941.
3. Hart RG, Easton JD: Hemorrhagic infarcts. Stroke 1986; 17:586–589.
4. Hart RG, Halperin JL: Atrial fibrillation and stroke: Revisiting the dilemmas. Stroke 1994; 25:1337–1341.

PATIENT 13

A 35-year-old man with progressive leg weakness, hand incoordination, deteriorating vision, and progressive cognitive problems

A 35-year-old man was admitted to hospital because of inability to walk. The patient and his family reported that he was normal as a child and a young adult. He was an accomplished athlete in high school, but did notice some numbness and clumsiness of his right leg at age 19. These symptoms gradually progressed; however, the patient was able to serve in the military for 2 years and carry out his duties satisfactorily. Nevertheless, by age 25 he had lost all sensation in his lower extremities and had started to develop urine and bowel incontinence. In the subsequent decade his legs became increasingly weak; he also described a loss of visual acuity and poor coordination. His family members mentioned difficulties with memory and concentration. There was no history of neurologic disorder in the family, including nine siblings.

Physical Examination: Vital signs: normal. General: normal. Mental status: marked difficulty with specifying the date, recall of three objects, calculations, and complex concepts. Speech: mild dysarthria. Cranial nerves: profound diminution in visual acuity; pallor of optic discs. Motor examination: severe spastic paraparesis. Sensory examination: subjective diminution of sensation to all primary modalities below the chest. Muscle stretch reflexes: pathologically brisk (grade 4) in all extremities. Plantar reflexes: Babinski signs bilaterally. Coordination: markedly impaired fine motor skills in both hands. Gait: unable to walk, virtually bed-bound.

Stop and Consider: Which pathways and structures of the central and peripheral nervous system are likely to be involved?

Laboratory Findings: CBC, serum glucose, renal and liver function tests, electrolytes, ESR, urinary arylsulfatase A: normal. Baseline cortisol: normal, but did not increase after ACTH administration, indicating impaired adrenocortical reserve. Serum long-chain fatty acids: C_{26} fatty acid markedly elevated at 0.038% of total fatty acids (normal < 0.024). Cerebrospinal fluid examination: normal. Visual evoked potentials: profound slowing of conduction in the optic pathway bilaterally. Nerve conduction studies: severe sensorimotor polyneuropathy with mixed axonal and demyelinating features. Brain MRI: see figure.

Question: Can the abnormalities on the brain MRI and nerve conduction studies be related to abnormal metabolism of the long-chain fatty acids?

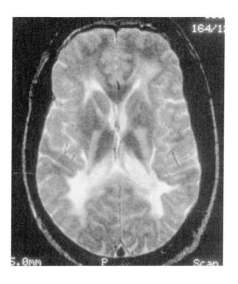

Diagnosis: Adrenoleukodystrophy

Discussion: The clinical exam was consistent with diffuse CNS involvement, including the optic nerves and tracts, cerebrum, and spinal cord. The nerve conduction study (NCS) confirmed coexisting severe involvement of the peripheral nervous system. The MRI scan showed diffuse and symmetric signal increase on T2 weighted images in the parietal and occipital lobes. Although multiple sclerosis had originally been considered because of the white matter abnormalities and increasing neurologic dysfunction, the relentlessly progressive nature of his disease, coupled with the very symmetric and extensive involvement of the white matter prompted reconsideration of the diagnosis. A form of adult-onset leukodystrophy was suspected. Elevated serum long-chain fatty acids were consistent with the diagnosis of adrenoleukodystrophy (ALD).

Leukodystrophies can be thought of as *dysmyelinating disorders*, in which there is metabolic disturbance affecting the white matter, causing formation of abnormal myelin. These disorders can be differentiated from demyelinating conditions, such as multiple sclerosis, in which myelin is formed normally, but is damaged by immunologic dysfunction.

The X-linked adrenoleukodystrophy is an inherited condition characterized by abnormal accumulation of saturated very-long-chain fatty acids, such as hexacosanoic acid ($C_{26:0}$). The mutation in the *ALD* gene on chromosome Xq28 appears to affect the import and degradation of the long-chain fatty acids in peroxisomes.

Adrenoleukodystrophy has a wide spectrum of clinical presentations. The most frequent phenotype is the childhood-onset cerebral ALD, but some patients may not develop symptoms until adolescence or adulthood. The childhood form of this disease typically affects boys 4 years of age or younger and is characterized by failure to develop, seizures, ataxia, and adrenal insufficiency. The course of the disease is rapidly progressive and devastating. In many cases when the genetic defect is mild, disease manifestations may not be apparent until late childhood or even adulthood. Adolescent-onset ALD is characterized by prominent spinal cord dysfunction and is therefore called *adrenomyeloneuropathy*. In these patients the dominant neurologic abnormality is myelopathy with some degree of sensorimotor, predominantly axonal, polyneuropathy. However, up to 50% of men who present clinically with adrenomyeloneuropathy have some degree of coexisting cerebral involvement on brain MRI. Very few patients present with isolated adrenocortical dysfunction without evident nervous system involvement. Up to 20–50% of female carriers may develop neurologic symptoms. Brain MRI may show white matter abnormalities in about 20% of carriers and in those patients multiple sclerosis is often the initial suspicion. Rare, neonatal form of ALD is autosomal recessive and caused by mutation in the PTS1 (peroxisomal targeting signal 1) receptor gene on chromosome 12p13.

The diagnosis can be established by analysis of long-chain fatty acids in serum. Genetic testing with mutation analysis is available and should be offered to patients and possible carriers. If no mutation at the Xq28 locus is detected, carriers can also be identified by linkage analysis or by immunofluorescence studies of X-ALD protein in cultured leukocytes or fibroblasts.

Several dietary treatments have been proposed (e.g., Lorenzo's oil), but there is no convincing evidence that they significantly delay the relentless progression of neurologic deterioration. Adrenocortical function should be closely monitored and steroid replacement therapy initiated if necessary. Bone marrow transplantation may have some therapeutic potential in patients with mild neurologic disability. Hopefully, increased understanding of the molecular basis of these diseases will lead to improved diagnosis and treatment, such as gene therapy.

The present patient, who was initially thought to have multiple sclerosis, has had a relentlessly progressive course of disease with severe disability.

Clinical Pearls

1. Consider ALD in the differential diagnosis of multifocal lesions affecting the white matter, especially in patients with a relentlessly progressive course.

2. Female carriers of ALD may be incorrectly regarded to have multiple sclerosis, because about 20% of heterozygotes may demonstrate white matter abnormalities in brain MRI.

3. Genetic testing and counseling should be offered to all patients and families with ALD.

4. Bone marrow transplantation may be beneficial in some patients with mild neurologic disability if a suitable donor is available.

REFERENCES

1. Boehm CD, Cutting GR, Lachtermacher MB, et al: Accurate DNA-based diagnostic and carrier testing for X-linked adrenoleukodystrophy. Mol Genet Metab 1999; 66:128–136.
2. Dodt G, Braverman N, Wong C, et al: Mutations in the PTS1 receptor gene, *PXR1*, define complementation group 2 of the peroxisome biogenesis disorders. Nature Genet 1995; 9:115–125.
3. Natowicz MR, Bejjani B: Genetic diseases that masquerade as multiple sclerosis. Am J Med Genet 1994; 49:149–169.
4. van Geel BM, Assies J, Wanders RJ, et al: X-linked adrenoleukodystrophy: Clinical presentation, diagnosis, and therapy. J Neurol Neurosurg Psychiatry 1997; 63:4–14.

PATIENT 14

A 68-year-old-man with increasing difficulty walking and poor balance

A 68-year-old right-handed man presented with a 1-year history of difficulty walking, imbalance, and frequent falls. Three months earlier his sister noted that the right side of his face was "drooping." He was told that he had "Bell's palsy" but his facial weakness did not improve and he complained that the right side of his tongue felt "heavy." During the previous few years he complained of numbness and burning in his feet. He denied any headaches, nausea, or focal weakness. Occasionally he would feel dizzy or lightheaded and sometimes experienced "spinning sensation." For the previous few years he had poor vision in the left eye and was told he had a cataract. His family also noted that he had some difficulty hearing. His medical history was significant for type II diabetes mellitus requiring insulin treatment, coronary artery disease, and depression.

Physical Examination: Pulse 80; blood pressure 132/70. HEENT: head normocephalic, skull nontender. Neck: supple, no bruits. Cardiac: normal. Spine: no deformity, nontender, good range of motion. Mental status: normal. Speech: mildly slurred. Cranial nerves: severe cataract in the left eye, the right eye visual field normal, fundus without papilledema, pupils equal, reactive to light and accommodation, bilateral horizontal nystagmus in the direction of gaze, severe bilateral nystagmus on vertical upward gaze, sensation on the right side of the face decreased to light touch and pain, right corneal reflex diminished, severe weakness of the right upper and lower facial muscles, markedly decreased hearing bilaterally, gag reflex absent, soft palate motion symmetric, trapezius and sternocleidomastoid muscles with normal bulk and strength bilaterally, tongue without atrophy or fasciculations. Motor examination: muscle bulk normal, spasticity in all limbs but most severe in the left lower extremity, mild fasciculations in distal muscles of both legs and the hands, strength reduced diffusely (grade 4) with more severe weakness in the left upper and lower extremity. Sensory examination: marked sensory loss to all modalities in glove and stocking distribution. Muscle stretch reflexes: very brisk, grade 3–4 throughout. Plantar reflexes: Babinski sign on the left. Coordination: slow but accurate finger-to-nose testing, rapid alternating motions diminished in all limbs. Gait/stance: wide-based gait, short steps, Romberg test negative.

Stop and Consider: What intracranial structures are involved, and where is the lesion?

Laboratory Findings: Fasting glucose 175 mg/dl (normal 70–110). CBC, renal and liver function tests, electrolytes, ESR: normal. Brain MRI with contrast: see figure.

Question: What is the likely pathology of the lesion demonstrated on the MRI?

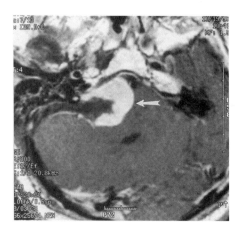

Diagnosis: Right cerebellopontine angle tumor (meningioma) and a coexisting sensorimotor polyneuropathy consistent with diabetic neuropathy

Discussion: The neurologic examination showed abnormalities consistent with a right cerebellopontine angle lesion. He also had symptoms and signs of peripheral neuropathy, most likely related to his diabetes. Because the neurologic exam demonstrated abnormalities involving the brain stem, the most appropriate diagnostic test was brain imaging. The MRI demonstrated a very contrast-enhancing mass in the inferior portion of the right cerebellopontine angle (arrow). This mass displaced the pontomedullary junction to the left and deformed the fourth ventricle. The imaging characteristics are most suggestive of a meningioma, although schwannoma could also have a similar MRI appearance.

The most common tumors in the cerebellopontine angle are acoustic neuromas. The second most common tumor in this location is a meningioma. The acoustic neuroma (schwannoma) usually causes enlargement of the internal auditory canal. It may be bilateral in patients with neurofibromatosis type 2. The meningioma typically shows a more uniform contrast enhancement, is more likely to be calcified, and may be associated with hyperostosis of the underlying bone. Other tumors in this location are relatively rare and include epidermoid cyst, metastatic cancer, chordoma, lymphoma, ependymoma, paraganglioma, lipoma, or arachnoid cyst.

Typical early symptoms of acoustic neuromas include hearing loss, dizziness, lightheadedness, and tinnitus. Patients may eventually complain of vertigo, facial numbness, difficulty walking, weakness, or headaches. By the time focal neurologic signs such as nystagmus, absent corneal reflex, facial weakness, or long tract signs are observed, the tumor is usually large in size. These signs are indicative of a space-occupying lesion in the cerebellopontine angle and are observed with any type of tumor in this location.

Management of patients with meningiomas may be complex and surgical risks are significant. Although these tumors are histologically benign, complete removal may not be possible because of localization near vital structures and tumor vascularity, which may be associated with severe intraoperative bleeding. If total resection is not possible, partial resection should be considered in order to reduce the mass effect. Some small tumors, especially in elderly patients, can be followed with serial MRIs. Radiation therapy is recommended in patients with partially removed or recurrent meningiomas, or meningiomas with anaplastic (malignant) features. Surgery, radiation, or chemotherapy may be necessary for cerebellopontine angle tumors of different histologic types.

The present patient underwent surgical treatment; however, because of the localization and the adherence of the tumor capsule to the brain stem, only approximately 60% of the tumor was resected. His postoperative period was complicated. The preoperative cranial nerve palsies did not improve. He also developed right vocal cord paresis with dysphonia and recurrent aspiration. Right thyroplasty was performed, but he continued to aspirate and a gastrostomy tube was placed. Because of high aspiration recurrence, a laryngeal tracheal diversion was performed. He was subsequently discharged to a nursing home. Radiation therapy was considered, but it was not initiated due to his overall poor medical condition.

Clinical Pearls

1. Consider acoustic neuroma in a patient with progressive unilateral or bilateral hearing loss and tinnitus.

2. Contrast-enhanced brain MRI is the best diagnostic test for evaluation of posterior fossa tumors.

3. Surgical excision is the treatment of choice for meningiomas, but radiation therapy should also be considered for partially resected, recurring, or malignant (anaplastic) meningiomas.

REFERENCES

1. Hasso AN, Smith DS: The cerebellopontine angle. Semin Ultrasound CT MR 1989; 10:280–301.
2. Morrison AW, King TT: Space-occupying lesions of the internal auditory meatus and cerebellopontine angle. Adv Otorhinolaryngol 1984; 34:121–142.

PATIENT 15

A 34-year-old man with a 20-year history of diplopia and headaches

A 34-year-old left-handed man was referred for a second opinion about possible multiple sclerosis. He reported having had intermittent diplopia in high school when he noted that visual images were separated horizontally on lateral gaze. These problems gradually increased, and the diplopia became more prominent. The patient was a self-described "hell of an athlete" in his younger years and remained an avid athletic fan. Because of the horizontal diplopia, he traded his 50-yard-line season tickets for end-zone seats so he could follow football games with his unaffected vertical eye movements rather than relying on horizontal eye movements. In his early twenties a diagnosis of multiple sclerosis was considered and he was treated with corticosteroids without appreciable effect. In the previous several years he developed progressive, pulsatile, occipital headaches.

Physical Examination: Vital signs: normal. Cardiac, chest, abdomen: normal. HEENT: head normocephalic, skull nontender. Neck: supple, no obvious deformity, no bruits. Spine: no deformity, good range of motion. Mental status: normal with good intellectual capabilities, emotional stability, and normal speech. Cranial nerves: normal pupils and visual fields, bilateral limitation of eye abduction and considerable end-point nystagmus, no eye muscle fatigability, no ptosis at rest or after exercise, other cranial nerve function normal. Red glass testing: maximally displaced image emanated from the abducting eye. Funduscopic examination: normal. Motor examination: normal bulk, tone, and strength, no fatigue with exercise. Sensory examination: normal. Muscle stretch reflexes: grade 2, symmetric. Plantar responses: flexor. Coordination: normal finger-to-nose and heel-sheen testing. Gait: normal.

Stop and Consider: What is the possible neuroanatomic localization of this patient's symptoms and clinical findings? Do these findings and pattern of presentation support the diagnosis of multiple sclerosis?

Laboratory Findings: CBC, chemistry, TSH: normal. Tensilon test: negative. Cranial CT scan: normal. Visual evoked responses: normal. Cerebrospinal fluid analysis, including protein electrophoresis: normal. Detailed testing in the neuro-ophthalmology laboratory: normal color vision and normal visual fields by tangent screen. Brain MRI: two small T2-intense periventricular lesions. Sagittal T1 weighted image (see figure). Cervical spine MRI: no evidence of syrinx or other intrinsic abnormality in the cervical cord.

Question: What diagnoses should be considered in this patient?

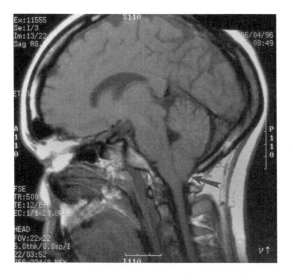

Diagnosis: Chiari type I malformation

Discussion: Differential diagnosis of intermittent diplopia includes numerous conditions relating to various neuroanatomic locations, including extraocular muscles. Consideration should be given to myasthenia gravis, but lack of muscle fatigability and lack of response to Tensilon do not support this diagnosis. Also, other conditions affecting eye muscles, such as mitochondrial myopathies, which are typically progressive, are rather unlikely given the static symptoms. The presence of bilateral lateral gaze paresis and nystagmus suggest an abnormality of the brain stem gaze pathways or bilateral sixth nerve dysfunction. The brain MRI showed downward displacement of the cerebellar tonsils below foramen magnum (arrow), consistent with Chiari type I malformation.

Multiple sclerosis (MS) was initially diagnosed in this patient. Certainly this disorder, which is relatively common in young adults, must be considered in a patient in the second or third decade of life who presents with diplopia. Typically, MS is characterized by events that are disseminated in time and space, i.e., recurrent attacks in which there is dysfunction of different white matter tracts in the central nervous system. Common manifestations of this disease include optic neuritis, cerebellar ataxia, nystagmus, diplopia, and myelopathy. With static symptoms of diplopia, this patient's course does not include relapsing/remitting multifocal symptoms and signs consistent with MS.

There are several types of structural hindbrain abnormalities that are referred to as Chiari malformations. Chiari type I malformation is the mildest and involves displacement of the cerebellar tonsils into the upper part of the cervical canal through the foramen magnum. It is usually asymptomatic but may be associated with headaches (usually occipital), neck pain, and unsteady gait. Rarely there are other symptoms, like dysarthria, dysphagia, or diplopia. More severe forms of Chiari malformations may be associated with abnormalities like hydrocephalus, cavitary changes of the brain stem or spinal cord, such as syringomyelia, or lumbosacral myelomeningocele.

Brain MRI is the best diagnostic test for evaluation of possible Chiari malformation, but it may show mild degrees of downward cerebellar tonsillar displacement of no clinical significance. Unless patients have symptoms and signs referable to dysfunction of the brain stem or upper cervical cord, there is no reason to pursue invasive investigations and treatment for a minor anatomic variant.

In the present patient, Chiari I malformation was clinically significant and accounted for his diplopia, probably by way of distortion and traction on the brain stem. Tonsillar herniation may have contributed to his headaches. The small abnormalities in the white matter of the cerebrum observed on the MRI were thought to be nonspecific and noncontributory. He underwent a suboccipital craniectomy, a C1 laminectomy, and placement of a dural patch graft. His headache improved postoperatively and over the next several years the diplopia remitted substantially.

Clinical Pearls

1. Atypical features in a patient with a diagnosis of multiple sclerosis should prompt diagnostic reevaluation and consideration of other etiologies.

2. Chiari type I malformation may appear as an incidental, clinically insignificant finding on the brain MRI.

3. Symptomatic patients with Chiari type I malformation can be successfully treated with suboccipital decompressive craniectomy.

REFERENCES

1. Madsen JR, Scott RM: Chiari malformations, syringomyelia, and intramedullary spinal cord tumors. Curr Opin Neurol Neurosurg 1993; 6:559–563.
2. Offenbacher H, Fazekas F, Schmidt R, et al: Assessment of MRI criteria for a diagnosis of MS. Neurology 1993; 43:905–909.
3. Rudick RA, Schiffer RB, Schwertz KM, et al: Multiple sclerosis: The problem of incorrect diagnosis. Arch Neurol 1986; 43:578–583.

PATIENT 16

A 28-year-old woman with headache and blurred vision

A 28-year-old woman was transferred from a community hospital for evaluation of severe headache and blurred vision. She was asymptomatic until 2 weeks prior to admission, when she developed a gradually worsening, pounding, predominantly occipital headache with nausea and vomiting. Subsequently the headache became more diffuse and was especially prominent behind the eyes. At that time, she also noticed a decreased vision in her right eye along with horizontal double vision when looking to the right. She was found to have bilateral papilledema. Brain MRI performed at that time was normal. She underwent serial lumbar punctures at the local hospital, and the opening cerebrospinal fluid (CSF) pressure ranged from 400–530 mmH$_2$O, with normal cell count, protein, and other CSF studies. She reported only transient improvement in symptoms after each lumbar puncture. Subsequently she was started on acetazolamide and referred to our department for further care. She denied any fever, chills, seizures, loss of consciousness, weakness, oral contraceptive intake, multivitamin therapy, exposure to tetracycline, or any trauma.

Physical Examination: Height: 5'1", weight 152 lbs. Temperature 36°; pulse 74, respirations 14; blood pressure 120/70. HEENT, cardiac, chest, abdomen, extremities, skin: normal. Neck: supple. Mental status, speech: normal. Cranial nerves: visual acuity 20/20 OS and 20/40 OD; pupils equal, reacting sluggishly to light; visual field examination with Goldmann perimetry: see figure, *top;* funduscopic examination: see figures, *bottom;* ocular motility: bilateral lateral rectus muscle weakness, worse on the right; the remainder of the cranial nerve examination: normal. Motor, sensory, reflexes, coordination, gait: normal.

Stop and Consider: What is the differential diagnosis of a patient presenting with symptoms and signs of increased intracranial pressure and negative neuroimaging?

Laboratory Findings: CBC, chemistry: normal. ESR: 11 mm/hr (normal 0–25). TSH: 1.24 IU/ml (normal 0.5–4.7). ANA: negative. Lumbar puncture: opening CSF pressure 320 mmH$_2$O, CSF cell count 1/μl, protein 30 mg/dl (normal), glucose 77 mg/dl (normal). Brain MRI and MR venogram: normal.

Question: What abnormality was demonstrated on the funduscopic examination?

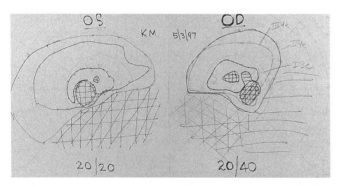

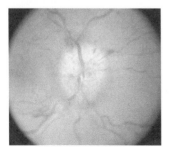
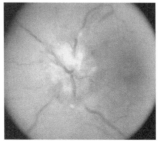

Diagnosis: Idiopathic intracranial hypertension syndrome

Discussion: The clinical presentation of this patient, with gradual onset of progressive headache, episodes of emesis, and blurred vision, is highly suggestive of increased intracranial pressure. The differential diagnosis includes intracranial tumors or hemorrhage (subarachnoid, subdural), cerebral venous thrombosis, infections (abscesses and meningitis, especially of chronic type), hydrocephalus, and idiopathic intracranial hypertension syndrome (IHHS), also referred to in the past as pseudotumor cerebri. The neuro-ophthalmologic abnormalities included severe bilateral papilledema, and both optic nerves were markedly swollen and elevated 3–4 diopters (figure, *bottom*). Visual field examination showed dense inferior nerve fiber bundle defects in both eyes, more severe in the right than the left eye (figure, *top*). The very high opening pressure on lumbar puncture confirmed the diagnosis of intracranial hypertension. The presence of papilledema, visual field defects, sixth nerve paresis, high intracranial pressure with normal CSF constituents, and negative brain MRI and MR venogram strongly suggest the diagnosis of IHHS.

The concept of "benign" or idiopathic intracranial hypertension syndrome (pseudotumor cerebri) emerged in the late 19th century. It has been typically diagnosed in patients with symptoms of increased intracranial pressure who have papilledema without a tumor, hydrocephalus, or infection. Some neurologists also include in this category patients with cerebral venous thrombosis presenting with intracranial hypertension. This syndrome is particularly common in obese young women and usually develops over a period of weeks or months. A generalized headache is the most common symptom, but in some patients headache may not be a presenting feature. Other frequent complaints include transient visual obscurations, diplopia, nausea, dizziness, and occasionally tinnitus. A typical patient usually has papilledema and the intracranial pressure is elevated in the range of 250–450 mmH$_2$O or higher. In early or mild papilledema the visual acuity is normal, and visual field testing shows only enlarged blind spots. With more severe and/or chronic optic disc swelling, nerve fiber bundle visual field defects develop secondary to ischemic insults to the optic nerves (as in the present case), and in some patients severe permanent visual impairment can ensue before the impact of the elevated intracranial pressure on the optic discs is reversed. Aside from unilateral or bilateral sixth nerve palsy or paresis as a nonspecific manifestation of raised intracranial pressure, the neurologic examination is usually normal.

Many types of endocrine abnormalities have been postulated as causative factors, but none have been substantiated. Oral contraceptives, hypervitaminosis, and tetracycline treatment have also been incriminated in the pathogenesis. However, the mechanism of increased CSF pressure remains obscure. It is possible that there is an increased resistance to CSF outflow, due to impaired absorptive function of arachnoid villi.

With regard to treatment, one must ascertain that there is no underlying pathologic process such as tumor, infection, or cerebral venous (sinus) thrombosis. Accordingly, appropriate neuroimaging (brain MRI and MR venogram) and a lumbar puncture should be done in every patient with suspected IIHS. Although proof of the ideal therapy for IIHS has not been established, most clinicians treat it initially with the carbonic anhydrase inhibitor acetazolamide (Diamox) in daily doses of 1 or 2 grams. Oral steroids, such as prednisone, at the initial dose of 40–60 mg/day, have also been advocated. In many cases withdrawal of an offending agent, weight reduction, and correction of an underlying endocrinologic abnormality may improve the condition. Some authorities also recommend repeated lumbar punctures and drainage of sufficient CSF, but this method is becoming less popular and in our opinion not feasible.

For patients whose visual function (acuity and visual fields) continues to worsen despite vigorous medical therapy, surgical intervention is usually required to prevent permanent impairment of sight. It should be noted that extensive visual field loss can occur before visual acuity impairment, and it is important for sequential visual field testing to be done to monitor the status of the optic nerves. When the major symptom is visual, optic nerve sheath fenestration can be effective, and in some patients a unilateral fenestration will succeed in relieving the headache and the papilledema of the other eye. In other patients, bilateral fenestrations are required. When headache is the major symptom and both eyes are similarly affected, decompressing the intracranial pressure by a lumbar-peritoneal or ventriculo-peritoneal shunt is another option. There has not been a good study to determine which of these three surgical procedures is best.

In the present patient, a right-sided optic sheath fenestration was performed 4 days after admission because of the worsening visual field deficits and increasing optic disc elevation. Postoperatively, the visual acuity and visual field of the right eye were worse, and the headache persisted. A ventriculo-peritoneal shunt was performed 3 weeks after the fenestration, followed by prompt resolution of the headaches and the papilledema of the left eye. Four months later, the visual acuity was only finger counting in the right eye and 20/30 in the left eye. The right eye had only an upper nasal island of visual field remaining, and the left had an inferior nasal defect. Although both optic discs were flat, there was marked atrophy of the right optic disc and mild pallor of the left. The relatively good visual acuity of the left eye enabled the patient to read, drive, and resume working.

Clinical Pearls

1. The diagnosis of pseudotumor cerebri or idiopathic intracranial hypertension syndrome should be made only after excluding all other causes of elevated intracranial pressure, especially tumors and chronic meningitis.

2. The term benign intracranial hypertension is a misnomer, since this condition can lead to severe visual loss.

3. Although the pathogenetic mechanisms are unclear, medical treatment is usually effective. For patients whose visual function worsens despite medical therapy, optic nerve sheath fenestration or ventriculo-peritoneal shunt surgery can be effective in preventing permanent visual deficits.

REFERENCES

1. Corbett JJ, Thompson HS: The rational management of idiopathic intracranial hypertension. Arch Neurol 1989; 46:1049–1051.
2. Johnston I, Hawke S, Halmagyi M, et al: The pseudotumor syndrome: Disorders of cerebrospinal fluid circulation causing intracranial hypertension without ventriculomegaly. Arch Neurol 1991; 48:740–747.
3. Radhakrishnan K, Ahlskog JE, Garrity JA, et al: Idiopathic intracranial hypertension. Mayo Clin Proc 1994; 69:169–180.
4. Scot IU, Siatkowski RM, Eneyni M, et al: Idiopathic intracranial hypertension in children and adolescents. Am J Ophthalmol 1997; 124:253–255.
5. Wolin MJ, Brannon WL: Disc edema in an overweight woman. Surv Ophthalmol 1995; 39:307–314.

PATIENT 17

A 62-year-old left-handed band instructor with tremor of the right hand

A 62-year-old musician reported that for about 10 years he had progressive difficulty playing the trumpet as a result of involuntary respiratory effort that produced an unwanted tremolo. Propranolol had improved this problem. He also developed a right-hand tremor during the previous year. It is apparent at rest but also causes him difficulty in performing fine motor tasks, such as playing an instrument. He reported no problems with gait or getting in or out of a car or bed. He denied autonomic symptoms and was athletically active. He had no exposure to carbon monoxide, manganese, or repeated head trauma, and there is no family history of tremor.

Physical Examination:　Vital signs: normal. Cardiac, spine, musculoskeletal: normal. Mental status: normal. Speech: fluent, no evidence of aphasia or dysarthria. Cranial nerves: normal with symmetric facial expressions. Motor examination: no wasting or fasciculations, mild cogwheeling in the right elbow but muscle tone normal, normal strength, resting tremor on the right side with a characteristic pill-rolling appearance, diminishing with intention or sustention. Sensory examination: normal. Muscle stretch reflexes: normal. Plantar reflexes: flexor. Coordination: rapid alternating movements generally fast, with a slight slowing on the right side, no significant bradykinesia. Gait and stance: normal except for reduced arm swing and tremor on the right, no retropulsion or propulsion.

Stop and Consider:　What is the differential diagnosis of tremor in this case?

Laboratory Findings:　CBC, chemistry: normal. Brain MRI: normal.

Question:　What pharmacologic treatment options can be considered in this patient?

Diagnosis: Parkinson's disease, most likely in the setting of pre-existing essential tremor

Discussion: This patient presented with a long history of involuntary respiratory movement with features of a vocal tremor, which manifested during attempts to play the trumpet. Vocal tremor may be due to abnormal movements of the diaphragm and other "bellows" muscles, or may have its origin in motor anomalies of the laryngeal musculature. In this case, the difficulty he has had playing the trumpet points to a likely bellows tremor. A vocal tremor of this sort is usually a form of essential tremor (ET), a common idiopathic disorder that is often familial. The association of this tremor with movement makes it an action tremor. Essential tremor may also be aggravated by sustained muscular effort, a so-called sustention tremor. The tremor may be less apparent when muscles are relaxed. In the case of a vocal tremor, it is not easy to assess its dependence on effort or relief with rest, because the involved muscles are not readily observed and are not under full voluntary control. The reduction of this patient's tremor with propranolol (a beta-blocking agent) is characteristic of ET.

In contrast with essential tremor, the tremor of Parkinson's disease (PD) is typically a resting tremor and usually starts in the hands rather than the head or voice. This patient developed just such a tremor. Resting tremor typically diminishes with sustention and intention. The tremor of PD often manifests initially in one hand and may not spread to the other hand for several years. Essential tremor may also be asymmetric, but more often starts symmetrically. The four cardinal signs of PD are tremor, rigidity, bradykinesia, and postural instability. The resting tremor of PD is typically relatively slow (3–4 Hz), high-amplitude tremor that is reduced with sustention or intention and may be obvious when the patient is distracted or relaxed. Rigidity is a characteristic increase of muscle tone with a uniform resistance throughout the range of movement of the limb. It may be associated with tremor, leading to a cogwheeling phenomenon. Bradykinesia is a shorthand for a variety of motor abnormalities, including hypokinesia (slowness and reduction of amplitude of movements), akinesia/freezing, or difficulty initiating movements. Two of the secondary manifestations of PD, reduced facial expression (also called masked facies) and micrographia (small handwriting), are both manifestations of hypokinesia. Postural instability is typically the most debilitating aspect of PD. This can cause problems with balance and walking, such as festination and retropulsion, and may manifest early in the course of the disease as difficulties with getting in and out of a car, bathtub, or bed.

The differentiation between essential tremor and Parkinson's tremor may be difficult in some cases, especially in patients with early PD. Parkinson's disease and essential tremor can also coexist, as demonstrated in the present patient. Proper diagnosis and classification is essential because treatment of the disorder is specific for the type of movement abnormality.

Parkinson's disease, essential tremor, and many other movement disorders are clinical diagnoses—currently there are no reliable laboratory tests to assist with the diagnoses. There is considerable variability in the signs of PD and not all patients will present with the same pattern of symptoms, signs, and the disease course. The lack of diagnostic tests further exacerbates the difficulty with differential diagnosis illustrated above. The anatomic localization of the defects that produce various signs of PD remains incompletely understood. Degeneration and loss of dopaminergic cells in the pars compacta of the substantia nigra are the major pathologic findings associated with PD.

Numerous pharmacologic agents are now available for management of PD. Replacement of the dopaminergic deficit with exogenous levodopa combined with a peripheral decarboxylase inhibitor (carbidopa/levodopa) is the mainstay of treatment. Anticholinergic medications (e.g., trihexyphenidyl, benztropine) and direct dopamine receptor agonists (bromocriptine, pergolide, pramipexole, ropinirole) are usually used as adjunctive drugs, although in some patients they may be prescribed as initial treatments. Selegiline (monoamine oxidase B inhibitor) may be neuroprotective and reduce the rate of cell loss in the pars compacta of substantia nigra, but this remains controversial. Selegiline treatment may suppress symptoms, but probably does not directly alter the underlying degenerative process.

Essential tremor typically occurs with posture or activity. It affects the hands most frequently, but in many patients it may affect the arms and the head. In about half of the cases there is an autosomal dominant inheritance pattern. The neuropathologic localization for ET is unknown. This type of tremor typically is not associated with parkinsonism or other neurologic disease. It may improve with small amount of alcohol. Propranolol (beta-adrenergic blocker) has been used effectively, although side effects may be significant in some patients. Primidone (antiepileptic agent) may also be effective, but higher doses may induce sedation. Other agents used in ET include benzodiazepines (clonazepam, alprazolam) and acetazolamide.

The present patient had a vocal tremor characteristic of ET and later developed a hand tremor characteristic of Parkinson's tremor. He was started on selegiline and trihexyphenidyl, which reduced the resting tremor. Propranolol was continued and seemed to reduce both the hand and the vocal tremor, particularly when the patient was anxious. Carbidopa/levodopa was not initially used, but may be considered in the event of disabling progressive symptoms and signs.

Clinical Pearls

1. The cardinal signs of Parkinson's disease are tremor, rigidity, bradykinesia, and postural instability.

2. Essential tremor is generally seen with sustention; Parkinson's tremor is usually seen at rest.

3. Parkinsonism may be secondary to drugs, toxins, or head trauma and may coexist with other neurologic conditions.

4. Different pharmacologic agents alone or in combinations may be useful in management of various stages of Parkinson's disease.

REFERENCES

1. Hely MA, MorrisJG: Controversies in the treatment of Parkinson's disease. Curr Opin Neurol 1996; 9:308–313.
2. Nutt JG: Management of parkinsonism and treatment of associated complications. Curr Opin Neurol 1995; 8:327–330.
3. Waters CH: Managing the late complications of Parkinson's disease. Neurology 1997; 49(Suppl 1):S49–S57.

PATIENT 18

A 58-year-old woman with a 3-year history of dizziness and numbness

This 58-year-old woman initially noticed numbness involving her left big toe several years earlier. The loss of sensation gradually spread to involve the whole of her left leg and has been present to a variable degree ever since. A year earlier she developed left facial numbness, which has also persisted. Finally, she has recently developed dizziness, which she described as lightheadedness and a "swimming" sensation in her head. All of these symptoms are exacerbated or triggered by episodes of severe anxiety. On further questioning, the patient indicated that 10 years earlier she was hospitalized for depression and anxiety. Over the years she has had recurrences of her anxiety and has been successfully treated with low doses of benzodiazepines. There is no family history of neurologic or psychiatric disease, except for a son who suffers from panic attacks and was successfully treated with benzodiazepines. The patient also has mild hypertension, which has been well controlled with diuretics.

Physical Examination: Vital signs: normal. Cardiac, chest, abdomen: normal. Head and neck: normal. Mental status: alert, oriented and cooperative, but very anxious, with manifest motor hyperactivity, easily distractable with a tendency to obsess on specific topics, mental status tests performed perfectly when urged to concentrate on a specific task. Speech: normal. Cranial nerves: optic nerve discs sharp and of normal color, normal pupillary reactions, normal extraocular movements without nystagmus, and intact visual acuity, other cranial nerves normal. Motor examination: muscle bulk, tone, and strength normal. Muscle stretch reflexes: normal. Plantar reflexes: flexor bilaterally. Sensory examination: normal, in spite of the patient's complaints of persistent paresthesias. Coordination and gait: normal.

Stop and Consider: What is the possible explanation of this patient's numerous symptoms and lack of objective signs on the neurologic examination?

Laboratory Findings: CBC, chemistry, electrolytes, thyroid function tests, and extensive serologic testing for infectious or rheumatologic conditions: normal. Audiogram and an electronystagmogram: normal. Brain MRI: see figure.

Follow-up Evaluation: On a subsequent clinical evaluation it was noticed that the patient experienced marked dizziness and numbness when she was hyperventilated. On further questioning, she indicated that these symptoms were identical to those she had during maximal periods of activity of her previous "disease." On further questioning she related a great variety of fears concerning her family and financial situation.

Question: How would you treat this patient?

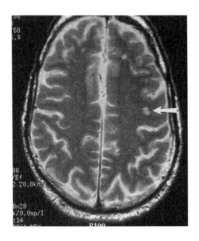

Diagnosis: Anxiety disorder with panic attacks

Discussion: Although this patient presented with a plethora of complaints, her detailed neurologic evaluation failed to demonstrate any objective abnormalities. Because of the persistence and disabling nature of her complaints, an MRI scan of the brain was obtained and showed few, small, scattered foci of increased signal on T2 weighted images in the deep periventricular white matter and in other subcortical regions (arrow). More prominent areas of increased signal were noted adjacent to the frontal and occipital horns of the ventricles. These abnormalities are nonspecific but in a patient of this age most frequently represent small-vessel ischemic changes, although they might be consistent with a demyelinating process. Her long history of hypertension would favor the possibility of white matter changes secondary to small-vessel ischemia. The possibility of cerebrovascular disease should be considered in any patient with significant neurologic symptoms and risk factors such as hypertension. Demyelinating diseases such as multiple sclerosis typically present in young adults, most frequently in the third decade of life, but some cases may present as late as the sixth or seventh decade of life.

The most remarkable features of this patient's evaluation were a normal neurologic examination, despite multiple symptoms, and her marked anxiety. Clinically significant cerebrovascular disease or demyelinating disease of 3 years' duration is usually accompanied by neurologic signs, such as hyperreflexia, Babinski sign, oculomotor abnormality, or optic nerve dysfunction. Given her prior history of psychiatric disease, the family history of panic attacks, and the dramatic improvement of her symptoms after counseling and pharmacologic treatment, it is quite likely that her primary disorder is one of anxiety with panic attacks.

Patients with primary psychiatric disease, such as depression, anxiety, panic attacks, borderline personality, and somatoform disorder, often will manifest symptoms that suggest primary neurologic disease. Differential diagnosis is made all the more difficult because many patients with absolutely typical and established psychiatric disease may show a subtle or even gross abnormalities during neuroimaging, creating a substantial possibility of incorrect diagnosis. For this reason it is essential to reassess the patient and keep an open mind with regard to the different possibilities. The key to managing patients who fall into the gray zone between disorders of neurology and psychiatry is careful follow-up and critical reassessment of the clinical and laboratory findings. The correct diagnosis is frequently clarified by prolonged observation and sometimes by therapeutic trials.

The management of patients with psychiatric disorders who present with nonorganic manifestations can be difficult and some patients resist the possibility that their symptoms may not be due to an underlying neurologic disorder. Such patients should be approached with tact and sympathy, and should not be confronted in a way that might encourage or promote anxiety. It is often useful to reassure the patient about the absence of evidence of a serious neurologic disorder and to emphasize that stress can manifest as psychophysiologic symptoms. A supportive approach to coping with neurologic symptoms is usually effective. In some patients counseling or psychiatric treatment may be helpful.

In the present patient the MRI abnormalities are nonspecific and could be related to her age and mild hypertension. She received counseling for stress reduction and was treated with alprazolam. She improved markedly on this regimen and her symptoms of numbness and dizziness disappeared. At a 3-year follow-up she reported no recurrent symptoms and her neurologic examination has remained within normal limits.

Clinical Pearls

1. Patients with multisystem complaints and nonlocalizing signs and symptoms are done a disservice by a casual examination and excessive reliance on neuroimaging studies, which may suggest etiologies that are not related to the clinical problem.

2. Failure to recognize and effectively manage patients with neurologic symptoms and coexisting psychiatric disorders may result in overuse of diagnostic tests, which can reinforce anxiety and exacerbate the symptoms. Unnecessary treatments in those patients may lead to serious iatrogenic complications.

3. Periodic reassessment and consideration of alternative diagnoses is essential in management of patients with neurologic symptoms related to stress and anxiety.

REFERENCES

1. Paulson GW: Pseudo-multiple sclerosis. South Med J 1996; 89:301–304.
2. Potts NL, Davidson JR, Krishnan KR: The role of nuclear magnetic resonance imaging in psychiatric research. J Clin Psychiatry 1993; 54(Suppl 12):13–18.

PATIENT 19

A 14-year-old mentally retarded boy with skin lesions, headache, seizures, and hemiparesis

A 14-year-old right-handed boy presented with pounding, unrelenting, diffuse headache that gradually worsened during 2 months prior to evaluation. The headache awakened him frequently from sleep and was markedly worsened by coughing and sneezing. His parents noted that over the previous year he had increasing difficulty using his right arm and leg, and tended to drag his right foot. His medical history was significant for a seizure disorder with onset at age 12. The seizures were initially manifest with movements in his right arm that would spread to involve the face and subsequently his entire body, and were well controlled with phenytoin. The boy was noted to be "developmentally slow" and received special education. His brother and a paternal uncle were also noted to be "slow" but the other family members were of normal intellect.

Physical Examination: Vital signs: normal. HEENT, cardiac, chest, abdomen, spine: normal. Skin: several white patches on the skin, focal thickening and disfigurement of nail beds, and an irregular patch of raised skin in the lumbar region that was rough to touch. Mental status: mild mental retardation. Cranial nerves: mild bilateral papilledema, otherwise normal. Motor: muscle bulk normal, increased muscle tone (spasticity) on the right and mild right hemiparesis. Sensation: normal. Muscle stretch reflexes: increased right biceps and knee reflexes (grade 3), right Achilles tendon reflex grade 4 with sustained clonus. Plantar reflexes: Babinski sign on the right. Gait: circumduction of the right hip.

Stop and Consider: How might the headache, seizures, and skin abnormalities be related in this patient?

Laboratory Findings: CBS, chemistry, electrolytes: normal. Cranial CT: see figures. EEG: focal slowing in the right frontal region.

Question: What is your interpretation of the cranial CT findings?

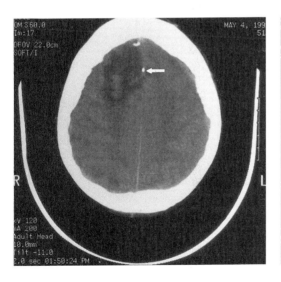
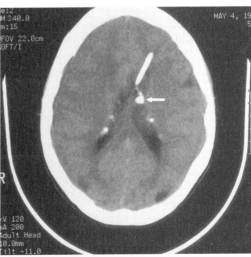

Diagnosis: Tuberous sclerosis with hydrocephalus secondary to the left cerebral hemisphere tumor, histopathologically diagnosed as giant-cell astrocytoma

Discussion: The headache on awakening with papilledema and progressive hemiparesis suggest a progressive CNS process associated with raised intracranial pressure. Important clues as to the nature of the patient's cerebral lesion can be obtained from skin examination. This patient had hypopigmented patches on his skin that were typical ash-leaf nevi. The lesion on the lower back was a shagreen patch, a connective tissue hamartoma. The presence of these lesions was very suggestive of tuberous sclerosis (TS). The cranial CT showed evidence of a large right frontal tumor (see figure, *left*) with obstructive hydrocephalus and the presence of multiple calcified nodules predominantly in the periventricular region (see figure, *right*). The findings from the neurologic examination, the skin abnormalities, and the abnormalities on the neuroimaging studies are typical of TS.

Tuberous sclerosis is an autosomal dominant disorder that is associated with lesions in multiple organs, including the skin, brain, retina, kidney, heart, and lung. The primary features of TS include facial angiofibromas, multiple ungual fibromas, retinal hamartomas, cerebral cortical tubers, subependymal glial nodules, and giant-cell astrocytomas. Other frequent features of TS are hypomelanotic macules, shagreen patches, gingival fibromas, bone cysts, dental enamel pits, cardiac rhabdomyomas, renal angiomyolipomas, and pulmonary lymphangiomyomatosis. Subependymal giant-cell tumors develop in the periventricular region and may grow sufficiently to obstruct the foramina of Monro, as in this patient, and cause obstructive hydrocephalus. Adenoma sebaceum, a synonym that refers to the cutaneous features, is a misnomer. Facial angiofibroma more accurately describes the lesions. White skin macules shaped like the leaf of a mountain ash tree are characteristically seen in patients with TS. In most cases these macules are present at birth and may allow early diagnosis, but can only be detected with a Wood's lamp. Kidney lesions are frequently seen in the form of angiomyolipoma.

The common manifestations of TS are seizures and mental retardation. The onset of seizures at a younger age is associated with higher risk of mental retardation. Infants with TS may present with infantile spasms, which are often associated with the pattern of hypsarrhythmia on the EEG. Older children frequently present with generalized tonic-clonic seizures or partial complex seizures. The development of hemiparesis or any other focal neurologic signs, papilledema, or other symptoms of increased intracranial pressure should always raise the suspicion of intracranial tumors, which are common in TS.

Two genetic loci for tuberous sclerosis complex (TSC) have been discovered in families with TS and mapped to chromosomal locations 9q34.3 (*TSC1*) and 16p13.3 (*TSC2*). About two thirds of TS cases are sporadic and represent *de novo* mutations. DNA testing with mutational analysis is currently available for mutations in both *TSC1* and *TSC2* genes. The wide spectrum of clinical presentations may be attributed to modifier genes. Embryologically, the skin and nervous system are both derived from the ectoderm; therefore, developmental abnormalities of the nervous system may be associated with skin lesions. Disorders involving the skin and nervous system, such as TS, are referred to as neurocutaneous syndromes. The most common neurocutaneous disorders are TS and neurofibromatosis.

Anticonvulsants may be effective in treatment of TS, but complete seizure control is not always possible. Infantile spasms may respond to adrenocorticotropic hormone (ACTH) or corticosteroids. Resection of intracranial lesions sometimes may improve seizure control. Surveillance for brain tumors and cardiac, pulmonary, renal, or ophthalmologic complications is necessary. Echocardiography is recommended to screen for cardiac rhabdomyosarcomas.

The present patient received a ventriculoperitoneal shunt for management of progressive hydrocephalus and subsequently craniotomy with resection of the left frontoparietal tumor. Two years following the initial presentation, his seizures were well controlled with anticonvulsants and the neurologic examination showed mild, nonprogressive hemiparesis and static cognitive deficits.

Clinical Pearls

1. Examination of the skin in a patient with a childhood-onset seizure disorder may reveal findings characteristic of a neurocutaneous disorder.

2. Surveillance for brain tumors is necessary in all patients with tuberous sclerosis.

3. Patients with tuberous sclerosis should have screening echocardiography to identify cardiac rhabdomyomas.

4. Tuberous sclerosis is an autosomal dominant condition; therefore, genetic testing and counseling should be offered to all affected patients and their families.

REFERENCES

1. Beauchamp RL, Banwell A, McNamara P, et al: Exon scanning of the entire *TSC2* gene for germline mutations in 40 unrelated patients with tuberous sclerosis. Hum Mutat 1998; 12:408–416.
2. Kuster W, Happle R: Neurocutaneous disorders in children. Curr Opin Pediatr 1993; 5:436–440.
3. Osborne J, Webb D: Seizures and intellectual disability associated with tuberous sclerosis. Dev Med Child Neurol 1993; 35:276.
4. Roach ES: Tuberous sclerosis: Function follows form. J Child Neurol 1997; 12:75–76.
5. Roach ES, Smith M, Huttenlocher P, et al: Diagnostic criteria: Tuberous sclerosis complex. Report of the Diagnostic Criteria Committee of the National Tuberous Sclerosis Association. J Child Neurol 1992; 7:221–224.

PATIENT 20

A 25-year-old woman with right-sided blindness and a family history of brain tumors

A 25-year-old woman presented for a consultation about the risk for a neurologic disorder. She had no complaints except for blindness of the right eye. She was diagnosed with retinal angiomatosis of the right eye at age 18, but her left retina has remained normal. Her medical history was otherwise unremarkable. Her family history was significant for brain and spinal cord tumors in her father and two of her siblings.

Physical Examination: Temperature and respiratory rate: normal; pulse 72 and regular; blood pressure 106/68. Skin, neck, cardiac, chest, abdomen: normal. Mental status, affect, speech, language: normal. Cranial nerves: complete blindness of the right eye with fixed nonreactive right pupil 6 mm in diameter; fundus, visual acuity, visual field, pupillary reflex, and gaze of the left eye: normal; muscles of facial expression: normal and symmetric; facial sensation: normal; oral and pharyngeal structures: midline. Motor examination: mild spasticity of the right upper extremity, bulk and power normal, mild intention tremor, dysmetria and difficulty with rapid alternating movements in the right hand. Sensory examination: area of sensory loss to pain and temperature with preserved vibratory sensation over the right shoulder; Lhermitte's sign referred to right upper extremity with neck flexion or extension. Muscle stretch reflexes: grade 3–4 in right upper extremity; otherwise normal. Plantar reflexes: normal. Coordination: normal except for mild incoordination of the right hand secondary to tremor. Gait: normal.

Stop and Consider: Can the neurologic abnormalities be explained by a single lesion? What is the likely diagnosis in a patient presenting with these symptoms and neurologic findings and a positive family history of CNS tumors?

Laboratory Findings: CBC, coagulation profile, platelet count, electrolytes, chemistry, serum B_{12} level, ESR: normal. Contrast-enhanced cervical spine MRI: see figure, *left*. Contrast-enhanced head MRI: see figure, *right*.

Question: What is the most likely histopathology of the contrast-enhancing lesions demonstrated on the head and spine MRI?

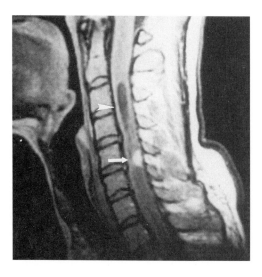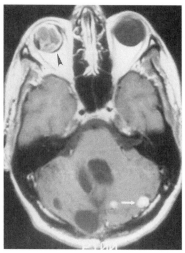

Diagnosis: von Hippel-Lindau disease with hemangioblastomas of the cervical spine and cerebellum, syringomyelia of the cervical spine, and retinal angiomatosis of the right eye

Discussion: The clinical presentation of this patient with retinal angiomatosis, increased muscle tone and reflexes of the right upper extremity, dissociated sensory loss over the right shoulder, and tremor and incoordination of the right hand, indicates multiple levels of CNS involvement. These include the right retina, the cervical spinal cord (with an intramedullary lesion), and probably the right cerebellum. The strong family history of brain and spinal cord tumors suggests a hereditary condition. Contrast-enhanced MRI of the cervical spine shows an intraspinal tumor at the fifth cervical level (arrow) with associated syringomyelia of the upper cervical cord (arrowhead). Head MRI with contrast shows several areas of cystic degeneration in the right cerebellum, at least two enhancing lesions in the left cerebellum (arrow), and an expanded fourth ventricle. The MRI also shows the angiomatosis of the right retina (arrowhead). The clinical and neuroradiologic findings and family history in this patient are typical of von Hippel-Lindau (VHL) disease.

VHL disease is a dominantly inherited neurologic disorder characterized by hemangioblastomas of the cerebellum and spinal cord and retinal angiomatosis, frequently associated with multiple cysts of the abdominal viscera, pheochromocytoma, renal cell carcinoma, and other malignancies, e.g., nonsecreting pancreatic tumors. VHL disease is caused by the mutation in the von Hippel-Lindau tumor suppressor gene that was isolated in 1993 and is localized on the short arm of chromosome 3. There is a wide phenotypic spectrum of disease, with patients presenting with different combination of malformations and malignancies. Coexisting mutations of other genes in the 3p25 locus may explain some other, nonvascular abnormalities in VHL disease. The *VHL* gene product inhibits the production of the vascular endothelial growth factor (VEGF). Mutation in the *VHL* gene enhances the VEGF production, leading to vascular proliferation.

Hemangioblastomas typically begin to appear between 8 and 12 years of age. Approximately 70–75% of patients with VHL disease have one or more CNS tumors, with involvement of the cerebellum in 52%, spinal cord in 44%, and brain stem in 18% of cases. In several large series, the mean patient age was 35 years and there was no specific age association between the appearance of CNS tumors and the expression of related symptomatology. Most authors agree that all patients at risk for VHL disease should be evaluated using contrast-enhanced MRI after 10 years of age, although careful ophthalmologic examinations should be initiated within the first 2 years of life. Careful inspection of retina, kidneys, ovaries, and testes over time is also indicated, as these structures may also develop angiomatosis. Some hemangiomas may be associated with pheochromocytomas. Genetic testing with mutational analysis should be offered to all patients with VHL disease and their families. It can reduce the necessity for costly and time-consuming screening programs and the screening can be directed at affected patients and family members at risk who carry the *VHL* gene mutation. However, the currently used DNA tests are not 100% sensitive; therefore, families with individuals affected by VHL disease in whom no mutations are detected should undergo periodic screening evaluations.

Only 10–20% of hemangioblastomas are associated with VHL disease. Hemangioblastomas of the brain are very rare (approximately 1–2% of all intracranial neoplasms). In some patients, especially with cerebellar hemangioblastomas, polycythemia may develop. These tumors usually contain large cysts filled with high-protein, yellow fluid with erythropoietin-like properties. Polycythemia improves after surgical removal of the tumor. The cystic cerebellar hemangioblastomas have MRI appearance similar to cystic astrocytomas with a mural nodule. The nodular component in hemangioblastoma is very vascular and displays strong contrast enhancement. Spinal cord hemangiomas are associated with syringomyelia. Those patients frequently present with central cord syndrome on neurologic exam with characteristic dissociated sensory loss.

Typically, hemangioblastomas are removed surgically, although some centers are using gamma-knife radiotherapy as a therapeutic option in patients with VHL disease. Some experts recommend that patients with VHL disease should have yearly contrast-enhanced cranial and spinal MRI and that staging of surgical procedures can be done electively and prior to hemangioblastomas presenting as frank CNS hemorrhages.

The present patient underwent successful surgical removal of the hemangioblastoma in the cervical spinal cord. During that procedure her syringomyelia was also treated with a shunt in order to decrease the progressive accumulation of fluid in the cystic spinal cord structures. To date, her cerebellar lesions have not been operated on because they have remained stable in size and number on yearly follow-ups with contrast-enhanced cranial and spinal MRI.

Clinical Pearls

1. von Hippel-Lindau disease may be associated with hemangioblastomas affecting the cerebellum, spinal cord, medulla, and, rarely, the cerebrum.

2. Early detection of symptomatic and asymptomatic tumors and other malformations associated with von Hippel-Lindau disease increases the chances of successful treatment and may enhance both the length and quality of life of affected patients.

3. Contrast-enhanced cranial and spinal MRI combined with abdominal CT, ultrasonography, and a thorough ophthalmologic examination should be performed regularly in affected patients and family members at risk.

4. Genetic testing and counseling should be offered to patients and their families.

REFERENCES

1. Choyke PL, Filling-Katz MR, Shawker TH, et al: von Hippel-Lindau disease: Radiologic screening for visceral manifestations. Radiology 1990; 174:815–820.
2. Filling-Katz MR, Choyke PL, Oldfield E, et al: Central nervous system involvement in von Hippel-Lindau disease. Neurology 1991; 41:41–46.
3. Filling-Katz MR, Choyke PL, Patronas NJ, et al: Radiologic screening for von Hippel-Lindau disease: The role of Gd-DTPA-–enhanced MR imaging of the CNS. J Comput Assist Tomogr 1989; 13:743–755.
4. Latif F, Tory K, Gnara J, et al: Identification of the von Hippel-Lindau disease tumor suppressor gene. Science 1993; 260:1317–1320.
5. Maher ER, Kaelin WG: von Hippel-Lindau disease. Medicine 1997; 76:381–391.
6. Martin RL,Goldblatt J, Walpole IR: Efficacy of gene testing for von Hippel-Lindau disease. Med J Aust 1998; 169:422–424.

PATIENT 21

A 25-year-old man with numbness and tingling of the right index and middle fingers

A 25-year-old man was evaluated for progressive loss of sensation over his right index and middle fingers. He became aware of numbness and tingling in the tips of these two fingers 2 years earlier. The initial symptoms gradually progressed to the point of near-total numbness of the whole middle and index fingers, with patchy numbness over the dorsum of his right hand. There was no history of weakness in the extremities, and he denied any problems with memory, speech, vision, hearing, or swallowing. Medical history was noncontributory for other diseases. The patient was born and raised in Bombay, India and came to the U.S. for studies 2 years earlier. He used no medications and denied tobacco or alcohol abuse. There were no other family members with similar symptoms.

Physical Examination: Pulse 68; blood pressure 125/75. Cardiac, chest, abdomen: normal. Skin: no abnormal pigmentation; the right index and middle fingers appeared swollen, possibly secondary to hypertrophic digital nerves in these fingers; the superficial radial sensory nerve was also markedly thickened in the right forearm. Mental status, cranial nerves, motor exam: normal. Sensory examination: decreased over the right index and middle fingers for pinprick, vibration, and position sense; area of patchy loss of sensation over the dorsum of the right hand. Muscle stretch reflexes: 1–2/4 in the upper and lower extremities and symmetric. Coordination and gait: normal.

Stop and Consider: What is the differential diagnosis in a patient with patchy sensory loss and thickened peripheral nerves?

Laboratory Findings: CBC, chemistry, electrolytes, sedimentation rate, ANA: normal. DNA analysis for mutations associated with Charcot-Marie-Tooth disease type 1: normal. Brain MRI: normal. Nerve conduction study/electromyography (NCS/EMG): no motor abnormalities, but small amplitudes of sensory nerve action potentials recorded from the digital nerves to the second and third fingers in the right hand and from the right radial sensory nerve. Nerve biopsy (electron microscopy) of the digital nerve to the right middle finger: see figure.

Question: What abnormality was observed on the sural nerve biopsy?

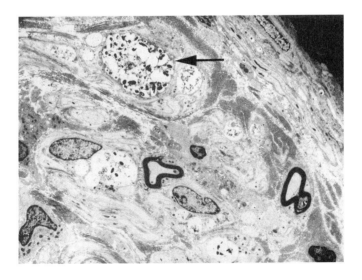

Diagnosis: Hypertrophic lepromatous neuropathy

Discussion: The findings of a hypertrophic neuropathy should always raise the possibility of an inherited demyelinating neuropathy (Charcot-Marie-Tooth type 1 disease). This diagnosis was unlikely, given the normal genetic studies and negative family history. The focal, patchy distribution of sensory signs would be extremely unusual in a hereditary polyneuropathy. Clinical and electrodiagnostic findings showed a multifocal axonal neuropathic process. This pattern of abnormalities in an individual from India was suggestive of leprosy. The nerve biopsy confirmed diagnosis by showing axonal degeneration and multiple Schwann's cells containing *Mycobacterium leprae* bacilli (arrow).

Leprosy is a common condition in the third world and is caused by *Mycobacterium leprae*. The disease typically affects cooler parts of the body. Infiltration is seen in the superficial nerves, the skin, the cornea, the upper respiratory tract, and the testes. Since the leprosy bacilli reproduce only in the cooler areas of the body (28–30°C), most vital organs are not affected. The World Health Organization estimated that there were more than 10 million cases of leprosy in the world in 1970, and these figures have changed little over the last 30 years. In the U.S. there are approximately 3,000–5,000 patients with leprosy. Most of these cases are seen in Florida, Louisiana, and Texas.

The body parts most commonly infected are the skin and the upper respiratory tract, but the pattern of clinical manifestation also depends on the immune status of infected patients. Susceptible patients with good T-cell responses to *Mycobacterium leprae* present with the clinical findings of tuberculoid leprosy. Patients with poor T-cell responses usually develop lepromatous leprosy. When features of both tuberculoid or lepromatous leprosy are present, the condition is classified as dimorphous (or intermediate) leprosy.

Skin lesions in patients with tuberculoid leprosy are sharply demarcated, often hyperpigmented, and tend to slowly enlarge with central healing. The border of the lesion is typically elevated and erythematous. The skin lesions typically affect the extensor surfaces of the limbs and face, or the buttocks, where the skin is exposed to cold. Biopsy of the skin lesions usually reveals epithelioid granulomata but few acid-fast bacilli. The superficial cutaneous nerves, most typically the cutaneous radial, digital, posterior auricular, and sural nerves, are commonly affected and clinically appear hypertrophic. The nerve damage is predominantly axonal and the nerve hypertrophy is the result of the granulomatous reaction within the nerve. The major nerves usually affected include the ulnar, medial, peroneal, and facial nerves. In lepromatous leprosy the skin lesions consist of macules, papules, nodules, and plaques, but some patients do not have skin abnormalities. A nodular infiltration of the face results in the so-called "leonine" facies that is a characteristic feature of leprosy. Granulomatous infiltration of the upper respiratory tract is common in these patients and results in nasal stuffiness and bleeding. Other findings include hoarseness, loss of sensation over the outer third of the eye, orchitic pain, and sterility. Biopsy of nerve and skin usually shows numerous bacilli, and the sensory nerve involvement in these cases usually has a stocking and glove distribution. Peripheral nerves are usually not hypertrophic. Dimorphous leprosy can present with a combination of the skin and nerve findings seen in classic lepromatous and tuberculoid leprosy.

The EMG studies in patients who develop neuropathy in the course of leprosy usually show axonal damage in the affected motor or sensory nerves. Patients with tuberculoid leprosy typically have a picture of mononeuritis multiplex. In lepromatous leprosy these changes are more diffuse, and the patients may appear to have distal motor and sensory axonal polyneuropathy. In some patients facial or glossopharyngeal nerves may be involved.

The antibacterial treatment of choice is sulfone drugs. A combination of dapsone and clofazimine, in conjunction with rifampin, is usually recommended for a period of 2–4 years. Longer treatments may be necessary in some cases. Treatment can result in unusual reactions, such as worsening of skin lesions, and erythema nodosum leprosum that may be associated with high fevers, myalgia, and prostration. Also, secondary amyloidosis can occur after many years of untreated leprosy. These reactions are treated with corticosteroids, despite the fact that the patients have an underlying infectious disease. Surgical treatment consists of abscess drainage and the treatment of contractures.

The present patient had an unusual appearance in the sense that he had pure neural leprosy, also referred to as polyneuritic leprosy. He returned to his native country shortly after the diagnosis, and was not seen in follow-up.

Clinical Pearls

1. The presence of hypertrophic neuropathy should always raise the possibility of leprosy, particularly if the changes are focal or patchy in distribution.

2. In the majority of patients with tuberculoid and lepromatous leprosy there is skin and nerve involvement. Patients can be classified based on the distribution and clinical features of the skin and nerve lesions.

3. Electrodiagnostic studies and nerve pathology in leprosy typically show axonal neuropathy.

4. Lepromatous neuropathy typically involves peripheral nerves in body areas with the lowest temperatures.

5. Leprosy is a common cause of neuropathy in the third-world countries.

REFERENCES

1. Job CK, Desikan KV: Pathologic changes and their distribution in peripheral nerves in lepromatous leprosy. Int J Lepr Other Mycobact Dis 1968; 36:257–270.
2. Mafoyane NA, Jacyk WK, Lotz BP: Primary neuritic leprosy in a black South African. Lepr Rev 1992; 63:277–281.
3. Sabin TB, Hackett ER, Brand PW: Temperatures along the course of certain nerves often affected in lepromatous leprosy. Int J Lepr Other Mycobact Dis 1974; 42:38–42.
4. Swift TR, Sabin TD: Neurologic manifestations of leprosy. Neurologist 1998; 4:21–30.

PATIENT 22

A 58-year-old man with deteriorating mental status after liver transplantation

A 58-year-old right-handed man with liver disease and alcoholism developed deteriorating mental status after orthotopic liver transplantation. Prior to surgery he had severe ascites and jaundice but was alert, followed commands, and moved all limbs symmetrically. Recovery was uncomplicated for 3 days postoperatively and he consistently followed simple commands. On the fourth postoperative day he became confused and delirious, and required mechanical ventilation for deteriorating oxygenation. Medications included methylprednisolone and FK506.

Physical Examination (postoperative day 8): Temperature 37°; pulse 75; blood pressure 140/80. Skin and sclera: mildly icteric, spider angiomata. Chest: bilateral basilar rales. Cardiac and abdomen: normal. Mental status: did not follow any commands. Speech: severely dysarthric. Cranial nerves: eyes spontaneously open, pupils equal, 3 mm in diameter, normal reaction to light; no papilledema or retinal hemorrhages; facial and oral structures symmetric; corneal and gag reflexes intact and symmetric; doll's-eye reflex: normal, with conjugate eye movements; cold caloric studies normal. Motor examination: diffusely reduced lean body mass, decreased muscle tone, no spontaneous or pain-induced limb movements observed, slight facial grimacing to sternal rub. Muscle stretch reflexes: hypoactive (grade 1) and symmetric, except for absent ankle reflexes. Plantar reflexes: minimal symmetric flexor movements.

Stop and Consider: Do these neurologic abnormalities suggest a diffuse or focal process?

Laboratory Findings: CBC: normal. Serum glucose (non-fasting): 153 mg/dl. Na+ (postoperative days 1–8) 132–148 mEq/L (135–144), ammonia 16 µmol/L (0–40), BUN 54 mg/dl (7–20), creatinine 7 mg/dl (0.6–1.3), total bilirubin 6.6 mg/dl (0–1.4), AST 27 IU/L (0–40), ALT 247 IU/L (0–65), GGT 447 IU/L (0–40), TSH 1.1 µIU/ml (0.5–4.7). Arterial blood gas studies with ventilator support (rate 12/min, PEEP 5 cmH$_2$O, 40% O$_2$): pO$_2$ 103 mmHg, pCO$_2$ 39 mmHg, pH 7.42. Cerebrospinal fluid analysis: protein 82 mg/ml (15–40), glucose 85 mg/dl, cell count < 1/µl. Electroencephalography: bilateral symmetric slowing in the theta and delta range, no epileptiform activity. NCS/EMG: mild sensorimotor, axonal polyneuropathy; repetitive stimulation test: normal. Brain MRI: see figure.

Question: What abnormality is demonstrated on the MRI?

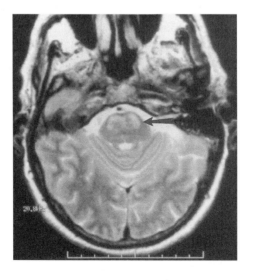

Diagnosis: Central pontine myelinolysis with coexisting polyneuropathy of critical illness

Discussion: The clinical presentation in this case with tetraplegia and severe mental status abnormality suggested involvement of the brain stem, although bihemispheric cerebral dysfunction also may produce similar abnormalities. The brain MRI confirmed the clinical suspicion, showing diffuse increase in signal intensity within the pons on T2 weighted images (arrow). The electrodiagnostic studies showed mild axonal polyneuropathy, which may have contributed to his weakness but was not sufficient to account for severe tetraplegia and mental status changes.

Central pontine myelinolysis (CPM) was originally described in association with alcoholism and malnutrition, but is now most commonly encountered while correcting hyponatremia. Recently recognized is the relatively high incidence of CPM in liver transplantation patients. This complication occurs during the postoperative period and may not be associated with large serum electrolyte fluctuations. The typical histopathologic feature of CPM is focal noninflammatory demyelination of the central basis pontis with relative preservation of axons and surrounding neurons. Extrapontine regions also may be affected, including the midbrain, thalamus, basal nuclei, and cerebellum. Because CPM has been causally associated with the rapid correction of chronic hyponatremia, it has been proposed that in regions of concentrated interdigitation of white and gray matter, such as the pons, cellular edema may compress adjacent fiber tracts sufficiently to cause demyelination.

Iatrogenic CPM has been typically reported in encephalopathic patients with hyponatremia treated rapidly with intravenous fluids. Correction of the electrolyte and fluid disturbance may initially produce improvement in mental status, but 48–72 hours later patients may deteriorate to coma with quadriplegia and bulbar abnormalities. Although a wide spectrum of neuropathologic findings has been reported, common to all cases is intense demyelination of the basis pontis revealed with MRI techniques, especially with T2 weighted scans that typically show increased signal intensity within the zone of demyelination. Patients with vertical ophthalmoparesis may show extension of the lesion into the midbrain. Delirium or coma may be associated with extension into the pontine tegmentum (reticular formation) and/or thalamic demyelination.

The extent of abnormal signal intensity on MRI may not correlate with neurologic findings. The scan may appear unremarkable in some patients with CPM, even with hyperactive reflexes, bilateral Babinski signs, and spasticity. In such cases brain stem auditory evoked potentials may help localize the lesion. The EEG of patients with CPM often demonstrates generalized symmetric bilateral slowing, which may be an effect of the initial electrolyte disturbance; however, in some patients the EEG abnormalities may persist for a few weeks. Status epilepticus may be a consideration in a patient with altered mental status after correction of hyponatremia. The EEG findings of generalized electroencephalographic slowing may be mistaken for a metabolic encephalopathy. The CSF studies frequently show elevated myelin basic protein.

Central pontine myelinolysis was found at autopsy in up to 29% of liver transplant cases and about two-thirds of these patients had significant (± 15–20 mEq/L) fluctuations of serum sodium during a period of 2–3 days. Liver disease, alcohol abuse, malnutrition, hyponatremia, and female gender are associated with susceptibility to CPM. Cyclosporine toxicity is associated with extrapontine myelinolysis and thus it may be prudent to reduce, if possible, the cyclosporine dosage in liver transplant patients with suspected CPM.

There is no specific treatment for CPM other than supportive care. Recovery may take weeks to months and surviving patients may be left with severe, permanent neurologic deficits, including coma, "locked-in syndrome," spastic paraparesis, tremor, or limb or gait ataxia. Prevention of metabolic abnormalities in critically ill patients and gradual correction of hyponatremia are crucial to avoid this devastating neurologic complication. The recommended rate for correction of hyponatremia is 10 mEq/L/24 hrs; rebound hypernatremia should be avoided.

The patient in this case was recovering well after liver transplantation but then developed deteriorating level of consciousness and increasing dependence on mechanical ventilation. His encephalopathy was initially attributed to metabolic derangements and possible infection. Because he had diminished extremity tone and hypoactive reflexes, and there was no evidence of sodium fluctuation, CPM was not initially considered. In his case the absence of hyperreflexia, spasticity, and Babinski signs may have been caused by coexisting polyneuropathy, demonstrated with nerve conduction/electromyography (NCS/EMG) studies. The pattern of electrodiagnostic abnormalities was consistent with critical illness polyneuropathy (CIN), although hepatic or renal failure also may be associated with predominantly axonal polyneuropathy. The critical illness polyneuropathy and critical illness myopathy (CIM) are now commonly recognized in ICU patients who present with respiratory failure or failure to wean from the ventilator and quadriplegia. The CIN typically develops in patients with multiorgan failure or sepsis, while CIM develops in patients receiving high-dose intravenous steroids concurrently with neuromuscular blocking agents. Some patients in early stages of CIM may have a characteristic, selective loss of myosin filaments on electron microscopy. In critically ill patients with evidence of both neuropathic and myopathic changes on NCS/EMG, the condition may be referred to as critical illness neuromyopathy.

The present patient slowly became more alert and interactive over the period of several months. After a year of physical therapy and other neurorehabilitative efforts, he was able to stand with assistance but was unable to walk and depended on a motorized wheelchair.

Clinical Pearls

1. Central pontine myelinolysis is a relatively common complication of liver transplantation and should be suspected in patients with mental status abnormalities and/or weakness.

2. Many cases of CPM are not associated with hyponatremia or significant fluctuations of serum sodium concentration.

3. Avoidance of rapid correction of hyponatremia is crucial to prevent CPM.

4. MRI is a diagnostic test of choice for evaluating patients with CPM and reveals pontine abnormalities.

5. Critical illness polyneuropathy and myopathy are relatively frequent causes of severe weakness and dependence on mechanical ventilation in patients with prolonged hospitalization in intensive care units.

REFERENCES

1. DeWitt LD, Buananno FS, Kistler JP, et al: Central pontine myelinolysis: Demonstration by nuclear magnetic resonance. Neurology 1984; 34:570–576.
2. Ghidoni P, DiBella C, Masini T, et al: Central pontine and extrapontine myelinolysis after orthotopic liver transplantation. Transplant Proc 1994; 26:3602–3603.
3. Illowsky-Karp B, Laureno R: Pontine and extrapontine myelinolysis: A neurologic disorder following rapid correction of hyponatremia. Medicine 1993; 72:359–373.
4. Laureno R, Illowsky-Karp B: Myelinolysis after correction of hyponatremia. Ann Int Med 1997; 126:57–62.
5. Singh N, Yu VL, Gayowski T: Central nervous system lesions in adult liver transplant recipients: Clinical review with implications for management. Medicine 1994; 73:110–118.
6. Zochodne DW, Bolton CF, Wells GA, et al: Critical illness polyneuropathy: A complication of sepsis and multiple organ failure. Brain 1987; 110:819–841.

PATIENT 23

A 53-year-old woman with severe headache, new-onset seizure, and a history of metastatic breast cancer

A 53-year-old woman presented to the emergency department with a severe occipital headache followed by a brief, generalized tonic-clonic seizure and emesis. She had a history of breast cancer treated 3 years earlier by a radical mastectomy with subsequent chest wall radiation and intravenous chemotherapy with cyclophosphamide and doxorubicin. Within the previous year she developed metastases in the peritoneum and ovaries that were treated with intravenous paclitaxel. During the course of therapy she developed anorexia and frequent nausea, which were regarded as chemotherapy side effects. Later she began to complain of progressive occipital headache and neck pain. She denied focal weakness or numbness, visual symptoms, or memory problems. Her medical history was otherwise noncontributory.

Physical Examination: Vital signs: normal. Neck: no adenopathy or thyromegaly, mild tenderness with flexion, Kernig's and Brudzinski's signs negative. Chest: left-sided mastectomy scar, lungs clear. Cardiac: normal. Abdomen: soft, nontender. Extremities: no edema. Mental status and speech: normal. Cranial nerves: mild bilateral papilledema, otherwise normal. Motor and sensory examinations: normal. Muscle stretch reflexes: grade 2 and symmetric. Coordination and gait: normal.

Stop and Consider: What are the possible causes of headache, elevated intracranial pressure, and seizures in a patient with a history of metastatic cancer and no focal neurologic abnormalities?

Laboratory Findings: CBC, chemistry including liver enzymes: normal. Electroencephalography: normal. Head CT scan: bilateral enlargement of the lateral ventricles. Head MRI with contrast: see figure.

Question: What is the significance of the abnormalities demonstrated on the MRI?

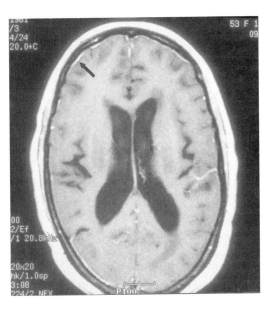

Diagnosis: Leptomeningeal metastases and hydrocephalus

Discussion: The clinical presentation of this patient with severe headache and a generalized seizure is consistent with several acute neurologic processes. A subarachnoid hemorrhage should be strongly suspected, but her head CT showed no evidence of intracranial hemorrhage. Although paclitaxel may induce encephalopathy, her cognitive status during hospitalization was unremarkable. The papilledema strongly indicated that her headache was related to a process associated with elevated intracranial pressure. In a patient with known metastatic disease, parenchymal, leptomeningeal, or epidural metastases are the most likely diagnostic considerations. These lesions may present with headache and other symptoms of intracranial hypertension, seizures, or focal neurologic signs. Hydrocephalus caused by leptomeningeal metastases or cerebral venous thrombosis with a hypercoagulable state were strongly suspected in this patient. The contrast-enhanced MRI showed hydrocephalus with some transependymal migration of the CSF, and focal areas of pial enhancement in the frontal, temporal, and parietal lobes, which were consistent with leptomeningeal metastases (arrow). Lumbar puncture was deferred because of signs of markedly increased intracranial pressure (papilledema) and hydrocephalus.

Neoplastic meningitis (NM) is a relatively frequent complication in patients with different types of neoplasms. Although the prognosis in NM is poor, prompt diagnosis and treatment may significantly prolong the survival and improve the quality of life. Based on autopsy studies, approximately 8% of patients with cancer, 10% with leukemia, and 4% with lymphoma develop NM at some stage of the disease. More than 70% of patients with solid tumors and NM have adenocarcinoma. Neoplastic meningitis in the course of lymphoma is typically associated with high-grade non-Hodgkin's lymphoma. In low-grade lymphoma and Hodgkin's disease this syndrome is very rare.

Leptomeningeal metastases of primary CNS tumors are common. Between 14–25% of adult patients with malignant gliomas and 30% of patients with primary CNS lymphoma develop metastases to the leptomeninges. In children, medulloblastomas and ependymomas are frequently associated with diffuse metastatic spread through the cerebrospinal fluid. Meningeal infiltration may occur by direct extension from subependymal and cortical metastases, by hematogenous spread via the choroid plexus, or from vertebral metastases. Flow disturbance of the CSF with hydrocephalus can occur in neoplastic meningitis without any apparent obstructive lesion on neuroimaging studies.

Mental status abnormalities and seizures may be a result of the parenchymal metastases, but also may be caused by diffuse infiltration of meninges and obstruction of the CSF flow. Meningeal spread within the spinal canal may be associated with radicular symptoms and signs of myelopathy. About one third of NM cases have cranial nerve involvement, but less than 50% of patients have nuchal rigidity, headache, nausea, or vomiting. Seizures and mental status changes may suggest cortical involvement.

The diagnosis of NM is usually made by the demonstration of malignant cells in the CSF, but there are biopsy-proven cases with persistently negative cytology. The yield of cisternal puncture is higher than lumbar puncture only when cortical signs are present. The CSF cell count, protein, and the opening CSF pressure on lumbar puncture are almost always abnormal. No other ancillary test is superior to CSF cytology.

Use of biochemical markers may increase the diagnostic yield of CSF examination in NM. Carcinoembrionic antigen (CEA) is frequently elevated in breast, lung, and gastrointestinal carcinoma. Other markers that may be increased in the CSF of some patients with NM include epithelial membrane antigen, beta-glucuronidase, beta-2-microglobulin, and lactate dehydrogenase. Measurement of the CSF levels of alpha-fetoprotein and beta subunit of human chorionic gonadotropin may help in evaluation of intracranial germ cell tumors that frequently metastasize to the subarachnoid space.

Brain CT scans with contrast are abnormal in up to 25–50% of investigated patients. Gadolinium-enhanced MRI scans are more sensitive than CT scans and can be as accurate as CSF cytology, whose sensitivity varies between 50–90%. The findings on both CT and MRI include leptomeningeal or ependymal enhancement, enhancing subarachnoid nodules, or hydrocephalus. There may be coexisting lesions in the brain parenchyma, spinal cord, or in the epidural space. Numerous cases have been reported in which MRI showed leptomeningeal infiltration with negative CSF cytology, and as many as 6 lumbar puncture studies may be required to obtain a positive CSF cytology.

With supportive treatment, the survival in NM is rarely more than 4–6 weeks. With aggressive treatment, including radiotherapy and systemic and intrathecal therapy, the median survival is 3–7 months, but up to 10% of patients can live more than 1 year. Agents most frequently used in intrathecal chemotherapy are methotrexate, thiotepa, and cytarabine. The CNS toxicity of chemotherapeutic agents may be significant and potentiated by concomitant use of brain radiation.

Breast cancer is the solid tumor most frequently associated with leptomeningeal metastases, also known as meningeal carcinomatosis. Between 2–5% of women with metastatic breast cancer develop meningeal carcinomatosis. The standard treatment for meningeal carcinomatosis from breast cancer is intrathecal chemotherapy (ITC), radiotherapy, or both. Methotrexate, thiotepa, or cytarabine are the drugs of choice. Single-drug ITC is less toxic and probably as effective as multidrug regimens. However, response rates are low, provide only brief improvement, and have not been shown to improve quality of life. In responding patients, ITC for longer than 6 weeks does not prolong response and is considerably more neurotoxic than treatment given for 6 weeks or less. ITC is usually not recommended in patients with very poor neurologic status, extensive metastatic visceral disease, and cranial nerve involvement. Radiation therapy to the affected area or to the whole brain can result in temporary disease stabilization or improvement of neurologic dysfunction.

The present patient was treated with radiation therapy to the whole brain with transient improvement, but her prognosis for long-term survival was poor.

Clinical Pearls

1. Contrast-enhanced head MRI is the most important initial diagnostic test in patients with suspected neoplastic meningitis.

2. A negative cytologic examination, even after more than one lumbar puncture, does not rule out leptomeningeal metastases.

3. Leptomeningeal metastases should be considered in patients with metastatic neoplasms who develop subtle, progressive cognitive or behavioral symptoms, or multifocal radicular abnormalities.

4. The life expectancy and prognosis of patients with carcinomatous meningitis are very poor. Palliative therapy with radiation and/or intrathecal chemotherapy are the mainstays of treatment.

REFERENCES

1. Boogerd W: Central nervous system metastasis in breast cancer. Radiother Oncol 1996; 40:5–22.
2. Chamberlain MC: Cytologically negative carcinomatous meningitis: Usefulness of CSF biochemical markers. Neurology 1998; 50 1173–1175.
3. Cosslett HB, Teja K, Sutula TP: Meningeal carcinomatosis 21 years following bronchiolo-alveolar carcinoma: Diagnosis by cisternal CSF examination. Cancer 1982; 49:173–176.
4. Fizazi K, Asselain B, Vincent-Salomon A, et al: Meningeal carcinomatosis in patients with breast carcinoma: Clinical features, prognostic factors, and results of a high-dose intrathecal methotrexate regimen. Cancer 1996; 77:1315–1323.
5. Freilich RJ, Krol G, DeAngelis LM: Neuroimaging and cerebrospinal fluid cytology in the diagnosis of leptomeningeal metastasis. Ann Neurol 1995; 38:51–57.
6. Lesser GJ: Neoplastic meningitis. Neurologist 1996; 2:11–24.

PATIENT 24

A 24-year-old woman with headache, visual disturbances, and left face and arm paresthesias

A 24-year-old woman was referred for evaluation of chronic headaches. She had had intermittent headaches since age 11. Some of the headaches were incapacitating and associated with visual obscurations with perception of flashing or shimmering lights. The headaches were infrequent and most of them were relatively minor, but approximately 18 months prior to evaluation they became more severe and frequent. She described more complex symptoms preceding her headache, which included an image of a bright line crossing diagonally from the right upper to left lower corner of the visual field, followed by numbness and tingling in the left face, arm, and to a lesser degree in her left leg. The paresthesias were always associated with the visual symptoms. Headaches were most frequently dull, but sometimes were throbbing and were most severe at the vertex. Some headaches were unilateral but many were diffuse and had a duration of several hours to a few days. On a few occasions the numbness persisted after resolution of the headache. She reported occasional episodes of visual obscurations accompanied by facial or arm numbness lasting 30 to > 60 minutes that were not followed by a headache. The headaches and other symptoms markedly interfered with her job and social life. Review of her headache and symptom diary revealed that most headaches occurred between the mid-cycle and during the first few days of menstruation. The review of systems was otherwise unrevealing and her medical history was unremarkable. Family history did not include migraine.

Physical Examination: Pulse 82 and regular; respirations 18; blood pressure 118/76. Chest and cardiac exams: normal. HEENT: normal, head nontender on palpation; neck supple, with good range of motion, no bruits. Mental status and speech: normal. Cranial nerves, including funduscopic examination: normal. Motor and sensory examinations: normal. Muscle stretch reflexes: normal and symmetric. Coordination and gait: normal.

Stop and Consider: What is the differential diagnosis in a patient presenting with a chronic headache and recurrent visual, sensory, or motor symptoms?

Laboratory Findings: CBC, chemistry with electrolytes, ESR, ANA: normal. Head CT, brain MRI on two occasions, and cerebral MR angiogram: normal.

Question: What is the most likely diagnosis in this patient?

Diagnosis: Classic migraine (migraine with aura) with features of complicated migraine (migraine with prolonged aura)

Discussion: The headache symptomatology in this patient was most suggestive of migraine. Her neurologic examination when she was not experiencing headache was normal and imaging studies of the brain and intracranial blood vessels revealed no abnormalities. Physical examination and laboratory tests showed no evidence of any systemic diseases that could cause headaches.

Migraine is a common disorder that affects about 6% of men and 15% of women. Migraine prevalence is highest between the ages of 25 and 55 years. There are two major types of migraines: migraine with aura (previously known as classic migraine) and common migraine (migraine without aura). The International Headache Society (IHS) classification defined the following criteria for diagnosis of both types of migraines: (1) headache duration of 4–72 hours; (2) headache fulfils at least two of the following four criteria: unilateral presentation, pulsatile quality, moderate to severe intensity, or aggravation by physical activity; (3) at least one of the associated features: nausea, vomiting, photophobia, or phonophobia; and (4) at least five episodes of headache without aura or two episodes of headache with aura.

A typical migraine aura may include transient paresthesias, numbness, homonymous visual disturbance, dysarthria, or dysphasia. As defined by the IHS, the aura should meet at least three of the following criteria: (1) one or more fully reversible symptoms of focal cerebral or brain stem dysfunction; (2) at least one aura symptom develops gradually over more than 4 minutes; (3) no aura symptom lasts more than 60 minutes; if more than one aura symptom is present, accepted duration of symptoms is proportionately increased; and (4) headache follows aura with a free interval of less than 60 minutes (it may also begin before or simultaneously with aura).

Migraine is diagnosis of exclusion and other organic diseases must be excluded by appropriate investigations. This is an important consideration in evaluation of all patients with headaches, and is emphasized in the IHS diagnostic criteria. Some patients may have attacks of short duration, but attacks shorter than 1 hour should prompt evaluation of other syndromes. Attacks longer than 72 hours are usually referred to as status migraine.

The migraine aura may be prolonged and can persist for extended periods after resolution of headache. Migraine attacks with prolonged neurologic deficit are usually referred to as complicated migraine, although the term "migraine with prolonged aura" (with the deficit lasting longer than 1 hour but shorter than 7 days) has been used in newer classifications. Migraine attacks have on rare occasions been associated with brain infarction. When auras are not followed by the headache phase, the symptoms are sometimes referred to as migraine equivalents.

The complex pathophysiologic events triggering migraine attacks have been a focus of intensive research over the last two decades but are still not well understood. It has been postulated that migraines may be the result of trigemino-vascular reflex abnormalities associated with sterile inflammation under the influence of serotonin receptor dysfunction. Menstrual migraines, posttraumatic migraine headaches, rebound analgesic and toxic migraines, and migraines associated with depression present special diagnostic and therapeutic circumstances. Pathophysiologically, all of these circumstances contribute to the susceptibilities of trigemino-vascular hyperactivity and, consequently, migraines.

Patients with migraines that easily respond to treatment and without neurologic abnormalities do not require further investigation. In the presence of complex history, poor response to treatment, or neurologic abnormalities, neuroimaging studies (brain MRI or CT with contrast) should be obtained. Other laboratory tests, including lumbar puncture with CSF analysis and measurement of the opening pressure, may be necessary.

Migraines may include a very wide range of presentations. They may be infrequent and easily treatable headaches, or may have a complex neurologic symptomatology and be frequent and intractable. Multiple headache types are frequently present in a given patient. This complexity presents a diagnostic and management challenge to clinicians, but with appropriate diagnosis and therapy most patients achieve marked and satisfactory control of headaches and associated symptoms.

Pharmacologic treatment of migraine can be divided into abortive (symptomatic) and prophylactic treatment. Nonspecific analgesics useful in migraine management include nonsteroidal anti-inflammatory drugs (e.g., ibuprofen, naproxen, aspirin) and acetaminophen. Antiemetic medications, sedatives, and opiates may be necessary in some patients with more severe migraine attacks. There is potential for addiction or opiate withdrawal symptoms when headaches are frequently treated with narcotics.

The most frequently used migraine-specific abortive agents are ergotamine and sumatriptan. Ergotamine is a strong vasoconstrictor but its antimigraine properties are also related to its action at the serotonin receptor. Sumatriptan and other triptans (zolmitriptan, naratriptan and rizatriptan) are relatively new agonists of the 5HT-1D receptor. More selective than ergotamine, they are most effective in treatment of pain, nausea, and other symptoms of migraine.

Frequent and severe migraines may require prophylactic therapy. Agents commonly used for prophylactic treatment are beta-blockers and tricyclic antidepressants. Valproic acid, an anticonvulsant, has been helpful in some treatment-resistant cases. Avoidance of migraine-triggering factors such as stress, sleep deprivation, caffeine or alcohol abuse, or dietary modification are very important measures for successful migraine management.

Sixty percent of female patients report that their attacks are linked to menstruation and 14% report that their attacks occur exclusively during the menstrual period. These women may be treated with the same preventive and abortive agents as other patients. Some women respond very well to a brief course of nonsteroidal anti-inflammatory drugs (ibuprofen or naproxen) or diuretics (acetazolamide) 2–3 days before and during the menstrual period. Hormone-related migraines have also been treated with estradiol transdermal patches or daily regimen of tamoxifen for days 7–14 of the luteal phase (ovulation to menstruation).

In the present patient, headaches were originally treated with acetazolamide without significant improvement. Inderal and naproxen were added, but her symptoms persisted and nortriptyline was initiated. The migraines continued despite increasing doses of nortriptyline, thus she received clomipramine, also without significant success. After consultation with a gynecologist and discussion of possible risks and side effects, a therapeutic trial with tamoxifen was initiated. Tamoxifen administered for 2 weeks each month, from midcycle to the second day of menstruation, has controlled the headaches and associated symptoms without significant side effects.

Clinical Pearls

1. The diagnosis of migraine can be reliably made in most patients by careful analysis of symptoms and exclusion of other causes of headache by thorough clinical examination and appropriate diagnostic studies.

2. Most patients with migraine can be successfully treated by a combination of abortive drugs, prophylactic agents, and preventive measures, including lifestyle and dietary modifications.

3. Hormonal manipulation can be successful in treatment of selected patients with menstrual migraine if other forms of therapy are ineffective.

REFERENCES

1. Freitag FG: Migraine headache variants. Clin J Pain 1989; 5:11–17.
2. Goadsby PJ: How do the currently used prophylactic agents work in migraine. Cephalalgia 1997; 17:85–92.
3. Headache Classification Committee of the International Headache Society: Classification and diagnostic criteria for headache disorders, cranial neuralgias and facial pain. Cephalalgia 1988; 8(Suppl 7):1–96.
4. Lance JW, Anthony M: Some clinical aspects of migraine: A prospective survey of 500 patients. Arch Neurol 1966; 15:356–361.
5. Lipton RB, Stewart WF: Prevalence and impact of migraine. Neurol Clin 1997; 15:1–13.
6. Marcus, DA: Serotonin and its role in headache pathogenesis and treatment. Clin J Pain 1993; 9:159–167.
7. O'Dea JPK, Davis EH: Tamoxifen in the treatment of menstrual migraine. Neurology 1990; 40:1470–1471.
8. Silberstein SD, Merriam GR: Estrogens, progestins, and headache. Neurology 1991; 41:786–793.

PATIENT 25

A 72-year-old man with progressive memory decline

A 72-year-old right-handed man presented with progressive memory decline over the previous year. His wife said that he would forget names of his coworkers, miss appointments, and could not remember what he had for dinner the night before or what he read in the newspaper earlier in the morning. His memory of remote events was preserved. He was a nonsmoker who did not indulge in alcohol. He was successful in the hotel construction and development business and otherwise has been in good health. Medical history was significant only for borderline hypertension. His mother suffered from poor memory in her old age.

Physical Examination: Vital signs: normal. HEENT: normal; neck supple, no bruits. Mental status: oriented to time, place, and person; mini-mental examination: score 21/30, missing points for registration, recall, and ability to abstract. Neuropsychological testing: high intellectual base with deterioration in cognitive-intellectual ability, causing memory deficits and language comprehension difficulties. Cranial nerves, motor, sensory, reflex, coordination, and gait examinations: normal. No frontal release signs.

Stop and Consider: Are this patient's abnormalities focal, multifocal, or diffuse, and how would you describe his disorder? What diagnostic work-up would you recommend?

Laboratory Findings: CBC, ESR, ANA, chemistry with liver and renal functions tests, serum vitamin B_{12} and folate, thyroid function tests: normal. *ApoE* DNA analysis: presence of *ApoE4* and *ApoE3* alleles. Head MRI: see figure.

Question: What is the diagnosis?

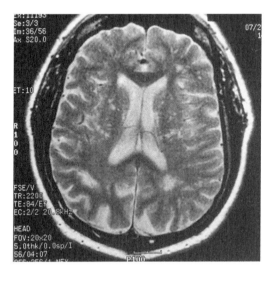

Diagnosis: Dementia consistent with Alzheimer's disease

Discussion: This patient presented with gradually progressive cognitive deficits. His neurologic examination otherwise did not show focal neurologic signs. Progressive dementia can result from many different pathologic processes. The diagnostic examination should focus primarily on potentially reversible causes of dementia, including structural abnormalities (brain tumors, subdural hematoma, normal-pressure hydrocephalus), metabolic conditions (e.g., vitamin B_{12} deficiency, hypothyroidism, hepatic or liver failure, electrolyte abnormalities), medication toxicity, chronic alcohol abuse, central nervous system or systemic inflammatory or infectious conditions, vascular lesions (multiinfarct dementia, vasculitis), and psychiatric conditions (depression). Chronic pulmonary and cardiac conditions may also lead to cognitive decline.

Extensive laboratory testing in this patient did not show evidence of a metabolic, inflammatory, or infectious process. Head MRI demonstrated mild generalized parenchymal volume loss and small-vessel ischemic changes involving subcortical white matter and basal nuclei. However, these changes were relatively mild, consistent with his history of hypertension, and were not sufficient to support a diagnosis of vascular dementia. His neuropsychological profile and otherwise negative laboratory testing for other causes of dementia strongly suggested the diagnosis of Alzheimer's dementia. The presence of the *ApoE4* allele provided additional support for this diagnosis.

Alzheimer's disease (AD) is the most common degenerative disease of the brain. It affects approximately 120 people per 100,000 population in the U.S. annually. The usual age of onset is ≥ 60 years, but patients have presented in their late 50s or younger. The familial occurrence of AD has been well documented in some families and several genetic abnormalities causing or predisposing to development of AD have been identified.

Typical AD patients show gradual development of forgetfulness, slow speech, deterioration of arithmetic skills, visuospatial disorientation, and personality changes. Common but late findings include apraxia, dysphasia, echolalia, anomia, agitation or apathy, self-neglect, incontinence, and unsteadiness of gait. With disease progression, frontal release signs like grasp, suck, or palmomental reflexes and motor, sensory, and autonomic deficits eventually develop. Affected persons eventually become wheelchair- or bed-bound.

In early stages, the diagnosis of AD may be difficult. Detailed history obtained from family members, neurologic examination, neuropsychometric assessment, laboratory tests and brain imaging (CT or preferentially MRI of the brain) in the majority of cases eliminate other treatable causes of dementia. Electroencephalography is useful to exclude conditions associated with periodic discharges, such as spongiform encephalopathies. Neuropsychological testing may help to identify subtle abnormalities, which otherwise can be difficult to detect on routine neurologic testing. In advanced cases diffuse brain atrophy involving frontal, parietal, and temporal lobes is observed. Histopathologic features include senile plaques, neurofibrillary tangles, granulovacuolar degeneration of neurons and Hirano inclusion bodies.

The *ApoE4* gene on chromosome 19 is associated with susceptibility to AD. Eighty percent of patients with familial AD and up to 64% of patients with sporadic, late-onset AD will have at least one *ApoE4* allele, compared with 31% of normal controls. The presence of this allele in a patient with dementia has a 97% positive predictive value for a diagnosis of AD. Other mutations have been associated with variants of AD. The amyloid precursor protein (APP) gene mutation on chromosome 21q21.1 is associated with early-onset AD but mutations in the *APP* gene account only for 5% of early-onset familial cases. Mutations in presenilin-1 on chromosome 14q24 and presenilin-2 on chromosome 1q31–42 have been found in rare cases of AD with autosomal dominant inheritance mode.

There is no preventive or effective treatment for AD. Acetylcholinesterase inhibitors with CNS action such as donepezil (Aricept) or tacrine (Cognex) may produce modest but usually temporary improvement. It has been suggested that estrogen (in elderly women), vitamin E, or anti-inflammatory drugs such as aspirin, ibuprofen, and indomethacin may possibly slow down the progression or delay the onset of AD. Behavioral symptoms (anxiety, depression, agitation, sleep disorders) may need to be alleviated with symptomatic pharmacotherapy. The side effects of medications in AD patients are significant and may have paradoxical effects, i.e., worsening of behavioral disturbances; therefore, any medications should be used with caution.

The present patient was started on vitamin E and donepezil (Aricept). His memory problems have been gradually progressive. With strong family support he has been able to function relatively well in his daily life, but had to retire from his professional activities.

Clinical Pearls

1. Alzheimer's disease is the most common neurodegenerative disease of the brain.

2. History obtained from family members may be essential in diagnosis of early Alzheimer's disease, because in early stages the patients may present with very subtle behavioral and personality changes.

3. Potentially treatable causes should be excluded through laboratory testing and brain imaging.

4. The presence of *ApoE4* allele with clinical evidence of dementia has a 97% positive predictive value for a diagnosis of Alzheimer's disease.

REFERENCES

1. Farrer LA: Genetics and the dementia patient. Neurologist 1997; 3:13–30.
2. National Institute on Aging/Alzheimer's Association Working Group: Apolipoprotein E genotyping in Alzheimer's disease. Lancet 1996; 347:1091–1095.
3. Saunders AM, Hulette C, Welsh-Bohmer KA, et al: Specificity, sensitivity, and predictive value of apolipoprotein-E genotyping for sporadic Alzheimer's disease. Lancet 1996; 348:90–93.
4. Small GW, Rabins PV, Barry PP, et al: Diagnosis and treatment of Alzheimer disease and related disorders. JAMA 1997; 278:1363–1371.

PATIENT 26

A 63-year-old woman with a 3-day history of fatigue and confusion

A 63-year-old previously healthy woman was admitted for evaluation of increasing fatigue and confusion. Her family reported that for the past 3 days the patient had not been her "normal self." Specifically, she had a decreased energy level, lost interest in her normal daily activities, and had episodes of confusion and disorientation when she did not know where she was and could not recognize familiar people. She complained of lightheadedness and poor appetite. There was no history of recent falls, fevers or chills, nausea or vomiting, headaches, visual changes, or weakness. Her medical, family, and social history was noncontributory.

Physical Examination: Vital signs: normal. Cardiac, chest, abdomen: normal. Neck: supple. Mental status: oriented to person and month, but not to place or time, unable to recall any objects after 3 minutes, marked difficulty with simple calculations. Speech: normal. Cranial nerves: normal, no papilledema. Motor examination: normal bulk, tone, and strength. Sensory examination: normal. Muscle stretch reflexes: normal throughout. Plantar reflexes: flexor. Coordination: normal in upper extremities. Gait: slightly wide-based.

Stop and Consider: What is the differential diagnosis in a patient presenting with subacute mental status changes and no focal neurologic abnormalities?

Laboratory Findings: CBC, chemistry, electrolytes: normal. Head CT on admission: normal. Lumbar puncture/cerebrospinal fluid: WBC 198/μl with 95% lymphocytes, 4% macrophages, 1% neutrophils; RBC 2/μl; protein 165 mg/dl (normal 15–45); glucose 58 mg/dl (serum glucose 113). EEG: periodic, lateralizing, epileptiform discharges in the right frontal-temporal area. MRI scan obtained the day after admission: see figure.

Question: What is your interpretation of the diagnostic studies? What other diagnostic tests should be obtained?

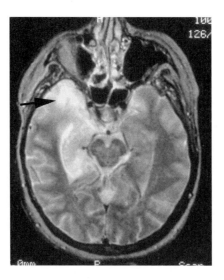

Diagnosis: Herpes simplex encephalitis

Discussion: This patient presented with a subacute onset of mental status changes but otherwise no significant focal neurologic findings or evidence of a systemic illness. An infectious or metabolic process affecting the central nervous system (CNS) was strongly suspected. The differential diagnosis for this clinical presentation includes structural abnormalities (e.g., tumor, subdural hematoma), toxic, metabolic, infectious, and immune vasculitic conditions. The CSF findings in this patient were consistent with an infectious, most likely viral process. The brain MRI showed an abnormally high signal on T2 weighted images and swelling within the right anterior-medial temporal lobe (arrow) and the right posterior-inferior frontal lobe. The MRI findings and the EEG abnormalities were typical of herpes simplex encephalitis (HSE). Polymerase chain reaction (PCR) CSF study for herpes simplex virus (HSV) was positive and confirmed the diagnosis in this patient.

Herpes encephalitis is the most common cause of fatal encephalitis in the U.S. and occurs with an annual frequency of 1 in 300,000 individuals. There is no seasonal, gender, or racial predilection. Patients who survive this infection are frequently left with severe, disabling neurologic deficits.

Primary infection with HSV type 1 occurs typically in children and adolescents through respiratory and salivary contact. As many as 90% of adults have antibodies against HSV type 1. The vast majority of HSE cases are caused by endogenous reactivation; only about 30% of cases appear to be a primary CNS infection. Although reactivation of the latent herpes infection in the form of herpes labialis is common, secondary involvement of the CNS is very rare. The factors that determine which individuals are susceptible to reactivation and development of CNS herpes infection are not known. Spread of HSV to the CNS from the trigeminal nerves or through the olfactory bulbs has been postulated.

Neonatal herpes encephalitis is usually caused by HSV type 2 infection. In this condition transmission to the CNS is hematogenous, involvement of the brain is diffuse, and systemic involvement with hepatitis and pneumonitis is relatively frequent.

Typical prodromal symptoms of HSE are fever and headache of relatively acute onset, followed by confusion, lethargy, focal or generalized seizures, aphasia, or hemiparesis. Behavioral symptoms such as personality changes or psychosis may develop early in the course. The pathology of HSE is characterized by acute inflammatory changes with hemorrhagic necrosis in affected brain areas. Eosinophillic intranuclear inclusions (Cowdry type A) are seen in about 50% of cases and may be present within the first week. Temporal lobes and inferior frontal brain regions are most commonly involved but in many cases the inflammatory changes are widespread. Progressive brain swelling, leading to uncal herniation and brain stem compression, is the most frequent cause of death in HSE.

Brain MRI or CT with contrast reveal focal or diffuse abnormalities in more than 60% of patients and MRI with T2 weighted images is more sensitive than CT. Focal EEG abnormalities are present in 80–90% of cases. The cerebrospinal fluid typically shows lymphocytic pleocytosis with increased protein. Moderately decreased glucose levels or red cells are sometimes observed. HSV is almost never cultured from the CSF but the rise in CSF anti-HSV titers may retrospectively establish the diagnosis. PCR amplification of the HSV DNA from CSF has revolutionized the laboratory diagnosis of HSE and can be used to monitor the response to therapy. The PCR for HSV detection appears to be highly specific and sensitive for HSE. This test can detect HSE cases as early as 24–48 hours from onset of symptoms and in suspected cases the CSF samples should be tested early and repeatedly if the first test is negative. The HSV PCR test remains positive for 2–5 days after initiation of therapy with acyclovir.

Before the introduction of the PCR test for HSV, brain biopsy with histopathologic and ultrastructural examinations, cultures, and immunocytochemical or immunofluorescent studies of the brain tissue to detect HSV particles were frequently done, especially in cases with atypical clinical presentations or atypical brain MRI or CSF findings. The HSV PCR test markedly reduced the number of patients who undergo brain biopsy; however, brain biopsy should be considered in all atypical cases, especially when alternative diagnoses are suspected.

Acyclovir is an effective treatment and should be initiated in all cases of suspected encephalitis when the PCR test for HSE or other diagnostic studies are pending. The intravenous treatment should be continued for at least 14 days with the dose adjusted for patient's renal function. Patients with suspected HSE should be closely monitored, preferentially in the intensive care units. Brain edema should be promptly treated by hyperventilation, osmotics, or other measures. If necessary, an intracranial pressure monitor may be placed. Prophylactic anticonvulsant therapy is usually not recommended, but if seizures occur, anticonvulsants (phenytoin) should be administered intravenously.

Improvement or recovery in most HSE patients treated with antiviral therapy usually occurs within a few weeks but some patients may have a fluctuating course and rare patients may have a relapse. Brain MRI and lumbar puncture should be repeated and repeat brain biopsy may be necessary if there is concern about relapse. In these patients a longer course of acyclovir (21 days) is recommended and addition of vidarabine may be considered. The use of steroids in viral encephalitis remains controversial.

Herpes simplex encephalitis may be difficult to diagnose in the initial stages and atypical presentations are relatively common. In some patients the evolution of clinical signs may be more chronic, with gradual onset of mental status or personality changes without significant focal findings or fever. The availability of the sensitive, specific, and noninvasive test employing the PCR technique for HSV detection enables early diagnosis in atypical cases, reduces use of invasive diagnostic procedures, and can facilitate prompt initiation of appropriate therapy.

The present patient was started empirically on acyclovir and ceftriaxone. Ceftriaxone was discontinued when the CSF PCR study for HSE was positive and the CSF cultures were negative. This patient presented at the time when the PCR test for HSV was just introduced to clinical practice and her clinical presentation was not very typical; therefore, a brain biopsy was performed and showed findings consistent with HSE. Despite acyclovir therapy, the patient's mental status never returned to normal and she continued to have episodic confusion. Because of her poor cognitive status, she was discharged to a rehabilitation center for further care.

Clinical Pearls

1. A significant proportion of patients with herpes simplex encephalitis may have an atypical presentation without headache or fever. Patients presenting with subacute or gradual deterioration of cognitive status or behavioral changes require a high index of suspicion for possible herpes simplex encephalitis.

2. PCR analysis of cerebrospinal fluid for herpes simplex virus provides diagnostic confirmation of suspected herpes encephalitis and is highly sensitive and specific.

3. Acyclovir therapy should be promptly initiated in patients with suspected herpes simplex encephalitis.

REFERENCES

1. Aurelius E, Johansson B, Sköldenberg B, et al: Rapid diagnosis of herpes simplex encephalitis by nested polymerase chain reaction assay of cerebrospinal fluid. Lancet 1991; 337:189–192.
2. Baringer JR, Pisani P: Herpes simplex virus genomes in human nervous system tissue analyzed by polymerase chain reaction. Ann Neurol 1994; 36:823–829.
3. Lipkin WI: European consensus in viral encephalitis. Lancet 1997; 349:299–300.
4. Meyding-Lamadé U, Lamadé W: HSV and the CNS. Neuroscientist 1996; 2:44–54.
5. Rose JW, Stroop WG, Matsuo F, et al: Atypical herpes simplex encephalitis: Clinical, virologic, and neuropathic evaluation. Neurology 1992; 42:1809–1812.

PATIENT 27

A 72-year-old man with a 1-month history of progressive leg weakness

A 72-year-old man was evaluated for progressive weakness that started 1 month earlier, shortly after he had received a pneumonia vaccination. Initially he complained of progressive weakness in his legs, especially when he was climbing stairs. About 3 weeks later he noticed difficulty in raising his arms above his head. He did not report any sensory disturbances, visual or hearing impairments, speech or swallowing difficulties, or hearing loss. His medical history was significant for coronary artery bypass surgery 3 years earlier and mild congestive heart failure. He was a heavy smoker all his life. He experienced a 20-pound weight loss during the previous 3 months. His current medications included aspirin and diltiazem. The family history was noncontributory.

Physical Examination: Vital signs: normal. Cardiac, chest, abdomen: normal. Extremities: mild distal edema in the legs. Mental status and speech: normal. Cranial nerves: normal except for sluggish pupillary reaction to light. Motor examination: muscle bulk and tone normal, mild (grade +4) proximal weakness in upper and lower extremities. Sensory examination: normal. Muscle stretch reflexes: absent in the upper and lower extremities. Coordination and gait: mildly impaired, as expected with his weakness.

Stop and Consider: What anatomic structures are producing this patient's weakness?

Laboratory Findings: CBC, chemistry, electrolytes: normal. ESR 80 mm/hr. Chest x-ray: mass in the right inferior lung lobe and prominent hilar lymphadenopathy. Nerve conduction study/electromyography: very low compound muscle action potential amplitudes at rest, conduction velocities normal. Repetitive nerve stimulation test: see figures.

Question: Are the results of the repetitive nerve stimulation test related to the chest x-ray findings?

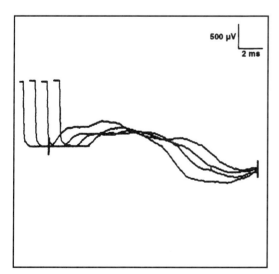 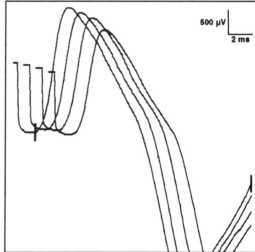

Repetitive nerve stimulation test: low-frequency (2 Hz) stimulation of the accesory nerve, recording over the trapezius muscle (at rest, *left*; after maximal voluntary exercise for 10 seconds, *right*).

Diagnosis: Lambert-Eaton myasthenic syndrome associated with small-cell lung cancer

Discussion: The findings from the neurologic examination suggest a pathologic process within the motor unit. The clinical history of this patient, who presented with subacute weakness without any sensory loss predominantly in the lower extremities, history of heavy tobacco use, and abnormalities on the chest x-ray, is suggestive of Lambert-Eaton myasthenic syndrome (LEMS). The electrodiagnostic testing showed small amplitudes of the compound muscle action potentials (CMAPs) at rest, and the repetitive nerve stimulation (RNS) test at low frequency (2 Hz) showed decrementing response (see figure, *left*). After maximal voluntary exercise for 10 seconds the CMAP amplitude increased by more than 100% in the distal hand muscles, the trapezius (see figure, *right*), and the distal leg muscles, and was followed by mild decrement with another train of 2 Hz RNS. This marked increase in the CMAP amplitude after exercise is indicative of a presynaptic neuromuscular transmission defect consistent with LEMS. The lung mass was biopsied and characterized as a small-cell lung cancer.

LEMS is a neuromuscular syndrome caused by a presynaptic defect in neuromuscular transmission. It occurs most commonly as a paraneoplastic syndrome in patients older than 40 years of age, usually in association with small-cell lung cancer, but may be associated with other neoplasms as well. Approximately two thirds of all cases are paraneoplastic and one third have underlying autoimmune diseases. Men predominate in the paraneoplastic group, whereas the association with autoimmune disorders is more common in women. Children can also present with this disease.

In addition to progressive motor dysfunction, the patients commonly have autonomic dysfunction that includes dry mouth, reduced accommodation, impotence, constipation, reduced sweating, and orthostatic hypotension. The sluggish pupillary responses, as seen in this case, are probably a sign of autonomic neuropathy. A history of easy fatigability is reported less frequently in LEMS than in myasthenia gravis, and patients with LEMS rarely present with respiratory failure. Sensory complaints are usually absent.

Electromyographic studies in LEMS reveal small amplitudes of the CMAP at rest in all clinically affected muscles, normal sensory nerve action potentials, and normal nerve conduction velocities. Low-frequency (2–3 Hz) RNS at rest induces a decrementing response similar to myasthenia gravis. After intense 10-second exercise there is a dramatic increase in the CMAP amplitude, typically more than 100% compared to baseline. High-frequency RNS at 20–50 Hz can be used instead of exercise to document the increase in the CMAP amplitude, but the exercise testing is much better tolerated by patients. The high-frequency RNS test is usually performed in patients who cannot cooperate.

LEMS is caused by antibodies directed against voltage-sensitive calcium channels in the presynaptic nerve terminal. The P/Q calcium channel–binding antibodies are detected in 90% of non-immunosuppressed patients with LEMS with or without evidence of cancer. The N-type calcium channel–binding antibodies are present in 73% of patients with a primary lung cancer and in 36% of patients with no evidence of cancer. Up to 13% of patients with clinical and electrodiagnostic findings typical of LEMS may have positive tests for nicotinic acetylcholine receptor–binding antibodies and striational antibodies.

Symptomatic treatment with diaminopyridine (3,4-DAP) or guanidine, which increase presynaptic acetylcholine release, may be helpful but side effects and toxicity are severe in some patients. Cholinesterase inhibitors may also improve neuromuscular transmission in patients with LEMS but the response is usually modest. Immunosuppressive therapy with prednisone, azathioprine, or cyclosporine has also been used. Plasmapheresis or high-dose intravenous immunoglobulin (IVIG) can be used in the short term for patients with severe weakness who can then be treated with oral immunosuppressors. The associated malignancy must also be treated, but the neuromuscular transmission defect may not improve in many patients.

The present patient received radiation therapy for lung cancer. His weakness responded moderately to oral treatment with pyridostigmine and infusion of IVIG. His general condition continued to deteriorate with metastatic spread of his cancer, and he expired 18 months later.

Clinical Pearls

1. The combination of muscle weakness and autonomic dysfunction is typical for LEMS. Not all patients with LEM have an associated malignancy, and in some patients, predominantly young women, a primary autoimmune etiology should be considered.

2. Electrodiagnostic studies with repetitive nerve stimulation should be performed in all patients with weakness of unknown etiology to rule out a defect in neuromuscular transmission.

3. A diligent search for malignancy is necessary in all patients diagnosed with LEMS.

4. LEMS may precede the detection of malignancy by 1–3 years in some patients.

REFERENCES

1. Bird SJ: Clinical and electrophysiological improvement in Lambert-Eaton syndrome with intravenous immunoglobulin therapy. Neurology 1992; 42:1422–1423.
2. Barr CW, Claussen G, Thomas D, et al: Primary respiratory failure as the presenting symptom in Lambert-Eaton myasthenic syndrome. Muscle Nerve 1993; 16:712–715.
3. Lennon VA, Kryzer TJ, Griesmann GE, et al: Calcium channel antibodies in Lambert-Eaton myasthenic syndrome and other paraneoplastic syndromes. N Engl J Med 1995; 332:1467–1474.
4. Oh SJ: Diverse electrophysiological spectrum of the Lambert-Eaton myasthenic syndrome. Muscle Nerve 1989; 12:464–469.
5. Pascuzzi RM, Kim YI: Lambert-Eaton syndrome. Semin Neurol 1990; 10:35–41.

PATIENT 28

A 69-year-old man with two episodes of right amaurosis fugax

A 69-year-old right-handed man reported two 30-minute spells of acute right monocular visual loss, which resolved with gradual restoration of normal sight over 2–3 hours. There were no associated changes in mental status, speech, or language. He did not report any weakness, numbness, diplopia, vertigo or dizziness, nausea, vomiting, sweats, chills, fever, dyspnea, or chest discomfort. During the preceding several months he experienced dull, bilateral headaches with frequent focal and sharp left-sided scalp pain, and constant neck and shoulder soreness. His medical history was unremarkable, with no history of stroke, coronary artery disease, diabetes, or ophthalmologic conditions. He quit smoking approximately 10–15 years earlier.

Physical Examination: Vital signs: normal. HEENT: scalp tenderness over the left temporal artery. Neck: supple, no carotid bruits. Heart, chest, abdomen: normal. Mental status, speech, language: normal. Cranial nerves: normal, including normal funduscopic exam and visual acuity (OD 20/25, OS 20/25). Motor and sensory examinations: normal. Muscle stretch reflexes: normal and symmetric throughout. Coordination and gait: normal.

Stop and Consider: What is the most likely diagnosis in an elderly patient presenting with a new-onset temporal headache and episodes of transient visual loss?

Laboratory Findings: CBC, chemistry with electrolytes: normal. Westergren erythrocyte sedimentation rate 60 mm/hr (normal 0–20). EKG: normal. MRI: minimal bilateral ischemic white matter disease. MR angiogram: normal intracranial and extracranial vessels. Echocardiography: no significant abnormalities. Temporal artery biopsy: see figure.

Question: What abnormalities does the temporal artery biopsy reveal?

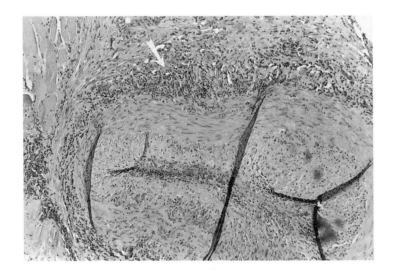

Diagnosis: Giant-cell arteritis (temporal arteritis)

Discussion: An elderly person with transient monocular blindness, elevated erythrocyte sedimentation rate (ESR), temporal artery tenderness, and headache most likely has temporal arteritis (TA). The temporal artery biopsy confirmed the diagnosis and showed typical severe perivascular inflammation (arrow) with invasion of superficial layers of the arterial wall and endothelial proliferation. In elderly patients, transient ischemic attacks with amaurosis fugax are most frequently caused by severe atherosclerotic disease of the carotid artery or its branches, usually as a result of emboli from the diseased artery. Other conditions that may cause transient or permanent monocular blindness include cardiogenic emboli or cardiogenic hypoperfusion episodes, hypercoagulable states, central retinal vein occlusion, thrombosis of the ophthalmic or retinal arteries, optic neuritis, or glaucoma. Visual loss in migraine is usually associated with scintillations or other "positive" phenomena rather than visual loss.

Temporal arteritis is a giant-cell arteritis (GCA) and shares pathologic features with Takayasu's arteritis, including inflammatory reaction in medium- and small-size arteries that involves granuloma formation with multinucleated giant cells deposited adjacent to fragmented internal elastic membrane, inflammatory cell infiltration, and intimal fibrosis. Although lesions may appear in any intermediate- or large-size artery, the most common are the temporal, ophthalmic, and vertebral arteries. Vasculitis of the posterior ciliary artery causes an ischemic optic neuropathy and blindness. Giant-cell aortitis is a rare complication and can cause aortic dissection. Diseased vessels become thickened and may develop thrombosis and complete occlusion.

Approximately 18 in 100,000 people older than 50 years develop TA. It is almost never seen in patients younger than this age and is twice as common in women. Juvenile TA is usually a relatively benign condition that affects only branches of the external carotid artery.

Headache, anorexia, weight loss, jaw claudication (due to masseter muscle ischemia), malaise, myalgia, fever, scalp tenderness, neck pain, and depression are common presenting complaints in TA. Any number of those relatively nonspecific symptoms may be reported early in the course of the disease, and the diagnosis can be difficult and mistaken for more common illnesses in the elderly. Amaurosis fugax occurs in up to 12% of patients with TA. Other symptoms of cerebral ischemia (e.g., cognitive problems) may develop in approximately 10% of patients and are related to involvement of large intracranial vessels. Vertigo, diplopia, and other symptoms of posterior circulation insufficiency may develop if the arteritis affects the vertebrobasilar system.

The examination of a patient with TA may reveal temporal artery or scalp tenderness, reduced temporal artery pulses and irregular thickening of the vessel, carotid bruits, encephalopathy, visual field defects, and abnormalities of the optic disc. Irreversible loss of vision occurs in up to 23% of untreated patients and is the most serious complication of TA. Different neurologic deficits caused by brain ischemia may develop depending on the blood supply distribution of the affected artery. Polyneuropathy, frequently presenting as mononeuritis multiplex or mononeuropathy, has been reported in up to 14% of patients with TA. Myelopathy caused by cervical cord ischemia is extremely rare.

Polymyalgia rheumatica (PR) frequently coexists in patients with TA. This syndrome includes morning aches and stiffness in back and proximal muscles and in shoulder and hip joints. Trigger points, fever, and malaise are often present, as well as an elevated ESR. About one-half of TA patients will develop PR and about one-seventh of PR patients will develop TA. Anemia (usually hypochromic type) is relatively frequent. There is an increased incidence of hypothyroidism in TA or PR patients; one study reported a prevalence of 5%.

Sensitive, though nonspecific serologic studies, useful in the diagnosis of TA are Westergren ESR and C-reactive protein (CRP). Typically, ESR is markedly elevated (> 50 mm/hr), but in some patients with typical TA it may be normal. It is reported that CRP is elevated in 100% of patients with biopsy-proven TA and that about 8% of those patients may not have an elevated ESR. ESR and CRP can be used to monitor disease activity in treated patients.

Patients with suspected TA should have a temporal artery biopsy to confirm the diagnosis and to justify prolonged steroid therapy. Because it is relatively common for affected vessels in GCA to have "skip areas" or regions of apparently normal histology, the entire length of the biopsy specimen is serially sectioned and examined if necessary. When the index of suspicion for the diagnosis of TA is relatively high and the first biopsy is negative or equivocal, it is recommended that the temporal artery biopsy be repeated on the other side. Up to 40% of patients who have classic signs of the disease and are responsive to treatment may have a negative biopsy.

Therapy for TA is oral prednisone with initial dosages of 60–80 mg/day followed by a gradual taper to maintenance dose that should be as low as possible. When significant neurologic deficits or encephalopathy have developed, initial treatment with intravenous methylprednisolone is recommended. The majority of patients will require steroid treatment for 1–5 years.

The present patient was treated initially with IV methylprednisolone and later with oral prednisone. His condition markedly improved and he had no further visual symptoms.

Clinical Pearls

1. Patients with suspected temporal arteritis require urgent evaluation, including temporal artery biopsy, because delay in diagnosis and treatment may cause visual loss and other neurologic deficits.

2. Temporal arteritis is unlikely in patients younger than 50 years.

3. Corticosteroids are usually very effective in treatment of temporal arteritis.

4. Most patients with temporal arteritis need treatment with corticosteroids for 1–5 years.

REFERENCES

1. Berlit PD: Giant-cell arteritis. In Lechtenberg R, Schutta HS (eds): Neurology Practice Guidelines. New York, Marcel Dekker, 1998, pp 51–62.
2. Caselli RJ, Hunder GG: Neurologic complications of giant cell (temporal) arteritis. Semin Neurol 1994; 14:349–353.
3. Hayreh SS, Podhajsky PA, Raman R, et al: Giant cell arteritis: Validity and reliability of various diagnostic criteria. Am J Ophthalmol 1997; 123:285–296.
4. Hellmann DB: Immunopathogenesis, diagnosis, and treatment of giant-cell arteritis, temporal arteritis, polymyalgia rheumatica, and Takayasu's arteritis. Curr Opin Rheumatol 1993; 5:25–32.

PATIENT 29

A 31-year-old woman with a new-onset seizure

A 31-year-old left-handed, previously healthy woman, was brought to the emergency department because of a new-onset seizure. She had been at work when she became suddenly lightheaded and developed vertigo and blurred vision. Her associates found her staring into space, unresponsive, with her fists tightly clenched and contraction of her facial muscles and head deviation to the right. She was subsequently described to be making "clicking noises" with her tongue, accompanied by brief clonic activity of the right upper extremity associated with extension of the right lower extremity. The total duration of the episode was approximately 20 minutes, and her responsiveness gradually improved.

Physical Examination: Vital signs: normal. Heart and chest: unremarkable. Mental status: drowsy, but improving ability to follow simple commands. Speech: slow but without aphasia or dysarthria. Cranial nerves: normal, no evidence of papilledema. Motor examination: normal bulk, slightly increased muscle tone in right upper and lower extremities, normal muscle power in all limbs. Sensory examination: normal to all modalities, including double simultaneous stimulation test and normal graphesthesia. Muscle stretch reflexes: asymmetric with mild hyperreflexia (grade 3) in right upper and lower extremities. Plantar reflexes: positive Babinski sign on the right and flexor plantar response on the left side. Coordination and gait: mild difficulty on tandem gait test.

Stop and Consider: What is the time course and localization of the neurologic dysfunction?

Laboratory Findings: CBC, chemistry with electrolytes, including calcium and magnesium: normal. Cranial CT scan: non-contrast (see figure, *top left*), contrast-enhanced (see figure, *top right*). Cerebral angiogram: see figure, *bottom*.

Question: What is your interpretation of the neuroimaging studies?

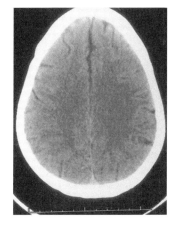
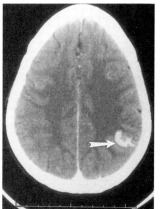
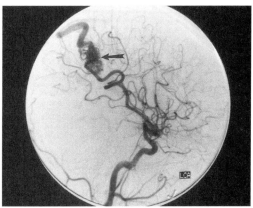

Diagnosis: Left cerebral hemisphere arteriovenous malformation presenting as a new-onset seizure

Discussion: This patient experienced a new-onset partial complex seizure with motor manifestations, including contraversive head movement to the right and tonic-clonic activity of the right extremities. The focal features of the seizure, along with the abnormalities observed on neurologic examination (increased muscle tone and reflexes and a positive Babinski sign on the right) indicate a structural lesion in the left cerebral hemisphere. Based on the well-characterized features of the episode provided by witnesses, other causes of episodic neurologic dysfunction such as transient focal brain ischemia, syncope, or hypoglycemia are unlikely. The emergent cranial CT demonstrated a contrast-enhancing lesion in the left parietal lobe (top figure, arrow). Additional studies included a brain MRI with contrast, which showed that the lesion most likely represented an arteriovenous malformation (AVM). A cerebral angiogram demonstrated left parietal-temporal AVM (bottom figure, arrow). The main arterial "feeder" of the AVM was the enlarged angular branch of the middle cerebral artery. The predominant venous drainage was through superficial veins into the superior sagittal sinus.

Partial seizures are seizures whose initial manifestations can be localized to a specific region of the cerebral hemisphere, in contrast to generalized seizure, whose manifestations are bilateral at onset. The term "complex" refers to the symptom of altered consciousness; "simple" seizures are those in which consciousness is normal. The differential diagnosis for new-onset partial seizures should include neoplastic processes (primary or metastatic brain tumors), stroke (infarction, hemorrhage of different etiologies), infectious processes (e.g., abscess), autoimmune conditions (e.g., lupus, primary CNS angiitis), or congenital malformations. Toxic and metabolic conditions may also present with focal neurologic signs.

Cerebrovascular malformations may be classified into five major types: (1) arteriovenous malformations; (2) venous malformations; (3) cavernous malformations; (4) telangiectasias; and (5) arteriovenous fistulas. They have distinct morphologic and pathophysiologic features and present with different clinical manifestations and natural history.

Arteriovenous malformations are abnormal connections between the arteries and veins that bypass the capillary system and typically consist of three morphologic components: a dysplastic vascular core usually referred to as nidus, feeding arteries, and draining veins. Most AVMs represent congenital anomalies but some may be caused by trauma or radiation. The largest AVMs often occur in the cerebral hemispheres in the distribution of the middle cerebral artery but may also occur in the branches of the anterior or posterior cerebral arteries. AVMs in the brain stem, cerebellum, or spinal cord are usually smaller and are observed in the branches of the vertebral and basilar arteries. There is a great variability in the patterns of feeding and draining vessels. Infratentorial feeding arteries may also supply some AVMs within the posterior cerebral hemispheres. The AVMs may drain into superficial or deep veins or to venous sinuses.

Approximately 50% of patients with AVM present with hemorrhage, about 25% with new-onset seizure, and the remainder present with headache (mimicking "typical" migraine) or focal neurologic signs. The location of the AVM has some predictive value with regard to presenting symptoms. AVMs located in the cerebellum, brain stem, and deeper regions of the hemispheres (basal ganglia, ventricles) or corpus callosum usually present with hemorrhage. Superficial AVMs in supratentorial cortex in 50% of cases present with a seizure and the location of the AVM in many patients correlates with a seizure type. Parietal and occipital AVMs frequently present with intractable headaches.

AVMs are prone to rupture and can produce an intracerebral or subarachnoid hemorrhage, or both. The prognosis of an AVM with hemorrhage at the time of diagnosis is worse compared to presentation with seizures, focal neurologic deficit, chronic headache, or other symptoms unrelated to bleeding. The annual risk of bleeding for a patient presenting with nonhemorrhagic symptoms is approximately 2%. The risk of rebleeding in the untreated group with hemorrhage is approximately 17.8%. Male sex and deep venous drainage seem to be associated with increased risk of subsequent bleeding but there is no significant association with age or size of the AVM. Pregnancy and childbirth increase the risk of hemorrhage from the AVM.

The initial diagnostic evaluation in a patient with suspected AVM should include an MRI or cranial CT with contrast. Non-contrast CT may not reveal even a large AVM in patients who present without hemorrhage. Intra-arterial cerebral (four-vessel) angiography is usually necessary to define the arterial and venous anatomy.

AVMs can be treated with surgical resection, embolization, or stereotactic radiosurgery. Surgical resection is the primary treatment for most AVMs, especially if the lesions are superficial and can be removed without significant neurologic deficits. Some lesions can be treated with embolization (alone or as an adjunct to surgical resection). Small AVMs can be successfully treated with radiofrequency ablation procedure.

The present patient received a loading dose of intravenous phenytoin and was monitored in the neuro–intensive care unit. She underwent surgical resection of the AVM and has done well postoperatively, without any further seizures.

This case illustrates the importance of urgent/emergent diagnostic work-up of patients with new-onset seizures and the benefit of appropriate neuroimaging studies to identify patients with treatable conditions.

Clinical Pearls

1. Clinical presentation of AVMs correlates to some degree with the location of the lesion.

2. Arteriovenous malformations presenting without a hemorrhage may be difficult to detect on non-contrast CT scan. Brain MRI or at least a CT with contrast should be obtained in all patients with suspected AVM.

3. Knowledge of natural history of different types of cerebral vascular malformations is important in decision making regarding therapeutic options.

4. Surgical resection, embolization, and stereotactic radiosurgery can be used alone or in combination in treatment of AVMs depending on the size, location, and other characteristics of the lesion.

REFERENCES
1. Brown RD, Wiebers DO, Forbes G, et al: The natural history of unruptured arteriovenous malformations. J Neurosurg 1988; 68:352–357.
2. Mast H: Young WL, Koennecke HC, et al: Risk of spontaneous haemorrhage after diagnosis of cerebral arteriovenous malformation. Lancet 1997; 350:1065–1068.

PATIENT 30

A 72-year-old man with recurring episodes of fleeting blindness in the left eye

A 72-year-old man with a history of hypertension, coronary artery disease, cigarette smoking, and diabetes mellitus experienced abrupt and recurring episodes of painless visual loss in his left eye, which usually resolved after 10–15 minutes. He described these as if "a curtain was being drawn over my left eye." He had experienced 8–10 of these episodes in the 2 weeks prior to presenting to an outpatient clinic for neurologic consultation. He denied any recent head or neck trauma, episodes of limb weakness or numbness, or any other neurologic symptoms.

Physical Examination: Temperature, respirations: normal; pulse 72 and regular; blood pressure 152/90. Cardiac: normal. Neck: loud systolic bruit over the left carotid bifurcation. Mental status, affect, speech, language: normal. Cranial nerves: pupillary reflexes intact, visual acuity 20/20 bilaterally, normal fundi, visual fields, and gaze; muscles of facial expression normal and symmetric; oral and pharyngeal structures midline. Motor examination: muscle tone, bulk, and power normal. Sensory examination: normal. Muscle stretch reflexes: grade 2 and symmetric. Plantar reflexes: flexor. Coordination and gait: normal.

Stop and Consider: What paroxysmal disorders should be considered in a patient presenting with recurrent episodes of painless visual loss?

Laboratory Findings: CBC, ESR, platelet count, PT, PTT, chemistry, electrolytes: normal. Head CT and MRI: normal. Carotid Doppler ultrasound: systolic flow velocity of the left internal carotid artery > 275 cm/sec (indicative of severe stenosis); right internal carotid flow measurements normal. Neck magnetic resonance angiogram (MRA): see figure.

Question: What treatment would you recommend for this patient?

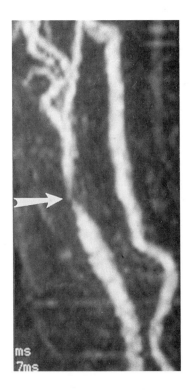

Diagnosis: Amaurosis fugax as a manifestation of recurrent transient ischemic attacks in the left internal carotid artery territory

Discussion: The clinical presentation of this patient with recurring episodes of fleeting, painless blindness of the left eye and a loud systolic bruit over the left carotid bifurcation indicates an abnormality of the left internal carotid artery circulation, more specifically intermittent ischemia of the left ophthalmic/retinal arterial circulation. Neck MRA (arrow) and carotid Doppler demonstrated severe stenosis of the left internal carotid artery, ipsilateral to the episodes of transient monocular blindness.

Amaurosis fugax (AF) or transient monocular blindness, usually suggests either an embolic process or temporal arteritis as a cause of transient ischemia in the vascular territory of ophthalmic or retinal arteries. In patients under the age 30, the heart is the leading source of emboli due to rheumatic valvular disease, bacterial endocarditis, cardiac myxoma, or other cardiac anomaly. In older patients, the source of the embolus may be cardiac or intra-arterial from atheromatous ulceration of the ipsilateral internal carotid artery or the aorta. Temporary thrombosis of small feeding arterial vessels supplying the optic nerve and retina is a less frequent cause of AF. This may develop in lipohyalinosis of small arterial blood vessels in patients with chronic hypertension or diabetes mellitus. Hypercoagulable states in the course of lupus erythematosus, malignancy, sickle cell anemia, and other conditions may also cause AF.

Transient ischemic attacks (TIAs) are usually defined as transient episodes of nonconvulsive focal neurologic dysfunction caused by a reversible interference in blood flow to a specific area of the brain, spinal cord, or retina. The transient nature of each event is usually explained by either rapid lysis of the occluding platelet thrombus or post-occlusion microcirculatory vasodilatation with increased blood flow. TIAs, by definition, resolve completely within 24 hours, but if symptoms persist for more than 1 hour, only 14% will resolve within 24 hours. The differential diagnosis of TIAs should include focal epileptic seizures, migraines with prolonged aura (complicated migraine), toxic or metabolic conditions (e.g., episodes of hypo- or hyperglycemia), and vestibulopathies. Structural lesions, such as brain tumors or subdural hematomas, may present with episodes of transient neurologic dysfunction.

TIAs are separated into those arising in the anterior cerebral circulation (carotid TIAs) or the posterior cerebral circulation (vertebrobasilar TIAs). Symptoms that favor a carotid TIA localization include: (1) contralateral weakness, clumsiness, or paralysis of the face and/or upper extremity or leg only; (2) contralateral numbness or loss of sensation in the face and/or upper extremity or leg only; (3) motor dysarthria or dysphasia; (4) transient monocular blindness or occasionally contralateral visual field loss; and (5) combinations of the above with or without hemicranial headache ipsilateral to the involved carotid artery. Intracranial and extracranial atherothrombotic occlusive disease of the large cerebral arteries is the most frequent cause of TIAs. Artery-to-artery emboli or cardiac emboli probably account for 80% of carotid TIAs and focal hypoperfusion is implicated in 20% of carotid TIAs.

Patients with both anterior and posterior circulation TIAs deserve rapid, thorough evaluations, including brain imaging, blood studies (including complete blood count and chemistries, erythrocyte sedimentation rate, coagulation profiles), cardiac evaluation, and noninvasive vascular studies, such as Doppler ultrasound and/or MRA. Some patients will still require intra-arterial angiography to clarify the underlying diagnosis. Treatment should be based on the nature, location, and severity of the specific underlying atherosclerotic lesion. Any identified risk factors should be treated or modified. Carotid endarterectomy was found to be beneficial in symptomatic patients who are good surgical candidates and have carotid stenosis greater than 70%. Medical therapy includes antiplatelet agents (aspirin, ticlopidine, clopidogrel) or anticoagulation with warfarin.

The present patient underwent successful left carotid endarterectomy. He was placed on aspirin following surgery and has remained free of cerebrovascular events during 5 years of follow-up.

Clinical Pearls

1. Transient monocular blindness, or amaurosis fugax, is often a specific premonitory symptom of impending stroke and its cause may be embolic, arteritic, localized hypoperfusion, or, rarely, an underlying coagulopathy.

2. Aspirin, ticlopidine, or clopidogrel (Plavix) are beneficial in the prevention of stroke following a TIA. Other treatment modalities (surgery or anticoagulation) may be necessary depending on the underlying etiology and mechanism of ischemic attacks.

3. Single or multiple transient ischemic attacks, irrespective of response to antiplatelet drugs, in the presence of high-grade ipsilateral carotid artery stenosis, in a good surgical candidate, are indications for carotid endarterectomy.

4. The goals of diagnostic tests are to identify or exclude etiologies of TIA requiring specific therapy, and to assess modifiable cerebrovascular and cardiovascular stroke risk factors.

REFERENCES

1. Culebras A, Kase CS, Masdeu JC, et al: Practice guidelines for the use of imaging in transient ischemic attacks and acute stroke: A report of the Stroke Council, American Heart Association. Stroke 1997; 28:1480–1497.
2. Feinberg WM, Albers GW, Barnett HJ, et al: Guidelines for the management of transient ischemic attacks: From the Ad Hoc Committee on Guidelines for the Management of Transient Ischemic Attacks of the Stroke Council of the American Heart Association. Circulation 1994; 89:2950–2965.
3. Levine R: Cerebrovascular disease: Occlusive stroke and transient ischemic attacks. In Lechtenberg R, Schutta HS (eds): Neurology Practice Guidelines. New York, Marcel Dekker, 1998, pp 117–158.
4. Moore WS, Barnett HJ, Beebe HG, et al: Guidelines for carotid endarterectomy: A multidisciplinary consensus statement from the Ad Hoc Committee, American Heart Association Stroke 1995; 26:188–201.
5. Wray SH: The management of acute visual failure. J Neurol Neurosurg Psychiatry 1993; 56:234–240.

PATIENT 31

A 19-year-old man with muscle pain and cramps

A 19-year-old man presented with complaints of severe exercise-induced muscle pain and cramps. His symptoms developed in early childhood. He was never able to run or even walk fast since he would almost immediately develop severe leg cramps. Any intense physical activity, such as carrying or lifting heavy objects or climbing stairs, caused painful muscle contractions. Typically, the episodes of muscle stiffness lasted a few minutes, but the affected muscles were sometimes very sore for many hours or days. Some episodes were followed by passing dark brown-red urine. Prolonged activities were tolerated relatively well if pursued at a slower pace. He was otherwise in good health and denied any permanent weakness or numbness, incoordination, or difficulty walking. He denied taking any medications or illegal substances and there was no family history of a similar condition.

Physical Examination: Vital signs: normal. HEENT: head normocephalic, skull nontender; neck supple, no bruits. Cardiac: normal. Spine: no deformity, nontender, good range of motion. Mental status, speech, cranial nerves: normal. Motor examination: muscle bulk, tone, and strength: normal. Sensory examination: normal. Muscle stretch reflexes: normal. Coordination and gait: normal.

Stop and Consider: What is the differential diagnosis in a patient presenting with exercise-induced muscle pain and cramps and a normal neurologic examination?

Laboratory Findings: CBC, ESR, chemistry, electrolytes: normal with the exception of creatine kinase 614 U/L (0–250). Muscle biopsy: scattered necrotic or regenerating fibers with some fibers containing subsarcolemmal vacuoles, positive for PAS reaction. Histochemical stain for myophosphorylase activity: see figure.

Question: What is the metabolic defect that produces painful cramps?

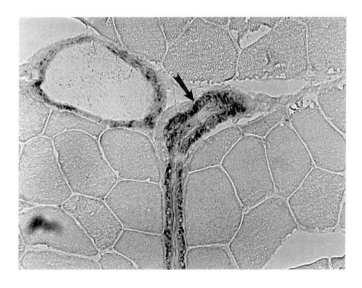

Diagnosis: Myophosphorylase deficiency (McArdle's disease)

Discussion: The symptoms of exercise-induced muscle pain and cramps strongly suggested a metabolic muscle disease. The muscle biopsy confirmed the suspected diagnosis. It showed evidence of glycogen storage and demonstrated absence of myophosphorylase activity in the muscle fibers, with preserved reaction only in the blood vessel walls (arrow). The isoenzyme expressed in the smooth muscle of the blood vessels is different from the isoenzyme in the skeletal muscle and is not affected in McArdle's disease. The quantitative biochemical assay confirmed the histochemical findings and showed only residual myophosphorylase activity at 0.17 µmol/min/g (normal > 12).

Myophosporylase deficiency (McArdle's disease) is an autosomal recessive metabolic muscle disease caused by mutation in the myophosphorylase gene located on chromosome 11. The enzyme deficiency causes disturbance in the process of energy delivery through the glycogenolytic pathway. The characteristic symptoms are exercise intolerance with severe muscle pain and stiffness (cramps) with physical activity. Typically, brief, very intense exercise (e.g., lifting heavy weights, fast run) or less intense but sustained activities (fast-paced walking, climbing stairs) may precipitate symptoms. Many patients report a "second wind" phenomenon—taking a short rest at the onset of symptoms may enable them to resume activities, usually at a lower pace, with much less muscle pain or cramping.

Most patients have normal muscle strength except during episodes of cramps and pain; however, some patients may develop fixed, usually mild, weakness with age. The painful cramps may be accompanied by muscle swelling with myoglobinuria caused by muscle necrosis. Approximately 25% of patients will have at least one episode of myoglobinuria. This often leads to erroneous diagnosis of kidney disease since patients who develop this complication may pass a "coca cola–like," dark brown urine, which may be misinterpreted as hematuria. The onset of symptoms is usually in childhood, although there is significant clinical heterogeneity, most likely related to residual enzyme activity in some patients.

In contrast to many other metabolic muscle conditions, most patients with McArdle's disease have a mild elevation of creatine kinase at rest. The forearm exercise test, with serial measurements of lactate levels in the venous blood, is very useful in diagnostic evaluation of patients with possible metabolic myopathies. However, this test is nonspecific for myophosphorylase deficiency since any potential defect in the glycogenolytic or glycolytic

pathway can lead to impairment of lactate production. This test should not be performed under ischemic conditions since it may precipitate severe muscle necrosis with a compartment syndrome and myoglobinuria.

Muscle histochemistry usually demonstrates a vacuolar myopathy with excessive glycogen accumulation. If the biopsy is obtained during an episode of myoglobinuria, muscle fiber necrosis can be extensive. In some biopsies, chronic myopathic changes may be seen, especially in older patients. The stain for myophosphorylase activity typically demonstrates absence of enzyme activity in the muscle fibers with preserved activity in the blood vessels. Quantitative myophosphorylase assay typically reveals absent or just residual enzyme activity.

Several different mutations in the myophosphorylase gene have been reported. Most patients with McArdle's disease are homozygous for the most common nonsense point mutation at codon 49 in exon 1, with C→T transition that changes an encoded arginine (CGA) to a stop codon (TGA). Molecular studies in patients with myophosphorylase deficiency indicate that in approximately 90% of patients the diagnosis can be made by DNA analysis from leukocytes; in these patients, muscle biopsy may not be necessary.

Specific treatment for McArdle's disease is currently not available. Dietary modifications (e.g., high-protein diet) or pharmacologic attempts to bypass the metabolic block are usually ineffective. Most patients can function reasonably well by avoiding activities that precipitate symptoms. Patients who develop muscle breakdown with myoglobinuria during the course of a typical attack need close observation and treatment to prevent possible renal failure caused by tubular necrosis. Massive muscle necrosis with swelling can cause a compartment syndrome. The necrotic muscle may sequester calcium with subsequent hypocalcemia, which, in combination with hyperkalemia (from myoglobinuria-precipitated renal failure), can cause life-threatening cardiac arrhythmias.

The present patient was initially switched to a high-protein diet that produced weight gain but no significant relief of symptoms. He was doing relatively well by avoiding activities that might precipitate his symptoms. Unfortunately, one day, after carrying a computer monitor to the parking lot he developed excruciating pain in his left forearm. Upon presentation to the local emergency room he was found to have myoglobinuria and a very high creatine kinase level, presumably caused by severe muscle fiber necrosis in the forearm flexors. He developed an acute compartment syndrome in the left forearm and underwent emergent surgical treatment. On a follow-up visit 3 months later, he had mild residual weakness of the left wrist flexors.

Clinical Pearls

1. Patients suffering from metabolic muscle disorders may develop episodes of life-threatening myoglobinuria.

2. The forearm exercise test is a useful diagnostic test in patients with suspected defects in the glycogenolytic or glycolytic pathways, but may be hazardous if performed under ischemic conditions.

3. The diagnosis of McArdle's disease can be established by DNA analysis from leukocytes in more than 90% of patients.

4. Histochemical stain for myophosphorylase activity should be performed in all patients who undergo muscle biopsy for evaluation of recurrent episodes of exercise-induced myalgias and cramps, especially those with history of myoglobinuria or elevated creatine kinase.

5. Education about avoidance of activities leading to development of typical symptoms is important in management of patients with McArdle's disease.

REFERENCES

1. Braakhekke JP, de Bruin MI, Stegeman, et al: The second wind phenomenon in McArdle's disease. Brain 1986; 109:1087–1101.
2. El-Schahawi M, Tsujino S, Shanske S, et al: Diagnosis of McArdle's disease by molecular genetic analysis of blood. Neurology 1996; 47:579–580.
3. Kushner RF, Berman SA: Are high-protein diets effective in McArdle's disease? Arch Neurol 1990; 47:383–384.
4. Meinck HM, Goebel HH, Rumpf KW, et al: The forearm ischaemic test—hazardous to McArdle patients. J Neurol Neurosurg Psychiatry 1982; 45:1144–1146.
5. Servidei S, Shanske S, Zeviani M, et al: McArdle's disease: Biochemical and molecular genetic studies. Ann Neurol 1988; 24:774–781.

PATIENT 32

A 19-year-old man with acute unilateral neck and shoulder pain after sneezing

A 19-year-old man developed sudden, severe right-sided neck pain after sneezing. The pain radiated to the right shoulder and occipital head region and subsided within a few days, but recurred any time he coughed, sneezed, or engaged in more strenuous activities involving the use of upper extremities. Three weeks later he noticed numbness and tingling affecting his right cheek and the right side of his neck. He was treated for a "pinched" nerve with anti-inflammatory medications and physical therapy, but his sensory symptoms persisted and he was referred for neurologic consultation. He denied any leg weakness or numbness or difficulty with bowel or bladder function. Over the past couple of years he complained of frequent headaches, most of which would start in occipital head region and later become diffuse. Medical and family histories were noncontributory.

Physical Examination: Vital signs: normal. HEENT: head normocephalic, skull nontender; neck nontender, supple, no bruits. Spine: no deformity, nontender, good range of motion. Mental status and speech: normal. Cranial nerves: mildly decreased sensation to pain on the lower aspect of his right cheek, otherwise unremarkable. Motor examination: normal muscle bulk, tone, and strength. Sensory examination: diminished pain and temperature sensation over the neck and upper extremities involving the C3–T2 dermatomes bilaterally, with preserved vibration and proprioception; no significant abnormality on sensory examination below approximately T2 level. Muscle stretch reflexes: normal. Plantar reflexes: flexor. Coordination and gait: normal.

Stop and Consider: What type of a lesion could explain his sensory symptoms and the bilateral symmetric segmental loss of pain and temperature sensation?

Laboratory Findings: CBC and chemistry: normal. Cervical spine MRI: see figure.

Question: What is the abnormality revealed by the MRI? Does it explain the findings from neurologic examination?

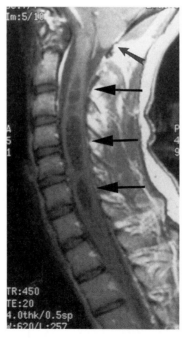

Diagnosis: Syringomyelia associated with Chiari type I malformation

Discussion: The bilateral "dissociated" sensory deficit (loss of pain and temperature sensation with preservation of vibration and position sensation) within the cervical dermatomes indicated a lesion affecting the central structures of the cervical cord. In this patient only the spinothalamic tract function was affected (pain and temperature sensation), whereas the dorsal column function (proprioception and vibration) was intact. This type of dissociated sensory loss is common in central spinal cord lesions, because these two tracts are widely separated and the axons that form the lateral spinothalamic tract decussate in the central cord anterior to the central canal. The patient's facial sensory abnormalities could also be explained by an intrinsic upper cervical cord lesion, since the fibers carrying pain and temperature sensations from the face descend to the cervical spine in the spinal tract of the fifth nerve to terminate on the spinal nucleus of the trigeminal nerve. The differential diagnosis of a patient with these neurologic deficits includes structural lesions affecting the central cord region, such as syringomyelia, neoplasm, and arteriovenous malformation. Demyelinating lesions are usually not associated with severe pain, as in the present patient. The MRI of the cervical spine showed a large syrinx within the spinal cord beginning at the level of C1–2 and extending caudally to at least the level of T3. The cerebellar tonsils extend below the foramen magnum, which indicates a Chiari type I malformation (arrow).

Syringomyelia is a chronic condition characterized by cystic cavitation (syrinx) of the spinal cord. If the cavitation extends to the brain stem, it is referred to as syringobulbia. The syrinx is typically filled with clear, low-protein-content fluid, similar to the cerebrospinal fluid (CSF). If the syrinx is related to a tumor, trauma, vascular malformations, or inflammatory processes, it may be filled with dense proteinaceous fluid. Syringomyelia may be associated with a variety of conditions, most frequently with Chiari malformations or other developmental hindbrain abnormalities, spinal cord tumors, trauma, cord ischemia, or some inflammatory processes. In many cases no coexisting conditions are identified. The most common type of syringomyelia is a cervical cystic cord lesion occurring in association with a Chiari I malformation. Based on pathologic studies, three major types of cavities are identified in non-neoplastic syringomyelia: (1) dilatations of the central canal that communicate directly with the fourth ventricle; (2) noncomunicating dilatations of the central canal that arise below the syrinx-free segment of the spinal cord; and (3) extracanalicular syrinxes that originate in the spinal cord parenchyma and do not communicate with the spinal canal.

The pathogenesis of syringomyelia is poorly understood and several different pathophysiologic mechanisms are likely to contribute to the formation of syrinx cavities. Syringomyelia with hindbrain malformations is probably related to the obstruction of the CSF flow at the foramen magnum. In syrinxes associated with Chiari type I malformation, the displaced cerebellar tonsils may prevent the normal flow pattern of the CSF across the foramen magnum, and increased pressure of the CSF may produce a caudally directed CSF flow that results in gradual growth of the cavity. Local tissue ischemia with impaired CSF absorption, or mechanical CSF flow obstruction may all contribute to syrinx formation in association with trauma.

The most common findings in syringomyelia are dissociated sensory loss, segmental lower motor neuron signs (muscle atrophy, fasciculations, weakness), and upper motor neuron signs below the level of the lesion. Sphincter disturbances, hyperhydrosis or anhydrosis, ataxia, and Horner's syndrome may also be observed. The clinical manifestation depends on the localization of the lesion. Syringomyelia is frequently associated with scoliosis. With medullary extension of the syrinx (syringobulbia) patients may complain of facial numbness, dysphagia, vertigo, or abnormal taste. Although symptoms of a syrinx are typically slowly progressive, a sudden onset or rapid deterioration of symptoms may occur. As in this case, some patients report onset or exacerbation of symptoms with cough or sneezing which may be related to a sudden rise in the intraspinal pressure secondary to the increased intrathoracic pressure.

MRI is the diagnostic test of choice for evaluation of suspected syringomyelia. Once the presence of a syrinx is detected, further evaluation should include MRI of the brain and craniovertebral junction to identify the associated anomalies. If syringomyelia occurs without a Chiari malformation or prior spinal cord injury, a complete spinal MRI with contrast should be done to rule out an intramedullary spinal cord tumor. Two-dimensional phase-contrast cine MRI has recently been employed in several centers to evaluate CSF motion during the cardiac cycle.[5]

Most patients with untreated syringomyelia will have a progressive course with worsening of neurologic disability. Different surgical treatments may improve symptoms in the short term, but many patients continue to experience long-term slow progression. The goal of surgical treatment is to correct the anatomic abnormality that interferes with normal CSF flow or drain the syrinx by a shunt to the subarachnoid space or the pleural or peritoneal cavity. Many patients with syringomyelia associated with Chiari I malformation have been successfully treated with decompression of the foramen magnum by suboccipital craniectomy, sometimes with removal of the C1 arch. This is usually combined with placement of the dural graft. Recent reports indicate that this surgical procedure may be effective in some patients without hindbrain malformations. Syringostomy or shunting of the cavity has also been preformed, but results have been unpredictable. The proper selection of a specific surgical procedure is controversial; better understanding of underlying pathogenesis in different forms of syringomyelia may lead to more effective surgical procedures.

The present patient was treated with suboccipital craniectomy and placement of the dural graft to decompress the foramen magnum. Within a few months he noted significant improvement of numbness and his headaches got markedly better. Follow-up MRI showed only a minimal, residual syrinx.

Clinical Pearls

1. Segmental dissociated sensory deficit with loss of pain and temperature sensation and preservation of touch, vibration, and position sensation is a sign of central cord lesions.
2. Syringomyelia is frequently associated with hindbrain malformations.
3. Acute presentations of cervical syringomyelia may mimic radiculopathy.
4. Childhood syringomyelia is frequently associated with scoliosis.
5. Some cases of syringomyelia can be successfully treated with surgical decompression of the posterior fossa.

REFERENCES

1. Iskandar BJ, Hedlund GL, Grabb PA, et al: The resolution of syringohydromyelia without hindbrain herniation after posterior fossa decompression. J Neurosurg 1998; 89:212–216.
2. Milhorat TH, Capocelli AL, Anzil AP, et al: Pathologic basis of spinal cord cavitation in syringomyelia: Analysis of 105 autopsy cases. J Neurosurg 1995; 82:802–812.
3. Oldfield EH, Muraszko K, Shawker TH, et al: Pathophysiology of syringomyelia associated with Chiari I malformation of the cerebellar tonsils. J Neurosurg 1994; 80:3–15.

PATIENT 33

A 73-year-old woman with a 1-year history of progressive weakness, numbness, and tingling in all limbs

A 73-year-old woman with an unremarkable medical history started experiencing burning pain in the left lower extremity 1 year prior to admission. Three months later she developed numbness and progressive incoordination of the right upper extremity. The numbness and tingling progressed to involve right lower extremity and right trunk, and over several weeks progressed to involve all four extremities. She denied facial sensory or motor symptoms, dizziness, dysphagia, visual difficulties, speech problems, or cognitive decline. She recently developed urinary incontinence, difficulty walking, and unsteady gait. She took no medications and denied recent head or neck trauma, or back pain.

Physical Examination: Temperature, respirations: normal; pulse 88 and regular; blood pressure 106/76. Skin, neck, cardiac, chest, and abdomen: normal. Mental status, affect, speech, and language: normal. Cranial nerves: normal. Jaw jerk: normal. Motor examination: normal muscle bulk, spasticity in the left upper extremity and both lower extremities, mild, bilateral, diffuse lower extremity weakness (grade +4). Sensory examination: decreased touch, pain, vibration, and joint position sensation below the clavicle level with the right trunk, right arm, and right leg more affected than on the left. Muscle stretch reflexes: hyperactive (grade +4) in all extremities, including brisk pectoralis reflexes with several beats of bilateral ankle clonus. Plantar reflexes: bilateral Babinski signs. Coordination: mild incoordination of right upper extremity and both lower extremities; no tremor. Gait: circumduction gait of the right foot with decreased arm swing bilaterally during ambulation. Romberg test: negative.

Stop and Consider: What is the time course and localization of neurologic dysfunction? What etiologies should be considered?

Laboratory Findings: CBC, coagulation profiles, chemistry, electrolytes, ESR: normal. Spine MRI with contrast: see figure.

Question: What abnormalities does the MRI show?

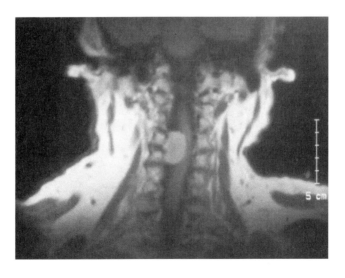

Diagnosis: Cervical cord (C3–4) meningioma

Discussion: The clinical presentation of this patient with chronic, progressive sensory and motor symptoms accompanied by evolving bladder dysfunction, signs of corticospinal tract involvement in all four extremities, without any symptoms and signs above the foramen magnum suggests a myelopathy. The absence of any brain stem or lower cranial nerve signs in the presence of spasticity and hyperactive reflexes in upper and lower extremities suggests an upper cervical or cervicomedullary junction lesion. With the slowly progressive time course the differential diagnosis includes neoplasms, cervical spondylosis, and other space-occupying lesions within the spinal canal. Cervical spine MRI revealed a contrast-enhancing extramedullary mass, consistent with a meningioma at the third and fourth cervical spinal levels anterior and to the right of the spinal cord, causing severe cord deformity (figure).

Tumors of the spinal cord are considerably less frequent than brain tumors. Typically, only 10–15% of primary tumors of the central nervous system are intraspinal. In addition, the majority of intraspinal tumors are benign and produce their effects mainly by compression of the spinal cord rather than by invasion of surrounding tissues. Neoplasms and other space-occupying lesions within the spinal canal can be divided into: (1) intraparenchymal tumors, which arise within the substance of the spinal cord and invade and destroy tracks and central gray structures, and (2) extramedullary tumors arising either in intradural structures, such as the leptomeninges and spinal roots, or extradural structures, such as vertebral bodies and epidural tissues. The most common extramedullary tumors are the meningiomas and neurofibromas, which together constitute at least 55% of all intraspinal neoplasms. Meningiomas are the most common intradural extramedullary tumors; over 80% of all spinal meningiomas occur in women.

Most spinal meningiomas that compress the spinal cord are found posteriorly or laterally and only 15–20% are anterior to the spinal cord. Spinal meningiomas may be associated with syringomyelia, which may appear with the development of the tumor or after its removal. In the cervical spinal cord region, as in this case, meningiomas are at least five times more prevalent than neurofibromas. Neurofibromas have a predilection for the thoracic spinal region, in contrast to meningiomas, which tend to be more evenly distributed along the spinal cord.

Patients with spinal cord tumors may present with a progressive myelopathy, with a painful radiculopathy and myelopathy, or with dissociated sensory syndrome when a central cord lesion is present. As in this case, the progressive sensory and motor symptoms and signs are typically caused by compression of the spinal tracts and less often by invasion and destruction of spinal cord structures. The onset of the compressive symptoms is typically gradual and the course is progressive over a period of weeks or months, but may rapidly progress to complete motor and sensory loss. The initial disturbance may be asymmetric in distribution. With cervical spinal cord tumors, a common sequence of motor impairment is first the arm, followed by the ipsilateral leg, contralateral leg, and finally the remaining arm. Sensory symptoms may also present with an asymmetric distribution. Development of bladder and bowel dysfunction is an advanced sign and may coincide with leg paralysis. If the compression is rapidly relieved, a variable recovery of the neurologic deficit may occur, which is a strong reason to emphasize the importance of early diagnosis and intervention that can prevent development of quadriplegia or paraplegia.

Surgical resection of meningiomas is curative in most patients. The outcome depends largely on the neurologic deficit prior to surgery. Patients with tumors that cannot be completely resected should be followed with serial MRIs every 6 months and reoperated or irradiated if recurrence is demonstrated.

The present patient underwent successful decompressive laminectomy and excision of a benign meningioma at the C3–C4 spinal level. Nine years postoperatively she has no ongoing neurologic problems.

Clinical Pearls

1. Slowly progressive bilateral motor and sensory symptoms in the extremities should raise the possibility of a myelopathy and prompt a definitive diagnostic investigation.

2. Neurologic examination usually allows accurate localization of the spinal cord lesions, but imaging studies are necessary to define the etiology.

3. MRI with contrast is the diagnostic test of choice for evaluation of progressive symptoms and signs of myelopathy.

4. Meningiomas are the most frequent intradural extramedullary tumors.

5. Early diagnosis of spinal tumors is crucial, since the outcome depends predominantly on the severity of the neurologic deficit prior to surgery.

6. Patients with incompletely resected meningiomas should be followed with serial MRIs and reoperated or treated with radiation if tumor recurs.

REFERENCES

1. Schutta HS: Spinal tumors. In Joynt RJ (ed): Clinical Neurology. Philadelphia, JB Lippincott, 1995, pp 1–175.
2. Woolsey RM, Young RR: The clinical diagnosis of disorders of the spinal cord. Neurol Clin 1991; 9:573–583.

PATIENT 34

A 68-year-old man with recurring episodes of lightheadedness, dizziness, visual distortions, and a "burring" sound in the right ear

A 68-year-old man with a history of atrial fibrillation and hyperlipidemia presented because of recurring episodes of sudden lightheadedness, dizziness, associated "black specks" in his vision, and a strange "burring" sound in his right ear. The spells lasted 1–2 minutes, were not associated with any alteration of consciousness, but were followed by fatigue lasting for about half an hour. The episodes occurred once or twice per month for 5 months prior to evaluation. In the 2 weeks prior to neurologic consultation the events had increased to 1–3 per day. There were no associated or precipitating factors for these events. With the most recent events he complained of difficulty with balance, veering to the right while walking, and feeling like he was going to "black-out during the spell." Review of his neurologic system was otherwise unremarkable.

Physical Examination: Temperature, respirations: normal; pulse 56 and irregularly irregular; blood pressure 130/92. Skin, cardiac, chest, and abdomen: normal. Neck: supple, no bruits. Mental status, affect, speech, and language: normal. Cranial nerves: normal fundi, visual fields, and gaze; normal pupillary reflexes; facial expressions normal and symmetric; normal facial sensation; oral and pharyngeal structures midline; Nylén-Bárány maneuver: negative. Motor examination: normal muscle tone, mass, and power. Sensory examination: normal. Muscle stretch reflexes: grade 2 and symmetric. Coordination: normal, no tremor. Plantar reflexes: flexor. Gait: normal.

Stop and Consider: What is the most likely classification of the patient's recurrent spells? What conditions should be considered in the differential diagnosis?

Laboratory Findings: CBC, ESR, platelet count, PT, PTT, electrolytes, chemistry: normal. EKG: atrial fibrillation. Head MRI: normal. Carotid/vertebral Doppler ultrasound: no hemodynamically significant stenosis in the internal carotid arteries, the left vertebral artery non-visualized or occluded. Head magnetic resonance angiogram (MRA): see figure.

Question: What abnormalities does the head MRA show? Can they explain the patient's symptoms?

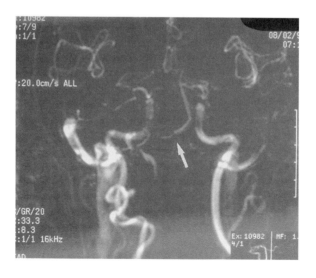

Diagnosis: Transient ischemic attacks secondary to vertebrobasilar insufficiency associated with severe occlusive disease of the vertebrobasilar circulation

Discussion: The clinical presentation of this patient with recurring brief events of lightheadedness, dizziness, gait ataxia, and visual and auditory distortions suggests a process within the posterior fossa structures (brain stem, cerebellum), with probable coexisting dysfunction of the occipital cortex (visual pathways). The most likely explanation is transient ischemic attacks (TIAs) secondary to the vertebrobasilar insufficiency. The differential diagnosis of episodes of transient neurologic dysfunction should also include focal epileptic seizures, complicated migraine, transient deficits caused by tumors or subdural hematoma, demyelinating disorders, or possible vestibulopathy. Metabolic conditions can also present with focal neurologic signs (e.g., hypoglycemia). Head MRA provided support for the suspected diagnosis by showing severe occlusive disease of the right intracranial vertebral artery (arrow), occlusion of the left vertebral artery, and slow flow through the basilar artery system. Atrial fibrillation was also a major risk factor for TIAs or ischemic stroke.

The diagnosis of a TIA is based on a careful clinical history. By definition, a TIA is a transient episode of focal, neurologic dysfunction caused by a reversible interference of blood flow to a specific area of the brain or the retina. The vast majority of TIAs resolve within 1 hour, with a median duration of 14 minutes in the carotid distribution and 8 minutes in the vertebrobasilar distribution. However, only 14% of TIAs lasting longer than 1 hour will resolve within 24 hours. If the initiation or resolution of transient symptoms is indistinct, the diagnosis of TIA should be questioned. Onset of a TIA is usually abrupt and typically unprovoked. The TIA symptoms are "negative" phenomena, such as loss of muscle power, vision, speech, or sensation in a focal pattern, which implies a vascular distribution. It is important to differentiate the anterior circulation TIAs (carotid TIAs) and the posterior circulation TIAs (vertebrobasilar insufficiency). Symptoms that are suggestive of vertebrobasilar insufficiency include: (1) bilateral or alternating motor weakness, clumsiness, or paralysis; (2) ataxia; (3) bilateral or alternating numbness or loss of sensation; (4) dysarthria; (5) diplopia or bilateral visual field disturbance; and (6) combinations of the above symptoms.

Artery-to-artery embolization of atherosclerotic plaque debris or plaque thrombi is thought to be the mechanism in 80% of carotid and 50% of vertebrobasilar TIAs. Local hypoperfusion is implicated in 20% of carotid and 50% of vertebrobasilar TIAs. A TIA caused by hypoperfusion requires hemodynamically compromised cerebral circulation or a precipitating factor, such as position change, orthostatic hypotension, or cardiac dysrhythmia. Atherothrombotic occlusive disease of the large intracranial and extracranial cerebral arteries is the most frequent cause of TIAs. Cardiac embolism is the next most common cause of TIAs. TIAs occur before 20–50% of atherothrombotic large vessel ischemic strokes, but before only 11–30% of cardioembolic strokes and 11–14% of small, deep strokes. The carotid TIAs often lead to brain infarction after just a single or a few events, while vertebrobasilar insufficiency events may be numerous and do not necessarily progress to infarction.

A TIA is a potentially serious symptom of impending cerebral infarction and demands rapid and thorough diagnostic evaluation to identify treatable conditions and prevent stroke. Patients with TIAs should undergo rapid, thorough evaluation, including brain imaging, blood tests, cardiac evaluation, and noninvasive vascular studies, such as ultrasound and MRA. If a surgically correctable lesion is suspected, a conventional angiogram may also be necessary. Treatment paradigms should be based on the TIA mechanism, location, and severity of the vascular occlusive disease. Most patients with TIAs caused by atherosclerotic disease of the vertebral or basilar arteries are initially treated with antiplatelet agents. Anticoagulation may also be considered, but may be hazardous, especially in elderly patients whose symptoms include ataxia or falls. Rare patients with severe, symptomatic vertebral artery stenosis who fail medical therapy may be candidates for angioplasty, although this treatment is still investigational.

The present patient was anticoagulated with warfarin (INR 2.5–3.0) and in 3 years of follow-up has remained asymptomatic with anticoagulation. His atrial fibrillation did not require treatment and he remained in a stable hemodynamic status. Possible cardiac emboli were not regarded as likely cause of the TIAs. Hypoperfusion episodes secondary to cardiac dysrhythmia were also very unlikely since his heart rate and blood pressure were unchanged during one witnessed event. Embolization from the right intracranial vertebral artery lesion and flow compromise caused by hemodynamically significant stenosis in the vertebrobasilar system were thought to be the pathomechanism of his TIAs.

Clinical Pearls

1. All patients with suspected TIAs require prompt diagnostic evaluation with adequate neuroimaging studies and identification of correctable stroke risk factors.

2. Intra-arterial embolization is the most common cause of posterior circulation ischemia. The most frequent sources of emboli are atherosclerotic lesions of the extracranial vertebral arteries, occlusive lesions of the intracranial vertebral arteries, or vertebral artery dissections.

3. In patients with posterior circulation TIAs and with minor atherosclerotic disease of vertebral or basilar arteries, antiplatelet agents are typically used. In cases with severe, hemodynamically significant stenosis, warfarin therapy may be used.

REFERENCES

1. Ausman JI, Schrontz CE, Pearce JE, et al: Vertebrobasilar insufficiency: A review. Arch Neurol 1985; 42:803–808.
2. Caplan LR: Vertebrobasilar disease: Time for a new strategy. Stroke 1981; 12:111–114.
3. Culebras A, Kase CS, Masdeau JC, et al: Practice guidelines for the use of imaging in transient ischemic attacks and acute stroke: A report of the Stroke Council, American Heart Association. Stroke 1997; 28:1480–1497.
4. Feinberg WM: Guidelines for the management of transient ischemic attacks: Ad Hoc Committee on Guidelines for the Management of Transient Ischemic Attacks of the Stroke Council, American Heart Association. Heart Disease Stroke 1994; 3:275–283.

PATIENT 35

A 19-year-old man with abrupt loss of consciousness following a lucid interval after a car accident

A 19-year-old man with an unremarkable medical history was involved in a motor vehicle accident. He was seated as a passenger in the front seat of the car and was thrown from the vehicle while it traveled at approximately 20 mph. The patient was unconscious when found, and was taken to a local emergency room where he regained alertness. Within 1 hour he became progressively lethargic and lapsed into coma. He was intubated, placed on a respirator, and transported via air ambulance to the local trauma center for further care.

Physical Examination: Temperature: normal; pulse 60 and regular; blood pressure 110/70; respiratory rate controlled on ventilatory system. Skin, neck, cardiac, chest, abdomen: normal. HEENT: head markedly swollen in the left periauricular area. Mental status: unresponsive to verbal stimuli. Cranial nerves: bilateral papilledema; left pupil markedly larger than the right and nonreactive to light; left eye deviated laterally and downward, full ocular motility on the right with doll's-eye maneuver (elicited after a cervical spine fracture was ruled out); symmetric facial grimacing to painful stimuli. Motor examination: increased tone (spasticity) in left lower extremity, no spontaneous movements; decreased movements on the left as compared to the right in response to painful stimuli. Sensory examination: withdrawal reaction bilaterally to deep painful stimuli. Muscle stretch reflexes: increased in the left upper and bilateral lower extremities (grade 3) with bilateral ankle clonus. Plantar reflexes: bilateral Babinski signs.

Stop and Consider: What is the localization of the intracranial injury based on the focal neurologic findings in this patient?

Laboratory Findings: CBC, electrolytes, chemistry: normal. Blood alcohol level: 220 mg/100 ml. Head CT scan: see figures (*left*, pre-treatment; *right*, post-treatment).

Question: What abnormalities are apparent on the head CT?

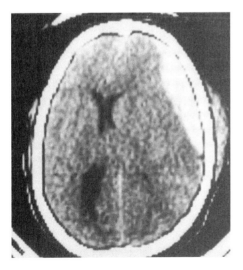 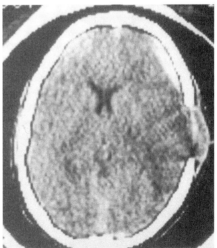

Diagnosis: Acute epidural hematoma compressing the left cerebral cortex, with brain displacement and transtentorial herniation syndrome

Discussion: The clinical presentation of this patient with altered mental status, bilateral papilledema, left third cranial nerve palsy, bilateral signs of corticospinal tract dysfunction, and cutaneous signs of head trauma are consistent with an acute mass lesion affecting the left cerebral hemisphere and temporal lobe-transtentorial herniation. Head CT (figure, *left*) confirmed the suspected diagnosis and revealed an acute epidural hematoma over the left cerebral hemisphere, accompanied by left-to-right shift of intracranial structures and an associated tissue swelling over the left scalp area.

Epidural hematoma (EH) occurs in 0.2–6% of patients with head trauma and is a life-threatening lesion. Early diagnosis allows rapid intervention, which is essential for successful outcome. Traffic accidents and falls account for most cases of EH. The EH is typically associated with skull fracture and laceration of meningeal vessels, diploic vessels, and dural sinuses. Bleeding from the middle meningeal artery is the cause of EH in over 50% of cases and approximately 30% of cases are caused by rupture of meningeal veins. Approximately 40% of cases are frontal or parietal, 50% are temporal, less than 10% are occipital, and approximately 3–13% are in the posterior fossa.

Approximately 40% patients with EH lose consciousness at the time of impact, but recover for a "lucid" interval progressing to obtundation and coma. Although the presentation with the lucid interval is the classic one, about 25% of EH patients are unconscious from the outset and do not regain consciousness; another 10% are awake despite the trauma and remain alert at the time of diagnosis. The larger the size of the hematoma, the higher the incidence of preoperative coma.

Complications of brain displacement and herniation are the major cause of death and acute neurologic deterioration. Expanding mass lesions produce pressure differences between intracranial compartments that shift intracranial tissues from compartments with higher pressure to compartments with lower pressures. Neurologic dysfunction produced by these shifts, which is often progressive and adds to the dysfunction produced by initial injury, is referred to as herniation syndrome. The three recognized herniation syndromes are temporal lobe–transtentorial herniation, subfacial herniation, and cerebellar–foramen magnum herniation. The present case is an example of the temporal lobe–transtentorial herniation. In this process the medial part of the temporal lobe (uncus and parahippocampal gyrus) is displaced contralaterally and caudally into the tentorial notch, which is adjacent to the third cranial nerve, the cerebral peduncle, midbrain, and the posterior cerebral artery.

The neurologic dysfunction and additional brain injury are related to compression of these structures against the relatively rigid tentorium. Compression of the third cranial nerve results in ipsilateral ptosis, pupillary dilation, and ophthalmoplegia. Compression of the ipsilateral cerebral peduncle produces contralateral hemiparesis. The signs of ipsilateral third nerve palsy and contralateral hemiparesis are classic manifestations of uncal herniation, but in many cases the pressure differences compress the contralateral peduncle, producing hemiparesis ipsilateral to the cerebral lesion—a "false localizing sign." Midbrain compression and ischemia from compression of the posterior cerebral artery may also contribute to the syndrome.

Age, location of the clot, and associated extracranial injuries influence the prognosis of EH. Posterior location of the hematoma and advanced age increase mortality and morbidity. Better neurologic status at the time of surgical intervention is associated with better outcome. Associated brain contusion, subdural hematoma, contralateral extradural hematoma, and diffuse brain swelling also occur in 30–50% of patients with EH and contribute to mortality and morbidity.

Cranial CT is the best diagnostic study for initial diagnosis of EH. Coexisting brain contusion or subdural hematoma is found in 24–76% of cases. In about 8% of cases an EH is not found on the initial head CT, but may become apparent on repeat CT with continuing deterioration of the neurologic dysfunction.

Acute extradural hematoma requires emergent neurosurgical intervention and management of elevated intracranial pressure. Rare patients with a small EH and no neurologic deficit may be managed conservatively and followed by frequent examinations and serial CT studies. Associated neurologic and systemic complications need to be recognized and treated aggressively. With rapid neurosurgical intervention 40–50% of patients can make a good recovery, 15–20% are moderately disabled, 7–10% are severely disabled, and the mortality is 10–30%. Availability of cranial head CT lowered the mortality rate to 0–5% in some series. Patients who have no focal neurologic signs can have a good recovery. Those who present with decerebration and decortication signs at the time of operation may still have a relatively good outcome, with moderate long-term disability in less than 50% of cases. Unfortunately, residual neurologic dysfunction after recovery from acute injury commonly includes impaired motor function, cognitive and neurobehavioral deficits, posttraumatic epilepsy, hydrocephalus, and chronic recurrent posttraumatic headache.

The present patient underwent emergent evacuation of the epidural hematoma (figure, *right*). He required prolonged hospitalization, but his neurologic recovery was relatively good. All signs of neurologic abnormality observed at the time of the acute injury resolved except for mild residual third nerve palsy.

Clinical Pearls

1. Acute epidural hemorrhage is usually caused by temporal or parietal skull fracture with laceration and hemorrhage from the middle meningeal artery and vein. Dural venous sinus lacerations contribute to the hemorrhage in some cases.

2. Rapid diagnosis and surgical treatment of epidural hematoma is the most important factor in preventing death and disability.

3. Outcome after head injury is improved by rapid evaluation, prompt surgical intervention, and aggressive management of increased intracranial pressure and its complications.

REFERENCES

1. Bricolo P, Pasut LM: Extradural hematoma. Toward zero mortality: A prospective study. Neurosurgery 1984; 14:8–12.
2. Cordobés F, Lobato RD, Rivas JJ, et al: Observations on 82 patients with extradural hematoma: Comparison of results before and after the advent of computerized tomography. J Neurosurg 1981; 54:179–186.
3. Katz DI, Alexander MP: Traumatic brain injury: Predicting course of recovery and outcome for patients admitted to rehabilitation. Arch Neurol 1994; 51:661–670.
4. Miller JD, Tocher JL, Jones PA: Extradural hematoma: Earlier detection, better results. Brain Inj 1988; 2:83–86.
5. Obana WG, Pitts LH: Management of head injury: Extracerebral lesions. Neurosurg Clin North Am 1991; 2:351–372.
6. Phonprasert C, Suwanwela C, Hongsaprabhas C, et al: Extradural hematoma: Analysis of 138 cases. J Trauma 1980; 20:679–683.

PATIENT 36

A 51-year-old woman with a chronic headache, memory decline, and a seizure

A 51-year-old woman presented with a long history of headaches that had increased in frequency and intensity during the previous 2 years. She was seen at the local emergency department for a recent episode of severe headache associated with a fall and loss of responsiveness for 10 minutes, which followed a similar episode of altered consciousness and transient left-sided weakness 6 months earlier. A head MRI taken at that time demonstrated ventriculomegaly and a small right pontine infarct, and an EEG showed occasional sharp-wave activity in the bitemporal region. She was placed on aspirin and phenytoin for a presumed partial complex seizure, but continued to have progressive headaches accompanied by episodes of confusion and altered responsiveness. She complained of unsteady gait, personality changes, particularly irritability, and poor attention, concentration, and short-term memory. Her medical and family history were otherwise unremarkable. She quit her real estate job 6 months earlier because of the headaches and memory problems. There was no history of alcohol or tobacco abuse.

Physical Examination: Vital signs, skin, HEENT, cardiac chest, abdomen: normal. Mental status: lethargic but easily aroused, oriented to person, place, and time; very poor attention and short-term memory. Speech: fluent, mild dysarthria. Cranial nerves: normal fundi, pupils 3 mm in diameter bilaterally and reactive to light and accommodation; extraocular movements full with mild, bilateral, end-gaze horizontal nystagmus. Motor and sensory examinations: normal. Coordination: slight dysmetria on finger-to-nose testing bilaterally. Muscle stretch reflexes: increased (grade 3) in all extremities. Plantar reflexes: Babinski signs bilaterally. Gait: wide-based, unsteady.

Stop and Consider: What systemic or neurologic conditions should be considered in a patient with chronic headache, seizures, bilateral corticospinal tract signs, and evidence of diffuse cortical dysfunction?

Laboratory Findings: CBC, chemistry including liver function tests, ANA, phenytoin: normal. ESR 58 mm/hr (0–25). Protein S, protein C, antithrombin III, angiotensin-1 CE: normal. Anticardiolipin antibodies: IgG 33 g/L (0–29); IgM negative. CSF studies: protein 244 mg/dl (15–45), glucose 8 mg/dl (8.7% of serum glucose level; normal 40–80%), WBC 60/μl with 95% lymphocytes. Repeated CSF study performed the next day: protein 210 mg/dl, glucose 19 mg/dl, WBC 33/μl. Gram stain: negative. Bacterial and fungal CSF cultures, cryptococcal antigen, VDRL, acid-fast bacilli, HSV 1 and 2, Lyme antibody, cytology: negative; fungal immunologic studies: *Blastomyces, Coccidioides:* negative; *Histoplasma:* yeast phase 1:16 (positive), mycelial phase < 1:8 (negative). Chest x-ray, gallium SPECT of the chest and abdomen, head MR angiogram: normal. Brain MRI: see figure.

Question: What is the relationship of the CSF abnormalities to the brain MRI findings?

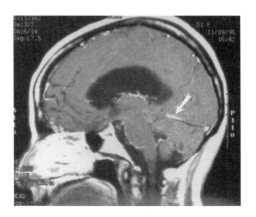

Diagnosis: CNS histoplasmosis with meningitis and hydrocephalus

Discussion: A slowly progressive encephalopathy with increasing headache, seizures, and cognitive impairment may be caused by systemic conditions or primary CNS disorders. Structural lesions such as tumor, subdural hematoma, sagittal sinus thrombosis, hydrocephalus, or brain abscess must initially be excluded by brain imaging, but pathologic conditions causing diffuse or multifocal abnormalities deserve primary consideration. Infectious conditions such as chronic meningoencephalitis should be evaluated by CSF examination after focal structural lesions are excluded by appropriate diagnostic studies. Meningeal or brain biopsy may be necessary in some cases. Immune-mediated processes that may cause multifocal or diffuse cerebral impairment, such as primary CNS vasculitis, lupus vasculitis or cerebritis, and Hashimoto's encephalopathy, may produce a similar clinical picture. Mitochondrial encephalopathies may present with cognitive decline, seizures, focal signs, and multisystem involvement. Carcinomatous meningitis, metabolic and toxic leukoencephalopathies associated with immunosuppressive agents (cyclosporine, tacrolimus), or encephalopathy associated with malignant hypertension should be considered in patients with these predisposing conditions.

In this patient, elevated CSF protein, markedly decreased glucose levels, and lymphocytic pleocytosis indicated chronic meningitis (CM). Low CSF glucose levels suggest the possibilities of tuberculous, fungal, or neoplastic meningitis or CNS sarcoidosis. The diagnosis of fungal meningitis was established on the basis of CSF immunologic studies. The MRI findings were also consistent with CM. There was marked enlargement of the lateral, third, and forth ventricles, indicative of communicating hydrocephalus and meningeal enhancement after gadolinium injection (arrow), consistent with a leptomeningeal process. The pontine infarct observed on prior brain MRI may have been caused by a local vasculitic process in the penetrating small pontine artery in the course of fungal infection.

CM is by convention defined as a meningoencephalitis with symptoms and associated CSF abnormalities persisting for more than 4 weeks. The differential diagnosis for CM is very broad and in many instances it may be difficult to establish an etiology even with extensive and repeated diagnostic evaluations. Headache, cognitive changes, focal neurologic deficits, and seizures are common, as illustrated by this case. Patients may also complain of chronic fevers, neck stiffness, and other nonspecific systemic symptoms caused by the infectious process.

The most common infectious agents causing CM are *Mycobacterium tuberculosis* and *Cryptococcus neoformans.* The most common noninfectious causes of CM are neoplastic meningitis, neurosarcoidosis, and vasculitis. The diagnostic evaluation of CM should include careful search for chronic systemic infection, including ophthalmologic and dermatologic examinations. Chest x-ray, PPD skin testing, blood, urine, and other fluid or tissue cultures, and abdominal and chest CT scans may be necessary. CSF examination is clearly a critical study and may need to be repeated if initial CSF examination is unrevealing. In addition to CSF protein, glucose, and cell count, CSF examination should include cytology, bacterial and fungal stains and cultures, antigen assays, and antibody titer (including viral) testing. Some infectious agents can be detected by PCR DNA analysis. Serial lumbar punctures with extensive CSF studies may be necessary to establish the diagnosis in some patients. Meningeal and brain biopsies should be considered if the etiology cannot be determined by other studies.

The mortality rate of CM depends on etiology, but can be as high as 27–35% in some series. Patients with an identified etiology who are treated may continue to suffer from severe neurologic disability. The mortality and morbidity is especially high in immunocompromised patients who are susceptible to systemic infections frequently associated with CM. Histoplasmosis is a rare cause of CM, especially in the absence of underlying immunosuppression. Meningitis occurs in 10–20% of patients with disseminated histoplasmosis, but CNS histoplasmosis may develop without evidence of systemic infection. CNS histoplasmosis may also present as a brain or spinal cord abscess. Patients with histoplasmal meningitis may have negative CSF and blood fungal cultures. Immunologic studies, as in this case, may significantly increase the diagnostic yield.

The standard therapy for histoplasmosis and other fungal meningitides is amphotericin B. A typical course of therapy is approximately 10 weeks, but longer courses may be necessary, especially in immunocompromised patients. Unfortunately, this drug has relatively poor blood–brain barrier penetration and relapses are common. A favorable response to therapy is indicated by decrease in CSF white blood cell count and protein, and an increase in CSF glucose.

The present patient received amphotericin B treatment and her improvement was relatively rapid and dramatic. At the 3-month follow-up visit her headaches completely resolved and the CSF abnormalities improved with the exception of persistently elevated CSF protein. She returned to full and successful management of her brokerage business.

Clinical Pearls

1. Chronic meningitis should be considered in patients with unexplained progressive headache, particularly in the presence of cognitive or behavioral changes and neurologic deficits.

2. The etiology of chronic meningitis can be difficult to identify and often necessitates repeated lumbar punctures and extensive CSF studies.

3. Brain and meningeal biopsy should be considered in cases of undiagnosed chronic meningitis or possible vasculitis if repeated CSF studies are unrevealing.

4. Brain MRI with gadolinium contrast for demonstration of leptomeningeal enhancement can be a valuable tool in confirming the chronic meningitis, but it does not identify a specific etiology.

REFERENCES

1. Cheng TM, O'Neill BP, Scheithauer BW, et al: Chronic meningitis: The role of meningeal or cortical biopsy. Neurosurgery 1994; 34:590–595.
2. Coyle P: Chronic meningitis. In Feldman E (ed): Current Diagnosis in Neurology. St Louis, Mosby-Year Book, 1994, pp 101–106.
3. Plouffe JF, Fass RJ: *Histoplasma* meningitis: Diagnostic value of cerebrospinal fluid serology. Ann Intern Med 1980; 92:189–191.
4. Wheat LJ, Batteiger BE, Sathapatayavongs B: *Histoplasma capsulatum* infections of the central nervous system: A clinical review. Medicine 1990; 69:244–260.
5. Smith JE, Aksamit AJ Jr: Outcome of chronic idiopathic meningitis. Mayo Clin Proc 1994; 69:548–556.
6. Zalduondo FM, Provenzale JM, Hulette C, et al: Meningitis, vasculitis, and cerebritis caused by CNS histoplasmosis: Radiologic-pathologic correlation. Am J Roentgenol 1996; 166:194–196.

PATIENT 37

A 68-year-old man with cognitive decline, gait difficulty, and myoclonus

A 68-year-old retired man was referred for evaluation of progressive difficulty with ambulation and balance and frequent falls of several weeks' duration. The initial symptoms were rapidly followed by impairment of fine motor skills and slurred speech. His wife initially observed sudden, jerky movements in his upper extremities while he was falling asleep, but later the movements were also observed when he was awake. She also reported that he had increasing difficulty with memory and had urinary incontinence on several occasions. He had a 10-year history of hypertension and 3-year history of diabetes mellitus type II treated with oral agents. There was no history of alcohol or drug abuse, or significant exposure to environmental or industrial toxins. His only prescription medications were those for treatment of hypertension and diabetes. His family history was noncontributory.

Physical Examination: Vital signs: normal. Cardiac: normal. Mental status: severe difficulty performing calculations, severe impairment of short-term memory and visual-spatial skills. Speech: mild dysarthria but no aphasia. Cranial nerves: normal except for irregular eye pursuit movements. Motor examination: paratonia in all limbs, normal bulk and strength, no fasciculations, rare myoclonic jerks in upper extremities. Sensory examination: normal. Muscle stretch reflexes: normal. Plantar reflexes: bilateral Babinski signs. Coordination: mild, bilateral dysmetria and dysdiadochokinesia in both upper extremities. Gait: wide-based, inability to perform tandem gait testing. Romberg test: negative.

Stop and Consider: What is the differential diagnosis of a rapidly progressive cognitive decline associated with myoclonus and multifocal neurologic findings involving the cerebral cortex, cerebellum, and corticospinal tracts?

Laboratory Findings: CBC, renal and liver function tests, fasting glucose, electrolytes, vitamin B_{12}, folate, thyroid function tests: normal. VDRL, Lyme titer, ANA, rheumatoid factor anti-Hu antibodies: negative. Head MRI and cerebral angiogram: normal. Cerebrospinal fluid (CSF): normal protein, glucose, cell count, and IgG index. CSF bacterial and fungal cultures and viral encephalitis panel: negative. Positron emission tomography (PET) of the brain: hypometabolism in bilateral frontal lobe, temporal lobe, left parietal lobe, caudate, thalamus, and putamen. EEG: occasional bifrontal and bitemporal low-amplitude theta slowing during wakefulness. No epileptiform abnormalities or periodic discharges were observed.

Hospital Course: The patient's condition rapidly deteriorated and he died several months later. Brain autopsy: see figure.

Question: What abnormality was demonstrated on brain autopsy?

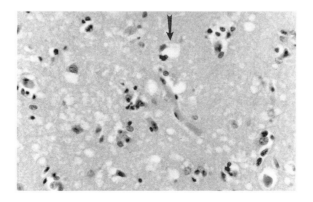

Diagnosis: Spongiform encephalopathy consistent with Creutzfeldt-Jakob disease (CJD)

Discussion: This patient presented with neurologic symptoms and signs indicative of multifocal CNS pathology, including diffuse bilateral cortical dysfunction, bilateral cerebellar involvement, and corticospinal tract involvement. Rapidly progressive dementia with focal neurologic signs may be caused by a variety of pathologic processes. Normal-pressure hydrocephalus may present with dementia, ataxia, and incontinence and in this patient was ruled out by negative brain MRI that also excluded structural lesions such as tumor, subdural hematoma, or brain infarction. There was no evidence for CNS vasculitis on the cerebral angiogram or MRI. Laboratory studies, including CSF examinations, showed no evidence of infectious or inflammatory conditions. The diagnostic evaluation did not reveal any metabolic, toxic, or endocrine abnormalities. A paraneoplastic syndrome was considered, but anti-Hu antibodies were not detected and there was no evidence of a neoplasm. Because of the rapidly progressive dementia associated with myoclonus, Creutzfeldt-Jakob disease (CJD) was strongly suspected. EEG did not demonstrate the typical finding of periodic discharges, which may be absent in some patients with CJD in early stages of the disease. The autopsy showed spongiform changes (arrow) in the cerebral and cerebellar cortex and the basal ganglia, which are characteristic of CJD.

CJD is a relatively uncommon neurodegenerative disorder that may present as a sporadic, genetic, or infectious illness. The pathogenesis of prion diseases is not fully understood, but according to the prion hypothesis these conditions are caused by an abnormal conformation of a naturally occurring prion protein (PrP^c) into a protease-resistant protein (PrP^{res}). The annual incidence is estimated at approximately one per million population. The genetic forms of CJD are caused by mutations in the prion protein gene (*PRPN*) located on the short arm of chromosome 20. About a dozen different mutations in the *PRPN* gene have been reported in association with familial CJD and there is significant clinical heterogeneity among individuals harboring the same mutation. The well-documented cases of human-to-human transmission of CJD have been related to exposure to infected CNS tissue during surgical or pathologic procedures (e.g., contaminated dura grafts or preparations of pituitary hormones). The possibility of bovine spongiform encephalopathy transmission to humans, causing a variant of CJD, is still controversial.

The average age at the time of onset is 60 years in sporadic cases, but the variants of the disease may affect teenagers and individuals older than 80 years.

The median duration of illness is approximately 4 months, but some familial cases have a longer course. The onset of the illness in the majority of patients is insidious, with rapid progression in weeks or months after the initial symptoms. Some patients experience a very rapid progressive course or sudden onset.

About one third of patients initially present with subtle behavioral changes followed by rapid cognitive decline, memory loss, and confusion. Another third of the patients present with focal abnormalities, such as gait ataxia, poor coordination, and disturbance of oculomotor or visual systems. The remaining third present with a combination of cognitive and focal abnormalities. Cases with rapid onset of hemiparesis or aphasia may initially be regarded as possible strokes. Many patients develop parkinsonian features, especially of hypokinetic-rigid type. About 25% of the patients describe nonspecific symptoms, such as asthenia, anxiety, and altered sleeping or eating patterns in the weeks before the onset of cognitive or focal abnormalities. Myoclonic seizures typically develop in advanced stages of the disease.

In the early stages the diagnosis of CJD may be difficult, but with rapid progression of multifocal signs and symptoms, dementia, and development of myoclonus, the evolving clinical picture is highly suggestive of CJD. Head CT may reveal diffuse cortical atrophy at the late stage of CJD, and brain MRI may be normal or show increased signal intensity on T2 weighted images in the basal ganglia, thalamus, and the cerebral cortex. The diagnostic yield of CSF examination usually is not very high. Some patients may have mild elevation of CSF protein, but radioimmunoassay for abnormal protein fraction termed 14-3-3, which was initially thought to be a marker of prion diseases, has also been reported in other CNS conditions. Positron emission tomography (PET) may be more sensitive than MRI, but is nonspecific. A characteristic but nonspecific EEG finding are periodic discharges consisting of approximately 1 cycle/sec biphasic or triphasic complexes, which may be unilateral or bilateral. In a patient with dementia, myoclonus, and periodic discharges, CJD should be strongly suspected.

The diagnosis of CJD can be conclusively established by pathologic examination of biopsy or autopsy of brain tissue. The brain exhibits spongiform encephalopathy with widespread neuronal loss and gliosis. Immunocytochemical staining or Western blot analysis for PrP^{res} are the most specific methods to establish the diagnosis.

Gerstmann-Sträussler-Scheinker (GSS) disease may resemble CJD, but the initial presenting symptom is usually cerebellar ataxia followed by cognitive decline and pyramidal signs. The clinical course of GSS disease is typically longer than that of CJD. All cases of GSS disease are associated with *PRPN* gene mutations. Patients suffering from fatal familial insomnia (FFI) have marked sleep abnormalities and develop dysautonomic symptoms, followed by ataxia, myoclonus, dysarthria, dysphagia, and cognitive decline. The main pathologic features of FFI are severe neuronal degeneration of thalamic nuclei with gliosis, but spongiform changes, in contrast to CJD, are typically not observed. Kuru is a prion disease transmitted by ritualistic cannibalism. In addition to cerebellar ataxia, spasticity, and extrapyramidal signs, patients may display exaggerated startle response and eventually develop severe, progressive cognitive decline.

In the present patient, as in all patients with prion diseases, management consisted of symptomatic treatment and supportive measures.

Clinical Pearls

1. Prion diseases should be suspected in patients with rapidly progressive dementia and focal neurologic abnormalities.

2. Aphasia, hemiparesis, ataxia, or visual loss may be presenting signs of CJD before dementia and myoclonus develop.

3. In cases of suspected CJD, a history of corneal transplants, growth hormone treatment, or neurosurgical procedures should be elicited since the incubation period of CJD can be several decades.

4. A definitive diagnosis of CJD can be made by brain tissue analysis for PrP[res] and associated spongiform degeneration.

REFERENCES

1. Brown P: The risk of bovine spongiform encephalopathy ("mad cow disease") to human health. JAMA 1997; 228:1008–1011.
2. Castellani RJ, Parchi P, Madoff L, et al: Biopsy diagnosis of Creutzfeldt-Jakob disease by Western blot: A case report. Hum Pathol 1997; 28:623–626.
3. Hsich G, Kenney K, Gibbs CJ, et al: The 14-3-3 brain protein in the cerebrospinal fluid as a marker for transmissible spongiform encephalopathies. N Engl J Med 1996; 335:924–930.
4. Kascsak RJ, Fersko R, Pulgiano D, et al: Immunodiagnosis of prion disease. Immunol Invest 1997; 26:259–268.
5. Korczyn AD: Prion diseases. Curr Opin Neurol 1997; 10:273–281.
6. Prusiner SB: Prion diseases and the BSE crisis. Science 1997; 278:245–251.

PATIENT 38

A 27-year-old woman with chronic pain and hyperalgesia following hand trauma

A 27-year-old right-handed woman presented for evaluation of chronic, excruciating pain in her right upper extremity. A year earlier she had fallen on the ice and hyperextended her right hand. She immediately experienced severe pain and paresthesias in her hand and wrist. X-rays of her hand, wrist, and forearm taken at the local emergency department were normal. Her pain persisted and worsened over the next several months. Nerve conduction study and needle electromyography (NCS/EMG) was performed a few months later and showed a mild median neuropathy of the wrist (carpal tunnel syndrome). After 3 months the patient had carpal tunnel release surgery without any improvement of her symptoms. The burning pain became progressively worse and spread to her forearm and arm. In addition to the pain, she developed swelling, increased temperature, and hyperemia in the affected extremity. She complained of depression and difficulty sleeping. At the time of her neurologic evaluation she rated her pain as 8 on a scale of 0–10.

Physical Examination: Vital signs: normal. Skin: warm to touch, the right arm skin temperature 3°C higher than the left; edema and hyperemia of right upper extremity. Mental status, speech, and cranial nerves: normal. Motor examination: marked dystonic posturing of the right hand and fingers (see figure), strength normal except for mild weakness (+4/5) in the right arm and hand. Sensory examination: marked allodynia and hyperalgesia in right forearm and dorsum of the hand. The sensory exam of the palmar aspect of the hand revealed hyperpathia (with pin stimulation at first she reported decreased sensation but after a few seconds reported severe pain). Muscle stretch reflexes: normal and symmetric. Coordination and gait: normal except for decreased motions of right upper extremity.

Stop and Consider: What is the differential diagnosis of the painful condition in this patient?

Laboratory Findings: CBC, chemistry, ESR, rheumatoid factor, ANA, EKG: normal. Quantitative sensory testing: increased vibratory and thermal thresholds in the right upper extremity. Somatosensory evoked potentials: normal for both median and posterior tibial nerve stimulations. Head and cervical spine MRIs: normal.

Question: What other diagnostic tests might be useful in evaluation of this patient's condition?

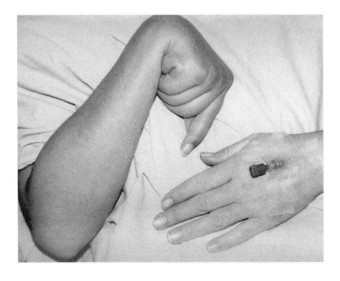

Diagnosis: Complex regional pain syndrome (CRPS) type I, previously also known as reflex sympathetic dystrophy (RSD)

Discussion: With persistent pain after trauma, skeletal or soft tissue injury and infection should be excluded. In this patient, imaging and other laboratory studies excluded the possibility of an unrecognized fracture or soft tissue injury. Radiculopathy was excluded by normal cervical spine MRI study and needle EMG. The distribution of the symptoms did not conform to a single dermatome or nerve pattern. The NCS/EMG showed mild median neuropathy at the wrist, but carpal tunnel release did not improve her pain. There was no evidence for any rheumatologic conditions. The pattern of evolution and distribution of the pain, as well as other features of vasomotor autonomic abnormalities on physical examination were consistent with a complex regional pain syndrome type I (CRPS I), also known as reflex sympathetic dystrophy (RSD).

CRPS I/RSD is a neuropathic pain syndrome that typically develops after an initial traumatic event. The pain is not limited to the distribution of a single peripheral nerve and is often disproportionate to the inciting event. The typical pain in CRPS develops within a few days to 3 months after the initial injury. This syndrome is closely related to causalgia (also known as CRPS type II), which develops after a well-defined peripheral nerve injury. In cases of CRPS I there is typically no evidence of a major nerve injury, but the clinical presentation is very similar to that of CRPS II.

The initial precipitating injury in more than 50% of patients who develop CRPS I is a fracture requiring immobilization by casting. Predisposing injuries involving the wrist and ankle are common. In some cases this syndrome follows a seemingly benign soft tissue injury, and rare patients cannot identify any injury prior to development of CRPS.

The International Association for the Study of Pain (IASP) proposed four major diagnostic criteria for CRPS: (1) the presence of an initial noxious event, often requiring immobilization; (2) continuing pain, allodynia, or hyperalgesia disproportionate to the inciting event; (3) evidence of edema, altered skin blood flow, or abnormal sudomotor activity in the region of pain; and (4) absence of other conditions that could cause pain and dysfunction. The last three criteria are required to make a diagnosis of CRPS.

The chronic and excruciating pain and associated sensory phenomena (numbness, dysesthesia, paresthesia, paroxysms of pain, allodynia, hyperalgesia, and hyperpathia), dominate the clinical picture of CRPS. Most patients develop motor impairment (weakness, dystonia, tremor, or dyskinesia) and autonomic abnormalities (edema, sudomotor, and thermoregulatory dysfunction).

Symptoms and signs of CRPS can evolve through several stages. Stage I is characterized by acute injury and may develop within a few hours to a few days from the initial injury. The pain is excruciating and diffuse, but most severe in the distal aspects of the extremity. It is exacerbated by motion, physical activity, change in temperature, or stress. Hyperalgesia and allodynia are frequently reported by patients. This stage of CRPS is usually associated with significant sympathetic component and in some patients symptoms may be at least transiently improved with sympathetic blocks. In this stage, which may last up to 6 months, the extremity is usually hyperthermic and hyperemic. In stage II, sometimes referred to as dystrophic stage, which may last from a few months to up to a few years, the pain may spread and is usually associated with sleep disruption and reactive depression. The affected extremity frequently becomes moist, hyperhydrotic, and cool, with associated trophic changes and skin discoloration. Bone x-rays frequently reveal cystic or subchondral erosion or early Sudeck's atrophy. In stage III the pain spreads proximally, and in some patients it may spread to the opposite limb. Patients may develop severe muscle spasms, tremors, and dystonic posturing, with the most severe hyperalgesia and allodynia. In this stage of the disease the sympathetic blocks are typically ineffective. Many patients in this stage have an abnormal bone scan.

The diagnosis of CRPS is based on the constellation of clinical symptoms and signs and depends on exclusion of other processes that may cause chronic pain. Differential diagnosis includes localized nerve pathology, such as entrapment or inflammation, rheumatologic conditions, such as infectious or inflammatory arthritis, or chronic musculoskeletal injuries. Bone scan and x-rays are not diagnostic but can be used to further delineate diagnostic possibilities. Relief by sympathetic nerve blocks supports the diagnosis, but failure to improve does not exclude the diagnosis of CRPS.

The etiology of CRPS is unknown and currently several different pathomechanisms have been postulated. Dysfunction of the sympathetic nervous system has been regarded as a major component of this syndrome but it now appears that the sympathetic system is just one component of the pathophysiology. Sympathectomies have been performed but typically do not produce long-lasting effects and some experts believe that they are contraindicated, since any surgical intervention in patients with CRPS may aggravate the pain.

The goal of therapy for CRPS is restitution of normal functional status and pain relief. Pain relief may be obtained by empirical trials of analgesics and adjuvant CNS-active medications, including tricyclic antidepressants and antiepileptics. Opioids are frequently required. Once satisfactory analgesia is achieved, rehabilitation therapy should be initiated. Psychological support, treatment of depression, and, if necessary, social assistance should be provided at the beginning of therapy since all those factors influence the successful outcome.

The prognosis of CRPS is unpredictable. Most patients are able to achieve long-term pain relief and can be rehabilitated to a level of function that allows gainful employment. Unfortunately, many patients continue to suffer from pain and disability, and some have progression of pain and vasomotor abnormalities to extremities that were not involved in the initial injury.

The patient in this case received a series of stellate ganglion sympathetic blocks, which did not produce sustained pain relief. Physical therapy was compromised by severe pain that was exacerbated with any use of the right hand and arm. Carbamazepine, phenytoin, amitriptyline, and nortriptyline had no effect on her pain, but modest pain relief was achieved by slowly increasing doses of extended-release morphine that produced severe sedation and constipation. She was subsequently treated with continuous subcutaneous infusion of lidocaine and physical therapy and during a period of 6 weeks achieved good pain control and gradual recovery of function in her right hand and arm.

Clinical Pearls

1. Hyperalgesia and allodynia are strongly suggestive of CRPS/RSD in a patient with a recent history of trauma or surgery.

2. In some patients CRPS may develop after relatively minor injuries like sprains or skin bruises, but in rare patients it may develop without apparent precipitating injury.

3. Adequate analgesia is usually required for successful physical therapy and rehabilitation.

4. Psychosocial management is important in the overall treatment plan of CRPS.

REFERENCES

1. Backonja M: Reflex sympathetic dystrophy (RSD)/sympathetically maintained pain/causalgia: The syndrome of neuropathic pain with dysautonomia. Semin Neurol 1994; 14:263–271.
2. Knobler KL: Reflex sympathetic dystrophy. In Johnson RT, Griffin JW (eds): Current Therapy in Neurologic Disease, 5th ed. St. Louis, Mosby-Year Book, 1997, pp 80–84.
3. Merskey H, Bogduk N: Classification of Chronic Pain, 2nd ed. Seattle, IASP Press, 1994.
4. Stanton-Hicks M, Janig W, Hassenbusch S, et al: Reflex sympathetic dystrophy: Changing concepts and taxonomy. Pain 1995; 63:127–133.
5. Wasner G, Backonja M, Baron R: Traumatic neuralgias: Complex regional pain syndromes (reflex sympathetic dystrophy and causalgia): Clinical characteristics, pathophysiologic mechanisms and therapy. Neurol Clin 1998; 16:851–868.

PATIENT 39

A 77-year-old woman with sudden speech difficulty

A 77-year-old right-handed woman was well until the day of admission, when her relatives noticed that she was very disconcerted during the telephone conversation. Her speech was confused and contained many repetitive sentences and phrases. When paramedics arrived at her apartment she was alert, but appeared confused, and was able to follow only simple commands. This was a sudden change as her family reported that she appeared completely normal the day before. She had no apparent weakness and walked without any difficulty. She had a 40-year history of hypertension and her current treatment included hydrochlorothiazide and propranolol. Her family history was noncontributory.

Physical Examination: Temperature 37°; pulse 70; respirations 14; blood pressure 150/90. Neck: supple, bilateral carotid bruits. Cardiac, chest, abdomen, and breast: normal. Mental status, speech, and language: alert, oriented to person but disoriented to time and place, impaired speech comprehension, able to follow only simple commands, unable to repeat the phrase "no ifs, ands or buts"; spontaneous speech included brief fluent phrases with severe anomia, paraphrasias, and neologisms, but overall was nonfluent and sparse; comprehension impairment precluded assessment of other cognitive functions. Cranial nerves: intact, no papilledema. Motor examination: normal bulk, tone, and power. Sensory examination: normal, no sensory neglect. Muscle stretch reflexes: normal. Plantar reflexes: flexor. Coordination and gait: normal.

Stop and Consider: What is the likely neuroanatomic localization of the neurologic deficit?

Laboratory Findings: CBC, chemistry, electrolytes, liver function tests, ESR, urinalysis: normal. Chest x-ray: moderate aortic atherosclerotic disease, otherwise unremarkable. Transthoracic echocardiogram: negative for mural thrombi or cardiac malformations. Magnetic resonance arteriography (MRA): Extensive bilateral carotid bifurcation plaques but no hemodynamically significant stenosis; normal flow in vertebral and basilar arteries. Head MRI scan with contrast: see figure, *left*. Stereotactic brain biopsy: see figure, *right*.

Question: Do the MRI abnormalities correlate with this patient's symptoms?

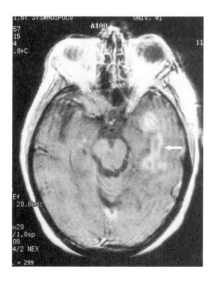 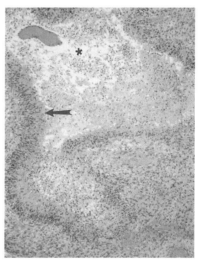

Diagnosis: Left temporal brain tumor histopathologically characterized as glioblastoma multiforme

Discussion: The neurologic examination in this patient was significant for a severe aphasia, which was characterized by relatively severe receptive language deficits compatible with Wernicke's aphasia, but also by nonfluent sparse speech. The abnormalities on mental status examination were most likely related to her language difficulties, which made it difficult to assess other cognitive functions. In a right-handed person these abnormalities indicate a left hemispheric frontotemporal lesion. The sudden onset of the neurologic deficit and bilateral carotid bruits in this patient initially suggested a vascular etiology (e.g., ischemic or hemorrhagic stroke). The MRI (figure, *left*) showed small hemorrhagic focus within the white matter of the left temporal lobe, but in addition demonstrated abnormal signal intensity throughout the entire left anterior and mesial temporal regions, including the regions irrigated by the middle and posterior cerebral arteries. There was edema and a mild mass effect, with temporal lobe uncus slightly displaced into the suprasellar cistern. After IV gadolinium contrast injection, nodular areas of enhanced signal in the left temporal white matter and along the insular cortex were observed (arrow), which were atypical for an acute ischemic or hemorrhagic stroke. The neuroimaging findings suggested a neoplastic process, but herpes encephalitis or brain abscess could also present with similar MRI abnormalities. Stereotactic brain biopsy was performed for further evaluation of the left temporal lesion. The pathologic examination (figure, *right*) showed a densely cellular neoplasm with extensive necrosis (asterisk) and palisading tumor cells (arrow) around the necrotic region. These features are typical of glioblastoma multiforme (GBM).

Brain tumors sometimes present with abrupt onset of symptoms that suggest infarction or TIA, and a high index of suspicion is necessary when evaluating such patients. Contrast-enhanced brain MRI or CT with contrast may be informative as the initial diagnostic tests but some cases of brain neoplasm may be difficult to differentiate from vascular lesions on the initial MRI. In equivocal cases, a follow-up MRI within a few weeks or an angiogram should be obtained to evaluate the evolution of the lesion on neuroimaging studies. Histopathologic examination of a stereotactic brain biopsy specimen is necessary to establish the etiology of the brain lesion when the presentation is acute but the MRI findings suggest a neoplasm.

Metastatic and primary brain tumors can bleed and mimic the presentation of a stroke. Intracerebral hemorrhages occur in approximately 10% of patients with metastatic brain tumors. The highest incidence of hemorrhage is observed in metastatic choriocarcinoma, malignant melanoma, lung, and renal cell carcinoma. Brain hemorrhage is also a recognized, although relatively infrequent, initial presentation of primary brain tumors. Approximately 5% of patients with GBM present with an intracranial hemorrhage. The most frequent type of hemorrhage in primary or metastatic brain tumors is intracerebral (83% of cases), but subarachnoid (15%) and subdural (2%) hemorrhages are also observed. Increased fibrinolytic activity associated with the tumor may contribute to the tendency to hemorrhage.

Glioblastoma multiforme, also referred to as grade IV astrocytoma, is the most malignant astrocytic brain tumor and is one of the most malignant of all neoplasms. It occurs predominantly in patients older than age 50. High-grade astrocytomas account for 33–45% of primary brain tumors in the U.S. and 50–80% of these astrocytomas are GBMs. GBM is characterized by markedly prominent cellularity with pleomorphism, endothelial proliferation, increased number of mitoses, necrosis, and hemorrhages.

Although the prognosis in GBM is poor, the therapeutic approach usually combines surgery, radiation, and chemotherapy. Maximum surgical resection should be attempted if at least 90% of the tumor can be removed without a significant neurologic deficit. Stereotactic biopsy to establish the histologic grade of the neoplasm should be done if the tumor cannot be removed safely. GBM is frequently associated with significant vasogenic edema that can be managed by corticosteroids, such as dexamethasone. Mannitol may be used in some acute clinical situations but loses its effectiveness within a few days. Radiation therapy is a useful adjunct to surgery and may produce some improvement. Conventional, external-beam fractionated radiotherapy to a total dose of 5500–6000 rads is typically administered.

The survival of GBM patients treated with surgery alone is approximately 14 weeks. If surgery is combined with radiation, the median survival may be extended to 9 months. Chemotherapy in GBM appears to have only a modest effect on prolongation of survival. The most frequently used agent is carmustine (BCNU), but lomustine (CCNU), procarbazine, and vincristine have also been used.

Because of the advanced age and poor prognosis, the present patient and her family decided against surgery. She was treated with palliative external-beam radiotherapy and was discharged in stable condition, but died several months later.

Clinical Pearls

1. Brain tumors may present with symptoms of abrupt onset and mimic transient ischemic attacks or stroke.

2. Because intracerebral hemorrhage is a relatively frequent initial manifestation of malignant brain tumors, neoplasm should be considered in the differential diagnosis of intracranial hemorrhages.

3. Glioblastoma multiforme is the most malignant primary brain tumor and frequently displays necrotic and hemorrhagic areas on histopathologic examination.

4. Histologic diagnosis is necessary to select appropriate therapy for brain neoplasms.

REFERENCES

1. Kyritsis AP: Evaluation and treatment of central nervous system neoplasms. In Lechtenberg R, Schutta HS (eds): Neurology Practice Guidelines. New York, Marcel Dekker, 1998, pp 473–496.
2. Nutt SH, Patchell RA: Intracranial hemorrhage associated with primary and secondary tumors. Neurosurg Clin North Am 1992; 3:591–599.
3. Oka K, Tsuda H, Sakamoto S, et al: Plasminogen activator and hemorrhage in brain tumors. J Neurooncol 1994; 22:183–187.
4. Whittle IR: Management of primary malignant brain tumours. J Neurol Neurosurg Psychiatry 1996; 60:2–5.

PATIENT 40

A 4-year-old boy with progressive weakness and a Gowers' sign

A 4-year-old boy was referred for evaluation of progressive difficulty with walking. He was the product of normal pregnancy and normal delivery. His motor developmental milestones were delayed, but he was able to walk independently by the age of 16–18 months. However, he was never able to run well. Over the previous year the parents noted progressive difficulty with walking or arising from the floor. He would stand up by "climbing his thighs." Cognitive development was normal. Family history was significant for a paternal great-uncle who developed difficulty with walking at about age 45 and was reported to have limb-girdle muscular dystrophy. The boy's parents and two siblings were normal.

Physical Examination: Vital signs: normal. Cardiac: normal. Head: normocephalic, skull nontender. Neck: supple. Spine: no deformity, nontender, good range of motion. Mental status, speech, cranial nerves: normal. Motor examination: muscle bulk diminished in both quadriceps muscles, muscle tone mildly diminished, strength in upper extremities grade +4 proximally and –5 distally, in lower extremities grade 4 proximally and –5 distally; arises from the floor with a typical Gowers' maneuver (see figure, *left*). Sensory examination: normal. Muscle stretch reflexes: depressed (1/4) and symmetric. Plantar reflexes: flexor. Coordination: normal. Gait: waddling. Clinical neuromuscular evaluation of both parents: normal.

Stop and Consider: What is the differential diagnosis in a child presenting with diffuse weakness, hypotonia, diminished reflexes, and a Gowers' sign?

Laboratory Findings: CBC, chemistry, electrolytes, ESR, creatine kinase (CK): normal. Nerve conduction study (NCS): normal. Needle electromyography (EMG): markedly decreased recruitment pattern with high-amplitude, prolonged, polyphasic motor unit potentials in all muscles tested. Biopsy of the quadriceps muscle (ATPase stain with preincubation at pH 4.6): see figure, *right*.

Question: What is your interpretation of the EMG and muscle biopsy findings? What other diagnostic test may confirm the suspected diagnosis?

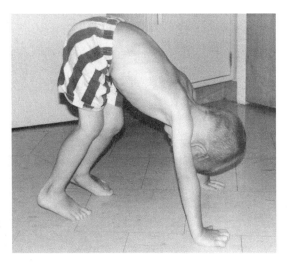 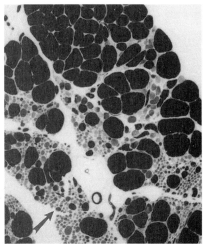

Diagnosis: Childhood form of spinal muscular atrophy (SMA type III, Kugelberg-Welander disease)

Discussion: The findings from the clinical examination, with muscle atrophy and weakness, hypotonia, hyporeflexia, and normal mental status and cranial nerve functions suggest that this boy's weakness is caused by dysfunction of the motor unit. The Gowers' sign indicated severe proximal lower extremity weakness but it is nonspecific and may be present in both myopathic and neurogenic conditions. Normal CK level excludes the possibility of Duchenne muscular dystrophy. Normal nerve conduction studies and sensory exam point away from a possible form of congenital polyneuropathy (e.g., Dejerine-Sottas disease) as the culprit of the weakness. The EMG findings strongly indicated anterior horn cell disease as the cause of the weakness by demonstrating chronic neurogenic changes on the needle examination. Muscle biopsy confirmed the severe neurogenic process, with large groups of atrophic fibers (arrow) and all hypertrophic fibers being histochemically type I. This pattern of histochemical abnormalities was strongly suggestive of spinal muscular atrophy (SMA). Subsequent DNA analysis showed homozygous deletions of exons 7 and 8 of the survival motor neuron (SMN) gene on chromosome 5q, which confirmed the diagnosis of SMA. The muscle biopsy from his great-uncle was reviewed and showed distinctly different findings, indicative of muscular dystrophy without evidence of a neurogenic process. The distinct clinical presentations and pathologic features indicated that they suffered from different neuromuscular disorders.

SMA is a hereditary disease affecting primarily the anterior horn cells of the spinal cord. In some patients there is also involvement of the motor neurons in the brain stem. The extraocular movements are spared and there is no involvement of the intellect. The mode of inheritance is autosomal recessive in a vast majority of cases. The incidence of SMA is 1 per 8,000 births and approximately 1.8% of population are carriers of this disease.

There is a wide spectrum of clinical presentations in patients with SMA, with differences in age of onset, severity, and rate of progression. On the basis of age of onset and rate of progression SMA has been classified into several subtypes. In SMA type I (Werdnig-Hoffmann disease) children present as "floppy infants," with severe hypotonia at birth and typically do not survive more than 1–2 years. Death is usually the result of respiratory failure. Infants affected by SMA type II (intermediate SMA) become symptomatic by age 6–12 months; some of them may learn to sit but typically none are able to walk. Death from respiratory failure typically occurs in early childhood, but some may

have prolonged survival. The childhood- or juvenile-onset SMA is referred to as SMA type III, also known as Kugelberg-Welander disease. The onset is typically between ages 2–30. Progression of weakness is relatively slow with prolonged survival. In some cases there is arrest of progression. Weakness is typically most severe in proximal muscles of lower extremities. Differentiation from limb-girdle muscular dystrophy is necessary and may be difficult as the CK level can be mildly elevated (up to 5 times normal) in SMA. EMG and muscle biopsy are usually necessary if no mutation in the SMN gene is found. Adult-onset SMA is classified as type IV. The onset is at age 30–60, with slow progression. As in cases of SMA type III, proximal muscle involvement may mimic limb-girdle muscular dystrophy. SMA type IV has a variable mode of inheritance and may be very difficult to distinguish from a lower motor neuron variant of amyotrophic lateral sclerosis.

The inheritance pattern in SMA is autosomal recessive, but in some families an autosomal dominant inheritance has been observed. The locus for autosomal recessive SMA was mapped to chromosome 5q region in 1990 and in 1995 a survival motor neuron (SMN) gene was isolated. The SMN gene exists in telomeric (tSMN) and centromeric (cSMN) forms and deletions in the tSMN gene have been found in approximately 95% of SMA type I–III cases. Some milder forms of SMA type II–III were found to be associated with conversion of the tSMN gene into its centromeric counterpart. Most adult-onset cases (SMA type IV) do not have a mutation in the SMN gene. The function of the protein product of the SMN gene is unknown but the association of the SMN gene mutation with the SMA types I–III is strong. Deletions in the SMN gene of normal control populations have not been detected; therefore, the presence of homozygous deletions in the SMN gene in a patient with clinical signs of SMA confirms the diagnosis of SMA. Rare cases of clinically normal siblings or parents of SMA patients with homozygous deletions in the SMN gene have been reported, which suggests that the SMN gene mutation may not be the only abnormality that produces SMA.

Other neighboring genes on chromosome 5q may also be deleted in some SMA patients. Deletions of the gene encoding the neuronal apoptosis inhibitor protein (NAIP) occur in approximately 50% of SMA type I and 20% type II and III patients. In clinically affected patients the NAIP gene deletions occur in addition to the tSMN gene deletions. In some studies the most severe phenotypes have been associated with deletion in the NAIP gene in addition to the *SMN* gene. There are many SMA variants that are not linked to chromosome 5, indicating that several other gene mutations may be associated with anterior horn cell degeneration.

SMA has some features that overlap with other motor system disorders. In the bulbospinal form of SMA (Kennedy's disease), bulbar involvement with dysarthria and dysphagia is observed in addition to proximal weakness and approximately 50% of patients have gynecomastia. This condition is caused by a mutation consisting of expansion of CAG repeats in the androgen receptor gene on chromosome Xq12. The Fazio-Londe syndrome, also known as progressive bulbar palsy of childhood, is an autosomal recessive condition with severe degeneration of brain stem motor neurons that presents with progressive facial weakness, ptosis, dysphagia, and respiratory stridor. In some patients with SMA, distal weakness may be more pronounced than proximal weakness. This disorder is usually classified as distal SMA or as a spinal variant of Charcot-Marie-Tooth (CMT) disease. In contrast to CMT disease, there is no sensory involvement. Both dominant and recessive modes of inheritance have been described in this entity.

Typically, the diagnosis of SMA is based on characteristic clinical findings, electrodiagnostic studies, and neurogenic changes in the muscle biopsy. However, in a child with clinical findings suggestive of SMA and normal or only mildly elevated CK, a DNA analysis for *SMN* gene mutation should be performed prior to muscle biopsy. If a typical deletion in the *SMN* gene is found, the muscle biopsy is not necessary. If no *SMN* gene mutation is documented, additional diagnostic studies including muscle biopsy should be strongly considered, since some children with different congenital myopathies may have clinical presentation that mimics SMA.

There is no effective treatment for SMA at the present time. Management is directed to treatment of musculoskeletal complications, such as scoliosis and contractures, and respiratory symptoms.

The present patient has had a slowly progressive course and at age 8 was still able to ambulate independently, but also used a motorized wheelchair for longer distances.

Clinical Pearls

1. Gowers' sign is caused by weakness of pelvic girdle muscles and may be observed in both myopathic and neurogenic conditions.

2. In a patient with clinical signs typical of SMA the presence of homozygous deletion in the survival motor neuron (*SMN*) gene on chromosome 5q confirms the diagnosis.

3. The rate of progression in SMA is variable and survival may be prolonged in patients with early childhood or even infantile onset.

4. Children with some congenital myopathies may have normal or mildly elevated CK and the clinical presentation may be similar to SMA. NCS/EMG, muscle biopsy, and genetic analysis may be required to establish the diagnosis.

REFERENCES

1. Morrison KE: Advances in SMA research: Review of gene deletions. Neuromuscul Disord 1996; 6:397–408.
2. Zerres K, Wirth B, Rudnik-Schöneborn S: Spinal muscular atrophy: Clinical and genetic correlations. Neuromuscul Disord 1997; 7:202–207.

PATIENT 41

A 61-year-old woman with hearing loss, imbalance, myoclonic jerks, and memory problems

A 61-year-old retired nurse complained of slowly progressive difficulty with balance and frequent falls during the last 3–4 years. Some falls were precipitated by brief, sudden jerking movements of her legs. There was no apparent loss or alteration of consciousness associated with the falls, but some episodes were accompanied by urinary incontinence. She also complained of progressive hearing loss, poor concentration, and memory problems. Her medical history was significant for depression, hypothyroidism treated with replacement, and recurring retinal detachments. Her 30-year-old daughter suffers from myoclonic epilepsy, hearing loss, and mental retardation. The patient reported that her mother and two older sisters also had brief jerking movements of arms and legs and that one of her sisters was diagnosed with myoclonic epilepsy.

Physical Examination: Vital signs: normal. Skull: normocephalic. Spine: nontender, good range of motion, no scoliosis. Cardiac: normal. Mental status: alert and oriented to place, person, and time, short attention span and some difficulty with recall (remembered 2/3 objects after 3 minutes), otherwise normal. Speech: normal. Cranial nerves: pupils equal, reactive to light and accommodation, visual acuity 20/200 OS, 20/400 OD; visual fields normal to confrontation; funduscopic examination: multiple retinal scars with areas of hyperpigmentation and hypopigmentation; severely impaired hearing bilaterally; other cranial nerves normal. Motor examination: muscle bulk, tone, and strength normal. Sensory examination: mild decrease of vibratory sensation in the toes, otherwise normal. Muscle stretch reflexes: brisk (grade 3) and symmetric. Plantar reflexes: flexor. Coordination: moderate bilateral dysmetria on finger-to-nose testing, diminished fine motor skills. Gait: wide-based with marked difficulty on tandem gait testing.

Stop and Consider: What central and peripheral systems appear to be involved? What is the significance of her family history and what is the most likely inheritance pattern in this family?

Laboratory Findings: CBC, chemistry panel, electrolytes: normal. Serum lactate 1.9 mmol/L (normal 0–2.0). ECG: normal. EEG: rhythmic, bifrontal slowing with occasional generalized bursts of spike and wave discharges without any clinical events. MRI, mild, diffuse volume loss, otherwise normal. Biopsy of the vastus lateralis muscle: numerous ragged red fibers (RRFs), cytochrome C oxidase (CCO)–negative fibers, and succinate dehydrogenase (SDH)–overreactive fibers. Muscle electron microscopy: see figure.

Question: How are the abnormalities observed in the muscle biopsy related to the other neurologic findings? What other diagnostic study may help confirm the diagnosis?

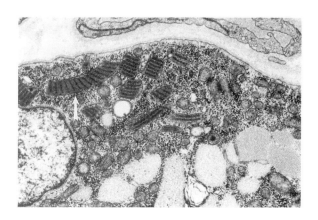

Diagnosis: Myoclonic epilepsy and ragged red fibers

Discussion: This patient presented with signs and symptoms of diffuse nervous system involvement including cortical, cerebellar, and cranial nerve dysfunction. The EEG abnormalities were consistent with possible myoclonic epilepsy. A hereditary disorder with maternal inheritance pattern was likely, with several family members affected by a similar condition. Because of the clinical presentation and maternal inheritance, a mitochondrial disorder was considered and a muscle biopsy performed. The light microscopy demonstrated mitochondrial abnormality (RRFs, CCO-negative fibers, and SDH-overreactive fibers) in the skeletal muscle and the electron microscopy showed large collections of morphologically abnormal mitochondria with numerous characteristic crystalline "parking lot" inclusions (figure, arrow). The finding of mitochondrial myopathy confirmed the clinical suspicion that the CNS abnormalities, including seizures, were caused by a mitochondrial encephalomyopathy. The clinical phenotype of this patient, with myoclonic epilepsy, hearing loss, psychomotor regression, ataxia, and presence of RRF in the skeletal muscle processed by modified Gomori trichrome stain were typical of a mitochondrial disorder known as myoclonic epilepsy and ragged red fibers (MERRF). The diagnosis was later confirmed with a mitochondrial DNA analysis of the DNA extracted from lymphocytes and muscle samples. The patient was found to have a mutation in the tRNA lysine gene (an A to G substitution at nucleotide 8344) known to be associated with the MERRF phenotype.

In addition to the myoclonus, ataxia, and mitochondrial myopathy with characteristic feature of RRFs in the muscle biopsy specimen, the MERRF syndrome frequently includes generalized seizures, optic atrophy, hearing loss, peripheral neuropathy, dementia, cardiomyopathy, pigmentary retinopathy, and lactic acidosis. Some patients may have pyramidal signs, some degree of ophthalmoparesis, and multiple lipomas. The mitochondrial myopathy in MERRF is associated with rather mild limb weakness. Brain MRI may show atrophy and basal ganglia calcifications. EEG may demonstrate generalized spike and wave discharges with slowing of the background activity. Nerve conduction studies and electromyography may reveal evidence of myopathy and coexisting polyneuropathy. Screening for possible cardiac involvement with an electrocardiogram should be performed in all patients. Lumbar puncture may show mild, nonspecific increase of protein content. Creatine kinase is usually normal or only mildly elevated. In typical cases muscle biopsy with the modified Gomori trichrome stain shows numerous RRFs, which contain large collections of morphologically abnormal mitochondria. Abnormal muscle fibers may overreact for SDH ("ragged blue" fibers) or display no CCO reactivity. Electron microscopy shows large collections of morphologically abnormal mitochondria, frequently containing crystalline inclusions.

Most patients with MERRF have family history of a mitochondrial encephalomyopathy, although there is a wide spectrum of clinical presentations in affected family members. There is a characteristic maternal mode of transmission in families affected by MERRF. Two different point mutations, both in the gene encoding the tRNA for lysine, have been associated with MERRF: an A→G substitution at nucleotide 8344 and a T→C transition at nucleotide 8356. Rare families with MERRF phenotype may not show typical mutations. The MERRF mutations are heteroplasmic with both the mutant and normal mitochondrial DNA (mtDNA) present in different tissues. The proportion of mutant mtDNA correlates with the disease severity. The pathogenetic mechanisms that produce the multisystem involvement associated with the mitochondrial mutations are uncertain. Patients with MERRF may have overlapping phenotypes with other mitochondrial disorders, such as MELAS (mitochondrial encephalopathy, lactic acidosis, and stroke-like episodes).

Muscle biopsy may not be necessary, but if performed demonstrates RRFs in a vast majority of patients with MERRF (90%). DNA analysis can be performed on muscle tissue if the leukocyte mtDNA analysis is inconclusive. Activity of mitochondrial enzymes may demonstrate defects in the respiratory chain system, especially in complex IV.

MERRF is one of many disorders in a rapidly expanding spectrum of mitochondrial cytopathies. When evaluating patients with suspected mitochondrial disorders, it is important to remember the rather characteristic pattern of recognition. Brain and muscle are particularly vulnerable to the dysfunction of mitochondrial metabolism because of their very high energy demands. The symptoms and signs of the nervous system involvement in those conditions include seizures, dementia, ataxia, myoclonus, strokes, cortical blindness, optic neuropathy, hemiparesis, dystonia, hearing loss, peripheral neuropathy, and muscle involvement (weakness, ophthalmoplegia, ptosis). The signs of diffuse systemic involvement include lactic acidosis, hypothyroidism, diabetes mellitus, growth retardation, cardiac involvement (conduction defects, cardiomyopathy), intestinal pseudoobstruction, cataracts, and retinitis pigmentosa.

The significant heteroplasmy of mitochondrial mutations has implications for selection of specimens for diagnostic DNA studies. For example, deletions of mtDNA in the Kearns-Sayre syndrome can be found only in the DNA extracted from the skeletal muscle and are not present in leukocytes.

RRFs in the muscle biopsies are not specific for mitochondrial disorders and may be observed in elderly patients, inflammatory myopathies, dystrophies, and other myopathies as a nonspecific finding. They are usually present in conditions associated with mutations affecting the intramitochondrial protein synthesis (point mutations, deletions, or duplications affecting tRNA genes), but in some mitochondrial disorder the RRFs may not be observed in muscle biopsies.

This patient was treated with valproic acid and experienced some improvement of the myoclonus, but she became progressively disabled by gait ataxia. Genetic counseling was provided to the family. This case illustrates how mitochondrial disorders may present with involvement of many organ systems, and how detailed investigation of family history may be necessary for diagnosis.

Clinical Pearls

1. Consider mitochondrial disorders in familial conditions with a maternal mode of inheritance.

2. There is a significant phenotypic overlap between MELAS, MERRF, and other mitochondrial syndromes.

3. The ragged red fibers in muscle biopsies are frequent in conditions associated with mitochondrial mutations in the tRNA genes.

4. Ragged red fibers are not specific for mitochondrial myopathies and may occur in numerous other myopathic, neurogenic, or toxic/metabolic conditions and their frequency increases with age.

5. DNA testing is currently available for several mitochondrial disorders.

REFERENCES

1. Fadic R, Johns DR: Clinical spectrum of mitochondrial diseases. Semin Neurol 1996; 16:11–20.
2. Hammans SR, Sweeney MG, Brockington M, et al: The mitochondrial DNA transfer RNA (Lys)A→G(8344) mutation and the syndrome of myoclonic epilepsy and ragged red fibers (MERRF): Relationship of clinical phenotype to proportion of mutant mitochondrial DNA. Brain 1993; 116:617–632.
3. Schon EA, Bonilla E, DiMauro S: Mitochondrial DNA mutations and pathogenesis. J Bioenerg Biomembr 1997; 29:131–149.

PATIENT 42

A 46-year-old man with a history of HTLV-1–associated myelopathy and subacute exacerbation of weakness

A 46-year-old man with an established diagnosis of HTLV-1–associated myelopathy (tropical spastic paraparesis, TSP) was referred for evaluation of a subacute exacerbation of weakness. The diagnosis of TSP was based on evidence of myelopathy, high titers of anti-HTLV-1 antibodies, and exclusion of alternative diagnoses with extensive diagnostic evaluations, including spinal MRI and cerebrospinal fluid examination. For the last 10 years he had a stable clinical course characterized by nonprogressive spastic paraparesis, neurogenic bladder, and sensory loss in his legs. A few moths prior to presentation he noted progressive increase in weakness, especially in upper extremities, which were previously not significantly affected. He had no cognitive or visual symptoms and denied back or neck pain. His medical and family history was otherwise unremarkable. He traveled to Africa 20 years ago but denied recent travel outside the U.S.

Physical Examination: Vital signs: normal. Head: normocephalic, skull nontender. Neck: supple, no bruits. Spine: no deformity, nontender, good range of motion. Mental status and speech: normal. Cranial nerves: normal. Motor examination: muscle bulk diminished diffusely, rare fasciculations in arms and thighs; severe spasticity in both lower extremities; marked symmetric proximal upper and lower extremity weakness (grade 4) with slight distal weakness. Sensory examination: decreased in lower extremities to pain, vibration and proprioception, but no sensory level. Muscle stretch reflexes: normal in upper extremities, pathologically brisk and symmetric in lower extremities (grade 4). Plantar reflexes: bilateral Babinski signs. Coordination: mild dysmetria in lower extremities. Gait: wide-based, with spastic features.

Stop and Consider: What is the significance of the symmetric proximal weakness in this patient with symptoms and signs of previously nonprogressive myelopathy associated with HTLV-1 infection? Should a second process be considered?

Laboratory Findings: CBC, chemistry panel, electrolytes, ESR, ANA: normal. Creatine kinase (CK) level: 1260 U/L (normal 0–250). MRI of the cervical and thoracic spine: small disc protrusion at the C4–5 level, otherwise unremarkable. CSF examination: mild elevation of the CSF protein with normal glucose and cell count; positive oligoclonal bands. Nerve conduction study (NCS): mildly decreased compound muscle action potential (CMAP) amplitudes in the lower extremities. Motor and sensory conduction velocities: normal. Needle electromyography (EMG): fibrillation potentials as well as a combination of small, short-duration, polyphasic motor unit potentials (MUPs) and long-duration, high-amplitude MUPs in different muscles in upper and lower extremities and cervical and thoracic paraspinal muscles. Serology: high levels of IgG anti-HTLV-1 antibodies in blood by Western blot with strong reactivities to *gag* (p19 and p24) and *env* (gp46 and rgp21) antigens. Muscle biopsy from the vastus lateralis muscle: see figure.

Question: Can the findings from the muscle biopsy and elevated CK level explain this patient's subacute deterioration of strength?

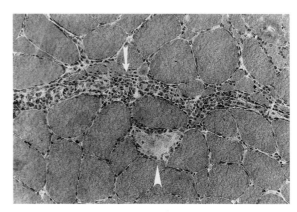

Diagnosis: HTLV-1–associated myelopathy (tropical spastic paraparesis) and coexisting HTLV-1–associated polymyositis

Discussion: Although the dominant neurologic abnormality in this patient was spastic paraparesis consistent with his well established diagnosis of TSP, the recent subacute increase in weakness with atrophy, especially in the upper extremities, suggested the possibility of a second process. Diffuse fasciculations and atrophy were consistent with anterior horn cell disease or motor axonal polyneuropathy. The neurogenic changes (long-duration, large-amplitude MUPs) on the EMG in three limbs and thoracic paraspinal muscles, with normal nerve conduction velocities, were consistent with either coexisting anterior horn cell involvement or diffuse polyradiculopathy. In addition, elevated CK, marked weakness of proximal muscles, especially in the upper extremities, and the presence of small, short-duration MUPs suggested a concurrent myopathic process. The inflammatory changes (figure, arrow) and necrotic muscle fibers (figure, arrowhead) in the muscle biopsy confirmed the clinical suspicion that the subacute deterioration was most likely caused by coexisting polymyositis, although progression of the myelopathy with anterior horn cell involvement could not be excluded. In addition to inflammatory cell collections with invasion of nonnecrotic muscle fibers, the muscle biopsy also showed evidence of coexisting denervation atrophy. The immunocytochemical studies in this patient showed that the immune attack against the skeletal muscle was primarily mediated by CD8+ T cells, with some contribution of CD4+ T cells and macrophages.

Inflammatory myopathy histologically indistinguishable from polymyositis may be a major feature of the spectrum of neurologic conditions that can develop in the course of HTLV-1 infection. Epidemiologic studies from Jamaica, where the HTLV-1 infection is endemic, have indicated that 85% of patients with polymyositis have IgG anti-HTLV-1 antibodies, whereas only 7.5% of patients with other neurologic disorders have antibodies to HTLV-1. Polymyositis may be the only clinical manifestation of HTLV-1 infection, but many patients with preexisting HTLV-1–associated myelopathy develop polymyositis.

HTLV-1 myelopathy/tropical spastic paraparesis (TSP) is a chronic or subacute condition characterized by prominent pyramidal signs, posterior column dysfunction (loss of vibration sense and proprioception), urinary bladder disturbance, impotence, and low back pain. Autopsy studies in TSP typically reveal severe myelin and axonal destruction with inflammatory infiltrates, mostly in the white matter of the thoracic spinal cord. In some patients anterior horn cell involvement produces severe muscle wasting and fasciculations. Weakness is typically most severe in proximal lower extremities. HTLV-1 infection may also be associated with peripheral neuropathy, polyradiculopathy, cranial neuropathies including optic atrophy and deafness, meningitis, cerebellar ataxia, and encephalopathy.

TSP has to be differentiated from other causes of myelopathy such as multiple sclerosis, compressive lesions (e.g., cervical spondylosis), neoplasms, vascular malformations, infectious and parainfectious conditions, or motor neuron disease with primarily or exclusively upper motor neuron involvement (progressive lateral sclerosis). Differentiation from multiple sclerosis may sometimes be difficult. In contrast to multiple sclerosis, the optic nerve involvement or eye movement disorders are very rare and most patients have a chronic progressive rather then relapsing-remitting course.

The diagnostic evaluation of HTLV-1–associated neurologic conditions is determined by features of the neurologic presentation. In patients with myelopathy MRI should be performed to exclude space-occupying lesions. In TSP the MRI frequently shows multiple foci of signal abnormality in T2 weighted images of spinal cord and sometimes in the brain. Cerebrospinal fluid analysis usually shows elevated protein, oligoclonal bands, and mild lymphocytic pleocytosis. CK levels may be elevated in patients with polymyositis. Nerve conduction studies and electromyography may be helpful in evaluation of coexisting polyneuropathy and myopathy. Detection of HTLV-1 antibodies in blood and cerebrospinal fluid is supportive of the diagnosis, but viral isolation is usually unsuccessful. HTLV-1 DNA can be detected by polymerase chain reaction (PCR) technique. Evidence of HTLV-1 infection by antibody titers, PCR analysis, or viral isolation should be correlated with the clinical picture since most patients infected with an HTLV-1 virus are asymptomatic carriers (up to 98%).

Deterioration of strength in a patient suffering from HTLV-1–associated myelopathy may create diagnostic dilemmas. Because of the deficits associated with the myelopathy, coexisting involvement of the skeletal muscle may not be recognized. However, neuromuscular evaluation suggesting the pattern of a myopathy (proximal > distal weakness) and electrodiagnostic, pathologic, and biochemical studies may provide clues about muscle involvement. The EMG may not reveal myopathic changes and the CK levels may be normal in some patients with HTLV-1–associated polymyositis; therefore, a high index of suspicion for coexisting myositis is necessary to rule out an inflammatory process that may be responsive to immunosuppressive treatment.

The present patient was started on prednisone 1 mg/kg/day. Within 2 weeks he showed marked improvement of his strength and his CK level normalized. His strength continued to improve and after 3 months a slow prednisone taper was initiated. After 6 months his strength in the upper extremities was normal and he had only mild to moderate weakness in the lower extremities. The upper extremity strength improved much more than the leg weakness and improvement was associated with CK normalization. These facts support the notion that the treatment of the inflammatory myopathy produced the improvement, but the anti-inflammatory effect of steroids on the spinal cord may also have contributed to his clinical improvement.

Clinical Pearls

1. A wide spectrum of neurologic syndromes may develop in the course of HTLV-1 infection, but most HTLV-1–infected patients are asymptomatic.

2. Consider coexisting polymyositis in all patients with HTLV-1–associated myelopathy (tropical spastic paraparesis) when weakness progresses or patients have abnormal serum CK levels.

3. Polymyositis may be a sole manifestation of HTLV-1 infection.

4. Muscle biopsy is essential to evaluate patients with suspected inflammatory muscle disease.

5. HTLV-1–related polymyositis can be successfully treated with corticosteroids.

REFERENCES

1. Evans BK, Gore I, Harrell LE, et al: HTLV-1–associated myelopathy and polymyositis in a U.S. native. Neurology 1989; 39:1572–1575.
2. Gabbai AA, Wiley CA, Oliveira ASB, et al: Skeletal muscle involvement in tropical spastic paraparesis/HTLV-1–associated myelopathy. Muscle Nerve 1994; 17:923–930.
3. Higuchi I, Montemayor ES, Izumo S, et al: Immunocytochemical characteristics of polymyositis in patients with HTLV-1–associated myelopathy and HTLV-1 carriers. Muscle Nerve 1993; 16:472–476.
4. Morgan OS, Rodgers-Johnson P, Mora C, et al: HTLV-1 and polymyositis in Jamaica. Lancet 1989; 2:1184–1187.
5. Rodgers-Johnson PE: Tropical spastic paraparesis/HTLV-1–associated myelopathy: Etiology and clinical spectrum. Mol Neurobiol 1994; 8:175–179.
6. Younger DS: Differential diagnosis of progressive spastic paraparesis. Semin Neurol 1993; 13:319–321.

PATIENT 43

A 31-year-old man with progressive memory complaints and recurring confusion, headache, and gait disturbance

A 31-year-old, obese, right-handed man with a history of chronic headaches and daytime sleepiness presented with a 1-month history of recurrent episodes of excruciating headache accompanied by confusion, disorientation, and staggering gait. The first two episodes lasted several hours and resolved spontaneously. After the second episode, a head CT scan was obtained and was normal. Following the third episode the patient was admitted for intractable headache, confusion, and imbalance lasting for 8 hours. The patient reported that he was experiencing progressive memory problems and difficulty with concentration for over a year. He and his wife denied preceding fevers, rashes, any focal weakness, or numbness. Medical, social, and family history were noncontributory with the exception of smoking two cigarette packs per day for the last several years and history of myocardial infarction in his father at age 52.

Physical Examination: Vital signs: normal, afebrile, significant obesity. Cardiac, chest, and abdomen: normal. Skin: normal. Neck: supple. Mental status: very anxious, alert, oriented to place and person but unable to state correct date, poor attention span, no recall after 3 minutes, unable to perform simple calculations. Speech: relatively short phrases but no convincing evidence of aphasia. Cranial nerves: normal, with normal funduscopic evaluation. Motor and sensory examinations: normal. Muscle stretch reflexes: mildly increased (grade 3) and symmetric. Plantar reflexes: flexor. Coordination and gait: normal.

Stop and Consider: What is the differential diagnosis of a patient presenting with progressive cognitive dysfunction and recurring episodes of headache, confusion, and gait disturbance?

Laboratory Findings: CBC, serum chemistries with liver and renal function tests, PT, PTT: normal. ESR: 93 mm/hr (normal 0–15) MRI: see figure, *left*. Cerebral arteriogram: see figure, *right*. CSF: 19 nucleated cells/μl (cytospin: 89% lymphocytes, no granulocytes), 64 RBCs/μl, no xantochromia, protein 51 mg/dl (normal 0–45), glucose 64 mg/dl (serum glucose 97). CSF bacterial and fungal cultures, cryptococcal antigen: negative. CSF IgG index: normal. Polymerase chain reaction (PCR) DNA analysis for herpes simplex virus: negative. ANA, C3, C5, HIV antibodies, ANCA, antiphospholipid antibodies, anti-SSA, anti-SSB, anti-RNLP, anti-Smith antibodies: negative. Protein S, protein C, and activated protein C resistance testing: normal. EEG: normal.

Question: What is the most likely cause of the abnormalities demonstrated on the brain MRI and cerebral angiogram?

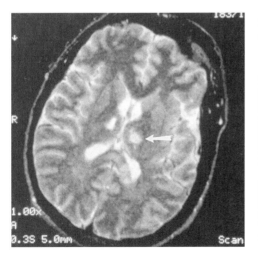 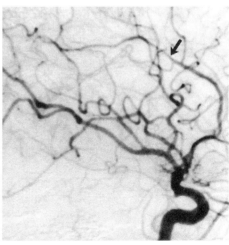

Diagnosis: Primary CNS angiitis

Discussion: This patient presented with slowly progressive cognitive symptoms and recurring episodes of severe headache, confusion, and gait disturbance. In the absence of significant focal or lateralizing abnormalities on examination, a fluctuating but progressive encephalopathy or subacute dementing process were considered as possible explanations for the fluctuating cortical dysfunction. Possible etiologies included recurring metabolic encephalopathies, subtle complex partial status epilepticus, or chronic infectious and inflammatory processes affecting the CNS, including CNS vasculitis. Typical causes of metabolic encephalopathy such as drug intoxication, hypoxemia, liver or renal dysfunction, and hypothyroidism were excluded by extensive laboratory studies. An infectious process was unlikely with negative CSF cultures and negative PCR for herpes simplex virus. Complex partial status epilepticus was excluded by the normal EEG. Episodes of complicated migraine would be rather unusual with such a prolonged encephalopathy and progressive course.

Structural lesions of different etiologies have to be ruled out by appropriate neuroimaging studies. In this patient the MRI showed multiple 1–2-cm areas of T2 signal hyperintensity in the posterior/medial thalamus bilaterally, the corpus callosum, and deep cerebral white matter (figure on the left, arrow). These multiple, small, nonenhancing lesions involving gray and white matter were consistent with small infarcts. More importantly, the cerebral angiogram strongly supported a diagnosis of CNS vasculitis by demonstrating abrupt changes in the caliber of the pericallosal arteries and their branches bilaterally (figure on the right, arrow). In a young person with normal cardiac examination and without peripheral signs of vasculitis, primary angiitis of the CNS (PACNS) was strongly suspected. The CSF findings in this patient, although consistent with a possible aseptic or viral process, were also consistent with PACNS.

Primary angiitis of the CNS was described infrequently prior to the availability of modern imaging techniques. It was also often assumed to be fatal, as it was usually discovered at autopsy. Many cases have been regarded as vasculitis based on cerebral angiography findings but have not been verified by histologic examination. CNS vasculitis may also develop in the course of infections (bacterial, viral, fungal, syphilis, borreliosis, rickettsiosis), lymphoproliferative disorders, and connective tissue diseases, or may be associated with drugs (amphetamines, cocaine, heroin, ephedrine, and phenylpropanolamine).

The most common presenting signs and symptoms of PACNS include focal CNS deficits (84%), headache (64%), and cognitive changes and depressed level of consciousness (56%). Spinal cord involvement is present in 15% of cases. CSF typically shows modest pleocytosis and elevated protein levels. Peripheral white blood cell count and ESR are abnormal in 58% and 35% of cases, respectively. The most common finding on MRI or CT is multiple bilateral, supratentorial infarcts in the cortex and deep white matter. Cranial CT or MRI may also reveal intraparenchymal or subarachnoid hemorrhages. In the spinal cord, increased signal on T2 weighted images may be evident within the cord.

Conventional angiography should be pursued in suspected CNS vasculitis, but it may be normal in about 40% of cases and findings typical of vasculitis (alternating areas of stenosis and ectasia in several vascular distributions) are absent in more than 60% of histologically proven cases. Angiographic findings, while supportive of the diagnosis, are nonspecific. Narrowing of the cerebral vessels can be seen in vasospasm (due to drug exposure, postpartum state, hypertension), CNS infections, or atherosclerosis. At the present time conventional angiography is superior to magnetic resonance angiography for detection of CNS vasculitis. Brain and leptomeningeal biopsies are often performed for diagnosis of CNS angiitis. In patients with absent focal lesions on neuroimaging studies, the temporal tip of the nondominant hemisphere is the preferred biopsy sight, but premortem biopsies are negative in 25% of autopsy-proven cases. Diagnostic histologic findings include granulomatous and necrotizing lymphocytic involvement of the small- and medium-size leptomeningeal and cortical arteries and veins.

Treatment of PACNS is complicated by lack of controlled clinical trials of different therapies. Typically high-dose corticosteroids and cyclophosphamide therapy is used in patients with definite CNS vasculitis. Some patients can be treated with corticosteroids alone.

The present patient was treated with a combination of cyclophosphamide and prednisone and experienced marked improvement within a few weeks and only mild residual memory problems. Reduction of the cyclophosphamide dose was followed by recurring symptoms and two new subcortical infarcts. Meningeal and brain biopsies showed necrotic changes without evidence of active vasculitis. He has been symptomatically stable for several years but developed diabetes and hypertension related to chronic use of corticosteroids.

Clinical Pearls

1. Suspect CNS vasculitis in patients with multiple small cortical and subcortical infarcts, even in the absence of systemic signs of vasculitis.

2. Primary CNS angiitis may be diagnosed on the basis of the characteristic clinical presentation with conventional angiography demonstrating multifocal microvascular abnormalities, but brain and leptomeningeal biopsies demonstrating vasculitis are more specific.

3. In many cases, CNS vasculitis is associated with nonbacterial meningitis, collagen vascular disease, lymphoproliferative disorders, or illicit drug use.

4. After exclusion of underlying causes, treatment with corticosteroids and cytotoxic agents is successful in many cases of CNS vasculitis.

REFERENCES

1. Calabrese LH, Duna GF, Lie JT: Vasculitis in the central nervous system. Arthritis Rheum 1997; 40:1189–1201.
2. Moore PM: Vasculitis of the central nervous system. Semin Neurol 1994; 14:307–312.

PATIENT 44

A 74-year-old man with a 5-day history of right-sided facial weakness, pain, vertigo, and imbalance

A 74-year-old previously healthy right-handed man awakened with severe pain in the right ear that extended to the right temporal area, face, and upper neck. During the next 12 hours he developed severe facial weakness and experienced decreased hearing and tinnitus in the right ear that was accompanied by dizziness, vertigo, and nausea. He also noticed an unusual taste sensation in the tip of his tongue. He denied weakness or numbness in his extremities, headache, or difficulty with bowel or bladder function. His medical, family, and social histories were noncontributory.

Physical Examination: Vital signs: normal, afebrile. HEENT: head atraumatic, vesicular rash with purulent drainage in right external auditory canal (see figure), ear lobe very tender to touch, right eye with redness of conjunctiva, no corneal abnormalities. Neck: supple, no lymphadenopathy or skin changes. Mental status: normal. Speech: mildly dysarthric. Cranial nerves: pupillary reflexes, visual acuity, visual fields, funduscopic examination normal; severe right facial weakness involving musculature of upper and lower face, inability to close the right eye; decreased hearing in the right ear, mild limitation of abduction in the right eye with some right end gaze nystagmus; other cranial nerves normal. Motor examination: normal bulk, tone, and power. Sensory examination: normal. Muscle stretch reflexes: normal. Coordination and gait: no limb ataxia, gait wide-based, unable to walk tandem, veers to right.

Stop and Consider: What is the significance of the vesicular rash in the right ear canal? On the basis of the symptoms and signs, what neural structures are involved?

Laboratory Findings: CBC and chemistries: normal. Head CT scan and noncontrast brain MRI: unremarkable.

Question: What is the prognosis for recovery of this patient's neurologic deficit?

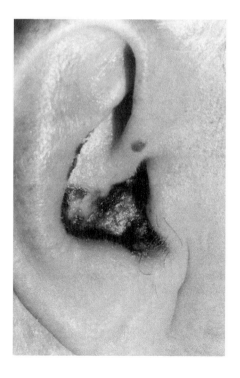

Diagnosis: Ramsay Hunt syndrome (herpes zoster oticus)

Discussion: The severe weakness of both the upper and lower facial musculature and taste dysfunction were typical of the peripheral seventh nerve palsy. The hearing loss, tinnitus, and vertigo indicated coexisting involvement of the vestibulocochlear nerve. The vestibular dysfunction may also explain his gait ataxia. He also appeared to have a coexisting right sixth nerve palsy. The vesicular skin changes in the external ear canal were typical of herpes zoster virus (HZV) infection and indicated that his neurologic deficits were most likely caused by HZV infection of the cranial nerves. There was no convincing clinical evidence of brain stem involvement and his brain MRI was unremarkable.

Ramsay Hunt syndrome (RHS), also known as herpes zoster oticus, is one of several neurologic syndromes that may develop in the course of varicella zoster virus infection. The incidence of RHS is approximately 5/100,000 population. This syndrome classically includes facial paralysis, hearing loss, tinnitus, hyperacusis, vertigo, dysgeusia, and decreased tearing. In some cases there may be coexisting involvement of the fifth, ninth, tenth, and other cranial nerves. In patients presenting with isolated facial nerve palsy in the course of HZV infection, the inflammatory process involves predominantly the geniculate ganglion. Involvement of the ganglia of Corti and Scarpa typically is accompanied by tinnitus, hearing loss, vertigo, and imbalance. In typical cases there is a vesicular eruption of the pina as well as external auditory canal. The rash may spread to involve the outer surface of the lobe of the ear, and when combined with cervical sensory ganglia involvement, vesicles are found on portions of the neck. The typical rash may develop before, during, or after the onset of the facial paralysis. Some cases of HZV infection may present without skin changes (zoster sine herpete).

The diagnosis of RHS is relatively easy in the presence of typical skin rash. In cases without skin rash a PCR DNA test from the CSF may be helpful. The CSF examination may also demonstrate some lymphocytic pleocytosis and elevated protein.

Some features of RHS overlap with Bell's palsy. The facial neuropathy in Bell's palsy is believed to be caused in most cases by herpes simplex virus infection. When patients present without any skin changes it may be very difficult to distinguish RHS from Bell's palsy. Facial paralysis caused by herpes zoster is frequently more severe, with complete paralysis and signs of acute denervation on electrodiagnostic studies. Patients with facial paralysis in the course of RHS are less likely to have complete recovery then patients with Bell's palsy. Patients with RHS frequently complain of severe balance problems. Brain MRI may show prominent facial nerve enhancement in both conditions. HZV may also involve the eye, and may be accompanied by zoster dermatitis on the forehead (herper zoster ophthalmicus). The eye involvement is especially frequent in patients who develop a rash in the distribution of the nasociliary nerve on the tip of the nose.

Postherpetic neuralgia is the most frequent long-term neurologic complication of HZV infection. Other neurologic complications of HZV infection include myelitis and encephalitis, thrombotic cerebral vasculopathy with acute ischemic stroke caused by HZV-associated vasculitis, acute ascending polyradiculitis, multiple cranial neuropathies, radiculopathy, plexopathy, motor neuropathy, or aseptic meningitis.

The varicella zoster virus persists for life in sensory ganglia after initial infection (varicella, chickenpox) that usually occurs in childhood or adolescence. Reactivation of the virus causes RHS, HZ ophthalmicus, and other neurologic syndromes. The immunologic and molecular events leading to virus reactivation are poorly understood.

Currently acyclovir is the antiviral drug of choice for herpes zoster. Typical treatment of RHS is oral acyclovir (400–800 mg 5 times/day for 7–10 days). A brief course of prednisone (7–10 days) may reduce inflammation. Many patients need pain management and a short course of opioids is frequently necessary.

The present patient presented with a classic RHS and was treated with acyclovir and prednisone. His symptoms gradually improved but after a few weeks he still had severe facial paralysis. He did not return for a follow-up evaluation.

Clinical Pearls

1. Herpes zoster infection is usually obvious from the vesicular rash in the distribution of cranial or peripheral nerves, but some cases may never demonstrate a rash, or the rash may develop several days after the onset of the focal neurologic deficit or pain.

2. The recovery of facial paralysis in Ramsay Hunt syndrome (herpes zoster oticus) is frequently incomplete.

3. Multiple cranial nerves may be involved in RHS, in addition to the cranial nerves VII and VIII.

4. PCR examination of the CSF may help with diagnosis of some cases of zoster infection, especially when the typical vesicular skin rash is not present.

5. Early treatment with acyclovir in Ramsay Hunt syndrome or Bell's palsy may be helpful.

REFERENCES

1. Adour KK: Otological complications of herpes zoster. Ann Neurol 1994; 35(Suppl):62–64.
2. Elliott KJ: Other neurological complications of herpes zoster and their management. Ann Neurol 1994; 35(Suppl):57–61.
3. Wood MJ: Current experience with antiviral therapy for acute herpes zoster. Ann Neurol 1994; 35(Suppl):65–68.

PATIENT 45

An 18-year-old woman with medically intractable seizures

An 18-year-old woman presented for evaluation of seizures that were not controlled by medical therapy. At the age of 6 months she was hospitalized with a fever and seizures, and was reported to have encephalitis. She lost motor and language developmental milestones, but these were gradually regained and she was treated for a year with phenobarbital and was without recurrent seizures. The phenobarbital was tapered at age 2 but at the age of 6 years she again experienced seizures, which occurred at low frequency until puberty, when the seizure frequency increased to two to three per day. The seizures were characterized by an initial aura of tightness in the head and chest and sweaty palms, followed by impaired consciousness, lip smacking, hand rubbing, and unresponsiveness. During a seizure she was unable to talk but could hear, and could not fully process information. She was treated with a variety of anticonvulsants, including phenobarbital, carbamazepine, phenytoin, valproate, and lamotrigine without significant success in seizure control. Her medical history was otherwise unremarkable. There was no family history of seizures.

Physical Examination: Vital signs: normal. Bedside mental status examination: no significant abnormalities. Neuropsychological testing: full-scale IQ of 97, performance IQ of 97 and a verbal IQ of 96; mild difficulty acquiring certain types of information and some difficulty with uncued recall. Speech: normal. Cranial nerves: normal with only minimal, unsustained nystagmus on lateral gaze. Motor and sensory examinations: normal. Muscle stretch reflexes: normal. Coordination and gait: normal.

Stop and Consider: What is the classification of her seizures according to the International Classification of Seizures? How should she be treated at this point?

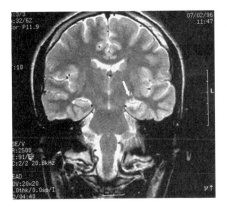

Laboratory Findings: CBC, serum chemistries with liver and renal functions, PT, PTT, ESR: normal. MRI: see figure, *top*. Interictal EEG: left temporal sharp and slow wave activity suggestive of left temporal onset of seizures. Continuous video-EEG monitoring: several seizures captured. EEG, see figure, *bottom*. Interictal positron emission tomography (PET) scan: hypometabolism of the left temporal lobe.

Question: What is the significance of the MRI and EEG findings with regard to considering surgical therapy?

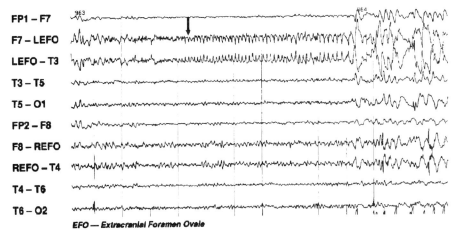

EFO — Extracranial Foramen Ovale

Diagnosis: Medically intractable partial complex seizures associated with hippocampal atrophy

Discussion: The clinical presentation of this patient's seizures with alteration of consciousness preceded by an aura of autonomic symptoms and evolution into altered consciousness with automatisms was typical of complex partial seizures, probably of limbic origin. MRI scan with coronal sections demonstrated atrophy of the left hippocampal formation as well as increased T2 signal in the left hippocampus (top figure, arrow). The continuous video-EEG monitoring, including recording from the mesial temporal regions with bilateral extracranial electrodes placed near the foramen ovale, demonstrated frequent left temporal spike or sharp wave discharges. Six complex partial seizures were recorded during monitoring. The seizures that were recorded while she was awake were preceded by a typical aura that developed after onset of an electrographic seizure arising from the left mesial temporal region (bottom figure, arrow). Four electrographic seizures were recorded during sleep and also appeared to begin in the left mesial temporal region.

Complex partial seizures (CPS) are the most common type of seizures and are observed in approximately 40% of patients with epilepsy. The term CPS refers to seizures that initially develop in a localized brain region and are accompanied by impaired consciousness and automatisms such as lip smacking, picking at clothes, or other semipurposeful motor activity. CPS are often preceded by an aura such as nausea, epigastric discomfort, fear, alteration of gustatory or visual perceptions, or abnormal cognitive phenomena. CPS often arise from the mesial temporal regions, but may also initiate from other brain regions including frontal, parietal, or occipital cortex. CPS may evolve into generalized tonic clonic seizures, and are then referred to as CPS with secondary generalization.

Temporal lobe epilepsy, defined by recurring CPS arising from limbic structures of the temporal lobe, is frequently associated with the characteristic lesion of hippocampal sclerosis. In these patients the neurologic exam is usually normal but neuropsychological testing may reveal a memory deficit that corresponds to the hippocampal neuronal loss. Medically intractable CPS with mesial temporal sclerosis frequently develop after complicated febrile seizures during childhood. As in this case, the initial seizures may be relatively easy to control with medications but become resistant to treatment during adolescence.

All patients with epilepsy should have an MRI scan performed at some time during their disorder. In cases of CPS, the MRI should include coronal views to allow examination of mesial temporal structures, which may reveal hippocampal atrophy.

A PET scan may reveal hypometabolism in the same region. Interictal EEG recording in typical cases reveals epileptiform discharges or focal slowing that corresponds in location to the regions of PET hypometabolism and hippocampal atrophy.

All patients with localization-related epilepsy, e.g., with partial seizures, should be considered candidates for surgical therapy if seizure control is not achieved with trials of two or three first-line anticonvulsants. Patients with as few as several seizures per year while receiving medication should be regarded as intractable, and there is urgency to consider early surgical intervention to prevent long-term cognitive impairment and disability. The identification of the site of the seizure onset can be established with noninvasive tests such as video-EEG, MRI, and PET. In patients with seizures that cannot be localized noninvasively, monitoring with foramen ovale, subdural strip, or depth electrodes may be necessary. Patients may be considered surgical candidates when the typical seizures arise consistently from a focal region.

Patients with bilateral interictal spike and sharp waves may have seizures that originate from one temporal lobe, usually associated with asymmetric and more significant hippocampal atrophy at the site of origin, and may still be candidates for surgery. As many as 70–90% of the patients with typical CPS of mesial temporal origin become seizure-free following surgery. Some patients can eventually be tapered from antiepileptic medications and are considered cured; others may achieve good seizure control but still require medication. In general, the prognosis for effective surgical treatment is usually improved by early recognition and surgery. The risks of anterior temporal lobectomy are minimal but include amnesia and mild superior quadrant visual field defect that is usually insignificant. Risk for postoperative memory dysfunction may be predicted from the intracarotid sodium pentobarbital (Wada's) test and preoperative neuropsychological testing that provide evidence of lateralized cognitive deficits or memory dysfunction.

In the present patient, MRI, prolonged video-EEG monitoring study, and PET scan were consistent with a left mesial onset of seizures and invasive recording was not necessary. Preoperative Wada's test demonstrated left hemisphere language dominance and adequate right hemisphere memory function. She underwent left anterior temporal lobectomy and did very well postoperatively in terms of memory function with no change from her baseline findings, and became seizure-free. An attempt to taper antiepileptic drugs was followed by breakthrough of seizures but reinstitution of antiepileptic medications again resulted in complete seizure control.

Clinical Pearls

1. All patients with complex partial seizures that have been refractory to medication therapy should be considered for surgical intervention, particularly when the history includes complex febrile seizures during childhood.

2. The MRI scan has improved and simplified the evaluation of patients with temporal lobe epilepsy for surgical therapy by noninvasively assessing for hippocampal atrophy. Concordant localization of abnormality by video-EEG, MRI, PET scan, and neuropsychological testing helps with selection of appropriate candidates for surgical treatment.

3. Surgical treatment may be performed safely and successfully in appropriately selected patients with intractable complex partial epilepsy and may result in cure or significant seizure control in as many as 70–90% of patients.

REFERENCES

1. Engel J Jr: Surgery for seizures. N Engl J Med 1996; 334:647–652.
2. French JA, Williamson PD, Thadani VM, et al: Characteristics of medial temporal lobe epilepsy: I. Results of history and physical examination. Ann Neurol 1993; 34:774–780.
3. Williamson PD, French JA, Thadani VM, et al: Characteristics of medial temporal lobe epilepsy: II. Interictal and ictal scalp electroencephalography, neuropsychological testing, neuroimaging, surgical results and pathology. Ann Neurol 1993; 34:781–787.

PATIENT 46

A 27-year-old woman with progressive cognitive impairment and difficulty walking

A 27-year-old woman presented with progressive cognitive impairment and difficulty walking for several years. Her first symptoms developed approximately 8 years previously when she started having memory problems. About 3 years later she started to make frequent "grunting noises" that her physician regarded as a tic disorder. At about the same time she noticed difficulties with activities requiring fine motor skills and her handwriting markedly deteriorated. During the last 2 years she developed emotional lability, with frequent crying spells followed by outbursts of laughing, and marked difficulties with bowel and bladder functions, including stool and urine incontinence. Medical history was noncontributory. She had two distant relatives who were diagnosed with possible multiple sclerosis.

Physical Examination: Vital signs: normal. Chest, heart, and abdomen normal. Mental status: very labile affect with outbursts of uncontrollable laughing or crying, oriented to place and person but unable to state correct date; memory impairment with inability to repeat more than one object immediately or to recall any objects after 2 minutes, unable to copy a design. Speech: normal. Cranial nerves: normal except for unsustained horizontal nystagmus at end gaze. Funduscopic examination: no papilledema or disc pallor. Motor examination: normal muscle bulk, increased tone (spasticity) in all four extremities, mild, diffuse weakness (grade + 4) in all limbs. Sensory examination: diminished vibratory sensation in the toes, diminished graphesthesia in both hands. Muscle stretch reflexes: pathologically brisk (grade 4) and symmetric throughout. Plantar reflexes: bilateral Babinski signs. Coordination: impaired on finger-to-nose testing with severe dysmetria and a mild intention tremor. Gait: severe truncal ataxia, unable to stand without assistance.

Stop and Consider: What is the time course and the localization of the neurologic dysfunction?

Laboratory Findings: CBC, chemistry panel, thyroid function tests: normal. Head MRI: see figure. Nerve conduction study: moderate, diffuse slowing of motor and sensory conduction velocities. Leukocyte arylsulfatase A activity: 0.5 U/10 cells (normal ≥ 2.5).

Question: What conditions may be associated with abnormalities demonstrated on the brain MRI and abnormal slowing of conduction velocities in the peripheral nerves on electrodiagnostic testing?

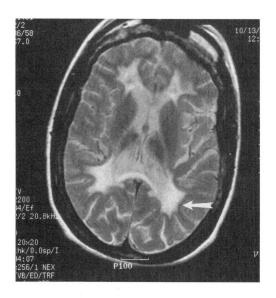

Diagnosis: Metachromatic leukodystrophy

Discussion: The clinical presentation of this patient suggested a chronic, progressive condition with diffuse bihemispheric dysfunction, global cognitive decline, emotional lability, long tract signs, cerebellar dysfunction, and peripheral neuropathy. Given the slowly and relentlessly progressive course without fluctuations or a pattern of relapse and remission, the differential diagnosis should include primarily metabolic and neurodegenerative processes. Inflammatory, autoimmune, and infectious conditions such as vasculitis or chronic meningitis, or focal structural lesions are less likely. The head MRI showed diffusely abnormal signal in the white matter of both cerebral hemispheres (figure, arrow) with relative sparing of subcortical arcuate fibers (U-fibers). These changes were very suggestive of a leukodystrophy. The finding of slow nerve conduction velocities, typical of demyelinating peripheral neuropathy, confirmed the suspicion of a leukodystrophy associated with both central and peripheral demyelination. The decreased level of arylsulfatase A activity in the leukocytes confirmed the diagnosis of metachromatic leukodystrophy.

Metachromatic leukodystrophy (MLD) is a hereditary, neurodegenerative, metabolic condition associated with widespread demyelination in the central and peripheral nervous system. The inheritance pattern of MLD is autosomal recessive. The metabolic abnormality is caused by a mutation in the gene coding for enzyme arylsulfatase A that is localized on chromosome 22. Deficiency of arylsulfatase A prevents the conversion of sulfatide to cerebroside, a major component of myelin, which results in sulfatide accumulation in oligodendrocytes, Schwann cells, and other tissues. In addition to deficiency of arylsulfatase A, sulfatide activator deficiency and the multiple sulfatide deficiency are also associated with abnormal sulfatide accumulation and can produce a clinical picture closely related to MLD.

The disease usually manifests between the first and fourth year of life, but the clinical presentation may vary depending on residual levels of the arylsulfatase A activity that most likely reflect different types of mutation in the causative gene. The most common form of MLD is the infantile form, but juvenile- and adult-onset forms are also observed. In the late infantile form, the onset is typically between the first and second year of life and is manifested initially by motor and later by mental regression. The child becomes ataxic, develops progressive limb weakness, and progresses to loss of ability to walk and quadriplegia with dystonic features. The reflexes are initially brisk but may diminish when polyneuropathy develops and may eventually be lost. Within several years from the onset most children are profoundly disabled, bedridden, blind, and unable to communicate. The juvenile form typically develops with an insidious onset of behavioral problems or learning disabilities, followed by progressive motor and cognitive disability. Adult-onset cases may present with subtle behavioral changes, memory problems, depression, or psychotic episodes, followed by development of quadriparesis, dementia, pseudobulbar palsy, sphincter dysfunction, and dystonia. In the adult-onset form the peripheral neuropathy may be mild and reflexes may be preserved. Optic atrophy is present in about one-third of patients. Some patients may develop abdominal symptoms related to sulfatide gallbladder stones.

Pathologic examination typically shows widespread degeneration of myelinated fibers in the cerebrum, cerebellum, spinal cord, and peripheral nerves. Despite the widespread demyelination, the U-fibers are spared. The presence of metachromatic granules in glial cells and Schwann cells is characteristic and the diagnosis can be made from a biopsy of peripheral nerve that also typically shows segmental demyelination. The stored material, sulfatase, stains brown-orange rather than purple with iodine dyes. The abnormal metachromatic granules are typically also present in the retina, kidney, gallbladder, and other tissues.

Brain MRI is the most helpful initial diagnostic test and typically shows diffuse increase of signal on T2 weighted images in cerebral white matter, especially in periventricular and subcortical regions. Nerve conduction studies show evidence of predominantly demyelinating neuropathy. Cerebrospinal fluid analysis may show nonspecific elevation of the protein content (60–200 mg/dl). Biochemical testing in MLD shows marked decrease or absence of arylsulfatase A in urine, white blood cells, or cultured fibroblasts. Differentiation from a pseudoarylsulfatase deficiency may be necessary in some cases by a sulfatide loading assay. MLD can be diagnosed by DNA analysis, which can also be used for screening of family members at risk and prenatal diagnosis. Multiple different mutations in the gene coding for arylsulfatase polypeptide have been reported.

Adult-onset MLD may be very difficult to diagnose in early stages, especially when patients present with subtle behavioral or cognitive symptoms. Many patients who demonstrate psychotic behavior may initially be misdiagnosed of psychiatric conditions or learning disabilities. MLD, especially of infantile onset, has to be differentiated from other leukodystrophies such as adrenoleukodystrophy, globoid cell leukodystrophy, lipidoses, and a variety of other metabolic and neurodegenerative conditions, including Wilson's disease and Leigh disease.

Treatment with bone marrow transplantation has been attempted in some young patients with MLD and may slow symptom progression, but is not effective in patients with advanced neurologic disability. Management of patients is focused on symptomatic measures. Families with MLD should receive genetic counseling and individuals at risk should be offered screening genetic and biochemical testing. Assay of sulfatase activity in cultured amniocytes allows prenatal diagnosis.

In the present patient, the condition has been relentlessly progressive. Genetic counseling and screening evaluation of potentially affected relatives was offered to the patient's family.

Clinical Pearls

1. Metachromatic leukodystrophy may present with a wide spectrum of clinical symptoms.

2. Peripheral nerve involvement is common in leukodystrophies and nerve conduction studies may help establish the diagnosis.

3. Diffuse confluent white matter changes on the brain MRI should raise suspicion of a metabolic dysmyelination disorder.

4. Diagnosis of MLD can be established by brain MRI and demonstration of arylsulfatase A deficiency. DNA analysis is also available.

5. Genetic counseling should be offered to all families with MLD. Identification of carriers and prenatal diagnosis of this disease is possible with DNA and biochemical testing.

REFERENCES

1. Barth ML, Fensom A, Harris A: The arylsulfatase A gene and molecular genetics of metachromatic leukodystrophy. J Med Genet 1994; 31:663–666.
2. Berger J, Loschl B, Bernheimer H, et al: Occurrence, distribution and phenotype of arylsulfatase A mutations in patients with metachromatic leukodystrophy. Am J Med Genet 1997; 69:335–340.
3. Eto Y, Tahara T, Koda N, et al: Prenatal diagnosis of metachromatic leukodystrophy: A diagnosis by amniotic fluid and its confirmation. Arch Neurol 1982; 39:29–32.
4. Gieselmann V, Zlotogora J, Harris A, et al: Molecular genetics of metachromatic leukodystrophy. Hum Mutat 1994; 4:233–242.
5. Kappler J, Leinekugel P, Conzelmann E, et al: Genotype–phenotype relationship in various degrees of arylsulfatase A deficiency. Hum Genet 1991; 86:463–470.
6. Kihara H, Ho CK, Fluharty AL, et al: Prenatal diagnosis of metachromatic leukodystrophy in a family with pseudoarylsulfatase A deficiency by the cerebroside sulfate loading test. Pediatr Res 1980; 14:224–227.
7. Krivit W, Shapiro, Kennedy W, et al: Treatment of late infantile metachromatic leukodystrophy by bone marrow transplantation. N Engl J Med 1990; 322:28–32.

PATIENT 47

A 23-year-old man with a sudden onset of left-sided weakness and confusion

A 23-year-old previously healthy man was admitted to the hospital after he had been found lying on his apartment floor in a confused state. Paramedics found him lethargic and noted weakness of the left face, arm, and leg. Six weeks prior to hospitalization he experienced low-grade fever, night sweats, malaise, and anorexia, which persisted despite oral antibiotic therapy with azithromycin. During those 6 weeks he lost approximately 20 pounds and developed severe occipital headache. Review of neurologic and other systems was otherwise unremarkable. Medical history was significant for an uneventful appendectomy 12 weeks earlier and uneventful dental root canal surgery 8 weeks prior to hospitalization. There was no history of drug abuse.

Physical Examination: Pulse 108 and regular, respirations 25, blood pressure 126/84, rectal temperature 38.3°. Skin: clean, no rash. Neck: supple, no carotid bruits. Chest and abdomen: normal. Cardiac: systolic ejection grade III/VI murmur heard best over the mitral valve region. Mental status: stuporous but easily arousable, able to follow only one-step commands. Speech: severely dysarthric. Cranial nerves: pupils of normal size with normal reaction to light, normal fundi; normal visual fields to confrontation; mild left horizontal gaze preference; normal facial sensation; mild left lower facial weakness; oral and pharyngeal structures midline. Motor examination: muscle tone and mass normal; severe weakness (3) in the left upper extremity and lower extremities. Sensory examination: normal. Reflexes: increased (3) in the left upper and lower extremities. Coordination: normal in the right-sided extremities, unable to test on the left. Plantar reflexes: flexor on the right, extensor on the left. Gait: unable to test.

Stop and Consider: What is the time course and localization of the neurologic dysfunction? What is the significance of fever, abnormal cardiac examination, and systemic symptoms lasting for 6 weeks?

Laboratory Findings: Head MRI: see figure, *left*. Head MRA: decreased flow signal in branches of the left middle cerebral artery. CBC: WBC 17,500/µl (normal 3,500–8,500) with 92% PMNs; otherwise normal. ESR: 98 mm/hr (normal 0–25). Platelet count, PT, PTT, electrolytes, chemistry panel, protein C, protein S, antithrombin III: normal. HIV antibodies, antiphospholipid antibodies: negative. Transesophageal echocardiography: see figure, *right*. Blood cultures: positive for S*treptococcus viridans*.

Question: What abnormalities were demonstrated on the head MRI and echocardiography?

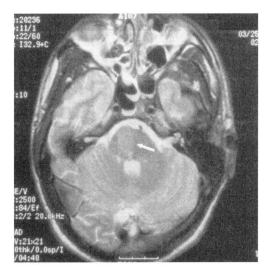
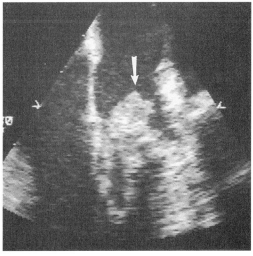

Diagnosis: Multiple cerebral infarctions caused by septic emboli in the course of *Streptococcus viridans* sepsis and subacute bacterial endocarditis with mitral valve vegetations

Discussion: The left hemiparesis and left lower facial weakness indicated involvement of the corticospinal and corticobulbar tracts that could be compatible with a right hemispheric lesion. The dysarthria could have been caused by a combination of corticobulbar tract involvement and his obtunded state. The left horizontal gaze preference was not compatible with a right frontal lesion and suggested a possible coexisting second lesion in the right paramedian pontine area or in the left frontal eye field. These findings in a patient with acute neurologic deficit associated with fever, cardiac murmur, and presence of malaise, fever, and weight loss strongly suggested cardioembolic stroke secondary to endocarditis. The brain MRI showed multiple areas of increased signal intensity on T2 images, including lesions in the right pons (figure on the left, arrow), left caudate, and putamen, consistent with multiple infarctions. His MRA showed a decreased flow signal in the left middle cerebral artery consistent with the underlying embolic stroke. The transesophageal echocardiography (TEE) showed a large, mobile strand attached to one of the mitral valve leaflets (figure on the right, arrow). The TEE results and positive blood cultures strongly supported the diagnosis of infectious endocarditis as the cause of this patient's brain infarctions.

The most common etiologies for multifocal acute ischemic lesions of the brain in young and middle-aged patients (ages 15–50 years) include evident sources for cardiac emboli, coagulopathies, and cerebral vasculitis. Cerebral infarcts associated with cardiogenic emboli often result in cerebral lesions situated in the junction between gray and white matter. With larger emboli, occlusion of larger-caliber cerebral vessels may result in infarctions in the territories of the middle or posterior cerebral arteries. Sometimes large emboli undergo thrombolysis and fragmentation into several smaller emboli, and depending on the adequacy of collateral circulation may result in distal secondary infarctions. Subcortical ischemic infarctions in the distribution of lenticulostriate vessels that are the deep irrigation zone of the middle, or less commonly the anterior, cerebral artery may also occur. In this patient, the subcortical infarction in the left basal ganglia and the abnormality of flow signal in the left middle cerebral artery branches are suggestive of a recent cardiogenic embolus to these brain regions.

The frequent association between CNS involvement and infective endocarditis (IE) has been recognized for more than a century and was first described by Sir William Osler. The disease is characterized by growth of microorganisms within a platelet-fibrin thrombus protruding from a cardiac valve leaflet with associated bacteremia and systemic arterial embolization. Risk factors for IE include surgical or invasive diagnostic procedures, intravenous drug abuse, recent dental procedures, neoplasms, and numerous cardiac conditions (especially valve replacement procedures).

IE should be suspected in the presence of a heart murmur and unexplained fever that persists for more than a week. The diagnosis of IE can be difficult because of the nonspecific systemic symptoms of endocarditis and the long latency between valve infection and neurologic events. The diagnosis of endocarditis requires a high index of suspicion supported by appropriate echocardiographic and blood culture findings. Echocardiographic study should be performed in all patients in whom infective endocarditis is suspected. Transesophageal echocardiogram (TEE) is much more sensitive than transthoracic echocardiogram (TTE) in detecting vegetations. Cranial CT and MR imaging have improved the detection of cerebral lesions that may not be accompanied by stroke-like events.

The incidence of neurologic events in infective endocarditis is approximately 30%, with the vast majority of these complications associated with left-sided cardiac valvular disease. Neurologic manifestations may be the presenting symptomatology in 16–23% of patients with infective endocarditis and may develop after the initiation of antimicrobial therapy in up to 30% of cases, usually within the first 2 weeks after the treatment has begun. Stroke or transient ischemic attacks are the most common neurologic complications occurring in association with infective endocarditis and occur in up to 20% of all patients with native valve endocarditis. The majority of these strokes or transient ischemic attacks occur before the diagnosis of IE is actually made. Because these emboli contain viable organisms, the CNS lesions may be ischemic, suppurative, or both. Further complications then arise, including aseptic or septic meningitis, brain abscess formation, or a nonspecific encephalopathy. Brain hemorrhage, either intracranial or subarachnoid, accounts for up to 7% of the neurologic manifestations of patients with IE; therefore, cerebral angiography should be considered in patients with a subarachnoid hemorrhage or if severe headache persists after control of infection. Brain hemorrhages are particularly common in patients with intravenous drug abuse and are most commonly associated with uncontrolled *Staphylococcus aureus* infection. Intracranial hemorrhage has traditionally been linked to the rupture of a mycotic aneurysm. Aneurysms may not develop until at least 7–10 days after the onset of focal neurologic symptoms. Aneurysm is not excluded if early angiographic findings are normal. Rupture of a mycotic aneurysm is associated with an 80% fatality rate.

The management of patients with IE is focused on rapid evaluation, appropriate antimicrobial therapy, and treatment of complications. The choice of antimicrobial therapy should be based on the isolation of the responsible microorganism on repeat blood cultures and aimed at eradication of all microorganisms from the vegetation. Broad antibiotic coverage may be initially necessary until specific microorganism is identified.

When curative antimicrobial therapy is not possible (e.g., in most cases of fungal endocarditis), when positive blood cultures persist during therapy, or when patients develop recurrent strokes despite appropriate antibiotic therapy, replacement of the valve should be considered. Immediate replacement is essential in patients developing heart failure secondary to severe valvular regurgitation. Neurosurgical intervention may be necessary for patients with symptomatic intracranial hemorrhages and for those with large or expanding mycotic aneurysms. Anticoagulants should be continued in patients with endocarditis who have prosthetic valves and there is no evidence of intracranial hemorrhage.

This patient's subacute bacterial endocarditis was probably a complication of either the recent appendectomy or dental surgery. Because of severe damage of the mitral valve, he underwent surgical valve replacement approximately 1 week after the stroke. Conventional cerebral angiogram was performed after the successful valve replacement surgery and was unremarkable, without any evidence of possible vasculitis or aneurysm. He was placed on long-term anticoagulation therapy with Coumadin and his neurologic function recovered to the extent that he was able to carry out activities of daily living without any assistance.

Clinical Pearls

1. Infective endocarditis is a relatively rare cause of stroke and may be a complication of diagnostic and therapeutic invasive procedures, intravenous drug abuse, cardiac disease, or neoplasms.

2. Development of a sudden neurologic deficit in a patient with systemic symptoms such as malaise, fever, and weight loss, and abnormal cardiac examination should raise suspicion of possible infective endocarditis.

3. A neurologic deficit may be the presenting symptom in over 20% of patients with infective endocarditis.

REFERENCES

1. Hart RG, Foster JW, Luther MF, et al: Stroke in infective endocarditis. Stroke 1990; 21:695–700.
2. Salgado AV: Central nervous system complications of infective endocarditis. Stroke 1991; 22:1461–1463.
3. Tunkel AR, Kaye D: Neurologic complications of infective endocarditis. Neurol Clin 1993; 11:419–440.

PATIENT 48

A 74-year-old man with a 6-week history of progressive disequilibrium, speech difficulty, and confusion

A 74-year-old man was admitted with a 6-week history of progressive gait unsteadiness, dysarthria, dysphagia, memory problems, and confusion. He also experienced episodes of vertigo and developed difficulty with fine motor skills. Two days prior to admission he developed fever, abdominal pain, and nausea. His medical history was significant for chronic lymphocytic leukemia that was diagnosed 5 years previously and treated with fludarabine. Fludarabine was discontinued 6 weeks earlier, after the onset of his neurologic symptoms that progressed nevertheless. He had a history of hepatic duct obstruction caused by leukemic infiltration that was treated with biliary stents. His medical history was also significant for coronary artery disease, atrial fibrillation, hypertension, and left carotid artery stenosis with episodes of amaurosis fugax, treated with carotid endarterectomy 5 years earlier. He had been receiving Coumadin for atrial fibrillation, but it was discontinued several weeks prior to this hospitalization because of frequent falls.

Physical Examination: Pulse 80, respirations 18, blood pressure 130/80, oral temperature 39.5°. Cachectic and ill-appearing elderly male, unable to follow commands. Cardiac: irregularly irregular rhythm and rate, no murmur. Chest exam: normal. Abdomen: diffusely tender but no peritoneal signs. Neck: supple, no carotid bruits, no lymphadenopathy. Mental status and speech: disoriented, confused, speech severely dysarthric, incoherent. Cranial nerves: pupils equal, normal and reactive to light; no papilledema, visual acuity and visual fields could not be assessed; oculocephalic reflexes normal; facial movements symmetric, gag reflex intact, tongue midline without atrophy. Motor examination: muscle bulk diffusely diminished without focal atrophy, spasticity in all four extremities, mild left hemiparesis. Sensory examination: stronger withdrawal reaction to painful stimuli on the right. Muscle stretch reflexes: brisk (grade 3) bilaterally and symmetric. Plantar reflexes: bilateral Babinski signs. Coordination and gait: not tested due to confusion.

Stop and Consider: What is the time course and localization of the neurologic dysfunction? What is the differential diagnosis of cognitive decline and multifocal neurologic abnormality in a patient with leukemia?

Laboratory Findings: WBC: 6,300/μl (3,500–8,500), hemoglobin 11 g/dl (13.6–16.8), platelets 84,000/μl (160,000–170,000). Electrolytes, PT, PTT, liver and renal function tests: normal. Brain MRI: see figure on opposite page, *left.* MRA: normal. CSF analysis: cell count: 7/μl (all lymphocytes), protein 47 mg/dl (0–45), glucose 64 mg/dl (serum glucose 104); PCR analysis for herpes simplex virus: negative; bacterial and fungal CSF cultures and CSF cytology: negative. Biliary drainage culture and blood cultures: positive for *Enterococcus* sp. and *Candida albicans.* Cardiac echo: no evidence of cardiac source of emboli.

Hospital Course: The rapid deterioration of mental status was presumably caused by biliary sepsis, but despite treatment with intravenous antibiotics he expired shortly after admission. Autopsy findings: leukemic infiltrates in numerous lymph nodes, hepatobiliary system, lungs, kidneys, and GI tract. Brain immunocytochemical stain with anti–JC virus antigen antibody: see figure on opposite page, *right.*

Question: What is the significance of the MRI abnormalities?

Diagnosis: Progressive multifocal leukoencephalopathy in a patient with advanced chronic lymphocytic leukemia

Discussion: The neurologic examination indicated diffuse cortical dysfunction with bilateral, asymmetric corticospinal tract involvement. Several conditions were considered in the differential diagnosis as possible explanations of his rapidly deteriorating mental status and focal signs. His progressive confusion could have been caused by biliary sepsis, but his neurologic deterioration started a few weeks before biliary tract infection had developed. Bacterial, fungal, or parasitic (e.g., toxoplasmosis) CNS infections are common in immunocompromised patients, but were unlikely because of negative CSF studies. Herpes encephalitis was ruled out with a negative PCR test. Multiple cerebral infarcts could possibly explain his neurologic status, but the step-like deterioration was not clearly elicited in this case. Neoplastic leukemic meningitis was unlikely with negative CSF studies, including cytology. Fludarabine neurotoxicity was initially considered, but the course of the illness was progressive despite discontinuation of the medication. Chronic subdural hematoma or cerebral hemorrhage due to bleeding diathesis were ruled out by neuroimaging studies. Other considerations included a paraneoplastic syndrome or Creutzfeldt-Jacob disease.

MRI of the brain showed extensive, multifocal areas of increased signal on T2 images in the periventricular white matter (figure on the left, arrow), centrum semiovale, and bilateral middle cerebellar peduncles. The diffuse white matter abnormalities were consistent with a demyelinating process or diffuse ischemic lesions; however, the abnormality in the cerebellar peduncles would be unusual for ischemic changes. The brain autopsy showed diffuse, multiple foci of demyelination and necrosis in the white matter extending into the gray–white matter junction, with relative preservation of axons and numerous abnormal oligodendrocytes with swollen, hyperchromatic nuclei. These findings were very suggestive of progressive multifocal encephalopathy (PML). Immunocytochemical stain with anti–JC virus antigen antibody showed strongly positive reaction in oligodendrocytic nuclei (figure on the right, arrow), confirming the diagnosis of PML. The electron microscopy demonstrated characteristic viral inclusions in the oligodendrocytes.

PML is caused by either a primary infection or reactivation of infection by JC virus in brain oligodendrocytes with impairment of myelin production. The JC virus is a double-stranded DNA virus that belongs to the *Papovaviridae* subfamily. Asymptomatic infection with JC virus is common and more then 75% of population develop antibodies against the JC virus by adulthood.

PML develops in association with conditions that compromise cell-mediated immunity, such as

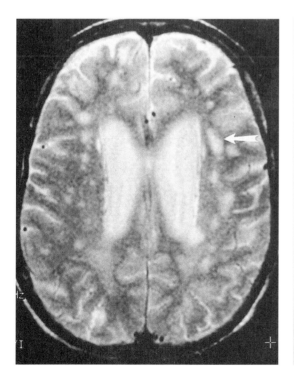
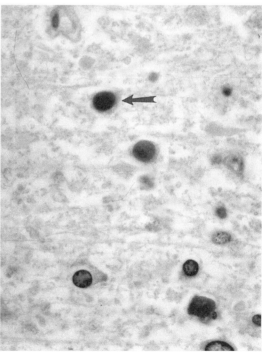

lymphoma, leukemia, multiple myeloma, sarcoidosis, tuberculosis, AIDS, connective tissue diseases treated with immunosuppressive drugs, or after renal transplants. Cases of PML also have occurred in patients with carcinoma and only a few cases of PML without underlying disease have been reported. AIDS is now the most frequent condition associated with PML. Cases of HIV-associated PML are usually more severe and progress more rapidly than PML associated with other conditions.

PML affects the white matter pathways of the cerebral hemispheres, cerebellum, brain stem, and rarely the spinal cord. The clinical manifestations depend on the neuroanatomic localization of the lesions. Patients typically develop cognitive deficits, memory problems, or behavioral and personality changes, which eventually progress to dementia, obtundation, and coma. Focal neurologic deficits such as hemianopia, hemiparesis, dysarthria, dysphasia, dysphagia, or gait abnormalities are common. Patients may also present with cranial nerve palsies or vertigo, but extrapyramidal signs are relatively rare. Seizures may develop in up to 20% of patients, especially in advanced stages of PML. The course is relentlessly progressive and most patients die within a few months to a year. Rare patients may stabilize or possibly improve.

Traditionally, brain tissue examination, either from biopsy or autopsy, has been necessary for definitive diagnosis of PML. Recently, CSF examination with PCR analysis has been introduced for JC virus infection and has been more than 90% sensitive. In a typical clinical setting of an immunocompromised patient with neurologic decline and brain MRI showing characteristic white matter changes, positive PCR for JC virus in CSF confirms the diagnosis of PML and brain biopsy is not necessary.

There is no effective treatment for PML, but cytosine arabinoside, alpha interferon, and other antiviral agents have been used. In patients who developed PML in the course of immunosuppressive treatment, remissions have been reported after withdrawal of immunosuppressive agents.

Clinical Pearls

1. PML should be suspected in immunocompromised patients with progressive cognitive decline or focal neurologic findings.

2. Brain MRI demonstrating multifocal demyelination in immunocompromised patients is suggestive but not specific for PML.

3. PML is a relatively common complication of advanced HIV infection.

4. Most patients with PML die within a few months to a year from the onset of neurologic symptoms.

5. In patients who present with clinical and MRI findings consistent with PML, PCR testing for JC virus in CSF can confirm the diagnosis and brain biopsy is not necessary.

REFERENCES

1. Aksamit AJ Jr: Progressive multifocal leukoencephalopathy: A review of the pathology and pathogenesis. Microsc Res Tech 1995; 32:302–311.
2. Krupp LB, Lipton RB, Swerdlow ML, et al: Progressive multifocal leukoencephalopathy: Clinical and radiographic features. Ann Neurol 1985; 17:344–349.
3. Richardson EP Jr: Progressive multifocal leukoencephalopathy 30 years later. N Engl J Med 1988; 318:315–317.
4. Weber T, Major E: Progressive multifocal leukoencephalopathy: Molecular biology, pathogenesis and clinical impact. Intervirology 1997; 40:98–111.
5. Weber T, Trebst C, Frye S, et al: Analysis of the systemic and intrathecal humoral immune response in progressive multifocal leukoencephalopathy. J Infect Dis 1997; 176:250–254.
6. Zu-Rhein GM: Association of papova-virions with a human demyelinating disease (progressive multifocal leukoencephalopathy). Prog Med Virol 1060; 11:185–247.

PATIENT 49

A 32-year-old man with sudden onset of dysphasia, headache, vomiting, and lethargy

A 32-year-old man presented with a 3-day history of progressive headache. On the day of the evaluation he also abruptly developed a speech disturbance characterized by inability to express himself, accompanied by tingling sensations on the right side of his body, nausea, vomiting, fatigue, and chills. He denied recent trauma, prior history of headache, other neurologic symptoms, or drug abuse. He had a history of mild depression in the past, but was not taking any antidepressants or other medications.

Physical Examination: Pulse 92 and regular, respirations 12 and regular, blood pressure 140/88, temperature 37.2°. Skin, neck, chest, and abdomen: normal. Cardiac exam: normal. Mental status and speech: lethargic but easily arousable, unable to follow multistep commands, difficulty with repetitions and naming, markedly reduced speech output. Cranial nerves: normal fundi; probable right inferior homonymous visual field loss; mild left conjugal gaze preference; pupillary reflexes intact; muscles of facial expression normal and symmetric; oral and pharyngeal structures midline. Motor examination: normal muscle tone and mass, slight pronator drift on the right but otherwise normal power, no tremor. Sensory examination: decreased sensation to light touch, vibration, and pain on the right side of the body. Muscle stretch reflexes: normal, symmetric. Coordination: normal. Plantar reflexes: flexor. Gait: mildly ataxic.

Stop and Consider: What is the time course and localization of the neurologic dysfunction? What is the differential diagnosis, and what is the significance of abnormal mental status accompanied by headache and a focal cerebral abnormality?

Laboratory Findings: WBC: 15,000/µl (3,500–8,500). Coagulation profile, electrolytes, chemistry panel: normal. Head CT scan with contrast: see figure. Skull, sinus, and chest x-rays: normal. Cardiac echocardiogram: normal. Blood and urine cultures: negative.

Question: What is suggested by the abnormality demonstrated on the head CT?

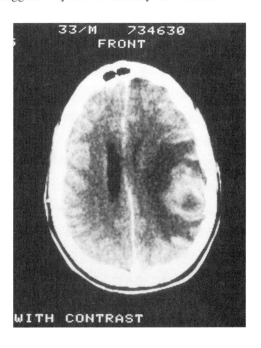

Diagnosis: Brain abscess in the left frontoparietal region

Discussion: The clinical presentation with headache, nausea, vomiting, and lethargy suggested elevated intracranial pressure. The left gaze preference (presumably due to impairment of the left frontal gaze center) and right hemisensory abnormalities with mild right-sided weakness suggested an acute process in the left cerebral hemisphere that could also account for his speech problems with both expressive and receptive dysfunction, but it is difficult to confirm dysphasia in the presence of abnormal alertness. The differential diagnosis should include acute mass lesions such as ischemic or hemorrhagic stroke, hemorrhage within a brain neoplasm, traumatic brain hemorrhage, or a localized CNS infection such as abscess. Head CT scan showed a large hypodense mass lesion with a pattern of ring enhancement in the left frontoparietal region and cerebral edema. Brain abscess, resolving cerebral hemorrhage, and malignant neoplasms such as gliomas may present as ring-enhancing lesions. In this patient, with the rapidly progressive course with fever, lateralized focal neurologic abnormalities, signs of increased intracranial pressure, and the ring-enhancing lesion on cranial CT, the diagnosis of a brain abscess was the most likely one.

Brain abscess occurs with incidence of 4 per million population. It may occur at any age but is most common in the third decade of life. Except for cases in which infection may be introduced through compound skull fractures or intracranial operations (about 10%), brain abscess usually results from seeding of infection from infectious sources that may not be apparent in some cases. At least 40% of all brain abscesses are secondary to infectious disease of the paranasal sinuses, middle ear, and mastoid air cells. Otogenic and rhinogenic brain abscesses may arise by direct extension into brain from middle ear or nasal sinuses infection and associated osteomyelitis. Spread of inflammation and bacterial penetration of the dura and meninges may occur directly or through venous structures. This mechanism helps explain how an abscess may spread sometimes form a considerable distance from the primary infectious source in the middle ear or paranasal sinuses. Hematogenic dissemination of infectious organisms can produce abscess formation from extracranial sources. Common risk factors include suppurative pulmonary infections, bacterial endocarditis, and dental infections. Brain abscesses in young children are frequently associated with cyanotic congenital heart disease. AIDS and other conditions associated with immunosuppression are also significant risk factors. In approximately 10–20% of all cases of brain abscesses the infectious source cannot be identified.

The most common organism causing brain abscess, especially in association with cranial sinuses or dental infections, is *Streptococcus vitadans*. Other relatively frequent microorganisms associated with brain abscess formation include *Proteus*, *Pseudomonas*, *Pneumococcus*, *Meningococcus*, and *Haemophilus* species and *Escherichia coli*. In many cases multiple microorganisms can be isolated. *Staphylococcus aureus* is frequently associated with penetrating trauma or neurosurgical procedures. Fungal abscesses may occur, especially in immunocompromised patients. The most common causes of brain abscess in patients with AIDS are toxoplasmosis or cryptococcosis.

Headache is the most frequent initial clinical symptom of an intracranial abscess. Other presenting symptoms include drowsiness, confusion, focal or generalized seizures, focal motor and sensory deficits, or speech disorders. The triad of headache, fever, and focal neurologic signs suggests brain abscess, but this typical presentation is observed in only a minority of patients. Stiff neck may accompany the generalized headache and suggest meningitis. Stroke is suggested by the rapid onset of focal neurologic deficit in some patients with brain abscess. The particular neurologic signs will depend on the location of the abscess. Frontal lobe abscess may present with headache, drowsiness, inattention, hemiparesis with unilateral seizures or a disorder of speech with involvement of the dominant hemisphere. An abscess in the parietal lobe may be accompanied by inferior contralateral quadrantanopsia, cortical sensory syndromes, or hemi-neglect. An occipital lobe abscess can produce a homonymous hemianopia. An abscess in the frontotemporal region of the dominant hemisphere may cause aphasia. In cerebellar abscess, headache may be localized to the postauricular or suboccipital region and be accompanied by cerebellar ataxia of the ipsilateral arm and leg and gaze dysfunction. Cerebellar abscesses may cause brain stem compression or obstructive hydrocephalus. Regardless of the focal signs, brain abscesses usually produce drowsiness, stupor, and inattentiveness, which may obscure other neurologic findings.

MRI with contrast or CT with contrast should be obtained rapidly in all patients with a suspected brain abscess. Early imaging findings include areas of localized abnormalities related to cerebritis, but after 4–5 days encapsulation occurs and results in ring enhancement with surrounding edema. Abscesses larger than 1 cm can be reliably detected, so for practical purposes an abscess is unlikely if the CT or MRI scan is normal. It may be difficult to exclude subdural empyema, cerebritis, brain infarction, herpes simplex encephalitis, and acute hemorrhagic leukoencephalitis on the basis of the appearances of the lesion on imaging studies. Lumbar puncture is contraindicated in patients with suspected brain abscess because of the risk of brain herniation.

Source of infection in the middle ear, mastoid, sinuses, lungs, or heart, or the presence of right-to-left cardiac shunt should be excluded in all patients. If there is no apparent source of infection, surgical exploration and bacterial cultures from the surgical specimen may be necessary to make a definitive diagnosis. The surgical treatment of brain abscess may involve aspiration or excision. Stereotactic, CT-guided aspiration is associated with less brain trauma than excision. Management includes treatment of increased intracranial pressure, identification of the responsible organism, and appropriate intravenous antibiotic therapy. Small abscesses (< 3 cm in diameter) in stable patients may be treated with IV antibiotics without surgery and followed with serial CTs or MRIs. Intravenous antibiotics should be started as soon as the diagnosis is suspected and should include broad-spectrum coverage until specific infectious agent can be identified.

The present patient was initially started on broad-spectrum intravenous antibiotics and acyclovir but infectious source was not identified. He underwent neurosurgical drainage and excision and the cultures from the abscess revealed mixed *Haemophilus* and *Streptococcus* strains, both sensitive to penicillin. The elevated intracranial pressure was treated with intravenous mannitol prior to surgery. Postoperatively he received intravenous penicillin for 6 weeks. With rehabilitation, he was eventually discharged with only a minimal expressive speech difficulties.

Clinical Pearls

1. Headache, nausea, vomiting, focal neurologic signs, and fever strongly suggest a brain abscess with elevated intracranial pressure.

2. In a patient with suspected brain abscess, a head MRI or CT with contrast and blood cultures should be rapidly obtained and broad-spectrum antibiotic coverage initiated until specific infectious agents can be identified.

3. Extensive diagnostic work-up for the primary infectious organisms should be undertaken in all patients with brain abscess, and the underlying condition should be appropriately treated.

4. Some patients with small brain abscesses and stable neurologic status may be treated with intravenous antibiotics alone with careful clinical monitoring and serial CT or MRI evaluations, but surgical excision or drainage is required for larger lesions.

REFERENCES

1. Ersahin Y, Mutluer S, Guzelbag E: Brain abscess in infants and children. Childs Nerv Syst 1994; 10:185–189.
2. Kaplan K: Brain abscess. Med Clin North Am 1985; 69:345–360.
3. Mamelak AN, Mampalan TJ, Obana WG, et al: Improvement of multiple brain abscesses: A combined surgical and medical approach. Neurosurgery 1995; 36:76–85.

PATIENT 50

A 71-year-old woman with progressive bilateral visual impairment and headache

A 71-year-old woman presented to the clinic with a 6-month history of slowly progressive, bitemporal, pounding, daily headache that increased noticeably with coughing or sneezing. She also complained of malaise, fatigue, and occasional bouts of nausea. Over the past 2–3 months she complained of slowly progressive bilateral visual impairment, which she described as recurrent "fogginess of vision." At other times she was unable to open her left eye. She had no history of headache and denied any recent head or neck trauma, limb weakness and numbness, or difficulty walking. Her medical history was otherwise noncontributory.

Physical Examination: Pulse 68 and regular, blood pressure 136/70, temperature and respirations normal. Skin: slightly pale, dry. Cardiac, chest, and abdomen: normal. Neck examination: normal, no arterial bruits. Mental status, affect, speech, and language: normal. Cranial nerves: normal visual acuity and pupillary reflexes, bitemporal hemianopsia; funduscopic evaluation: mild bilateral disc pallor; left-sided ptosis, left eye exotropia with diminished left eye adduction; facial expressions normal, hearing intact, oral and pharyngeal structures midline. Motor examination: normal muscle bulk, tone, and power. Sensory examination: normal. Muscle stretch reflexes: normal (2). Plantar reflexes: flexor. Coordination and gait: normal.

Stop and Consider: What is the time course and localization of the neurologic dysfunction?

Laboratory Findings: CBC, ESR, platelet count, PT, PTT, electrolytes, chemistry panel, urinanalysis: normal. Head MRI: see figure. Serum prolactin, growth hormone, and cortisol levels and thyroid function studies: normal.

Question: What abnormalities does the head MRI show?

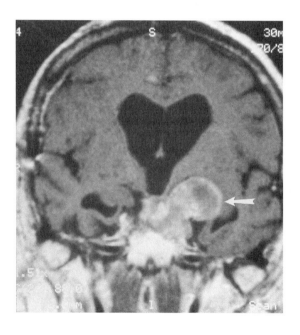

Diagnosis: Pituitary adenoma

Discussion: The clinical presentation of this patient with progressive headache exacerbated by coughing or sneezing and progressive visual impairment suggested an intracranial lesion associated with increased intracranial pressure. The presence of bitemporal hemianopsia indicated optic chiasm involvement. The third nerve palsy was most likely caused by compression of the nerve along its course in the cavernous sinus.

The diagnosis of a pituitary tumor compressing the optic chiasm and nearby structures was strongly suspected. The head MRI scan showed an expanding tumor arising from the sella turcica (figure, arrow), with surrounding mass effect and suprasellar extension into the left choroid fissure and mesencephalic cistern. The tumor was contrast-enhancing with solid and cystic components consistent with pituitary adenoma. There was also evidence of hydrocephalus. There were no clinical signs of acromegaly, Cushing's syndrome, or hyperprolactinemia and the unremarkable hormonal studies indicated that the pituitary adenoma was probably nonsecretory.

Pituitary adenomas (PAs) account for 10–50% of all intracranial neoplasms. They can cause pituitary hormonal disorders and deficits caused by invasion or compression of surrounding structures. Pituitary microadenomas may present exclusively with hormonal disturbances. Occasionally, the diagnosis is the result of an incidental finding on skull x-ray, head CT scan, or cranial MR imaging. Small pituitary tumors are also present in 6–20% of adults at autopsy.

The most common visual field defect observed in a patient with a pituitary macroadenoma is a variable pattern of bitemporal hemianopsia. About 8% of patients progress to complete loss of vision in one eye with a temporal visual field defect in the opposite eye. When PAs cause visual field defects, sellar enlargement is usually present. PAs may also extend laterally, invade the cavernous sinus, and cause third nerve palsy. Lateral extension may also involve the fourth and sixth cranial nerves, cause pain or numbness in the distribution of the fifth cranial nerve, or cause compression or obstruction of the ipsilateral carotid artery. Very large pituitary tumors may invade hypothalamus and may cause clinical signs related to hypothalamic dysfunction, such as hyperphagia, hypo- or hyperthermia, disturbances of consciousness, and personality changes. Obstructive hydrocephalus following the third ventricle compression is less common with pituitary adenomas than with cranial craniopharyngiomas. Tumor invasion into the temporal lobe may also be associated with partial complex seizures,

while invasion of the frontal lobe may cause various neurobehavioral changes. Headaches are common in patients with pituitary adenomas and are thought to be due to stretching of the diaphragm of the sella. The headache may be referred to the vertex of the skull or may be retro-orbital, fronto-occipital, frontotemporal, or radiate to occipital-cervical areas.

Prolactinoma is the most common pituitary tumor and most prolactin-secreting tumors are microadenomas. They may produce galactorrhea, amenorrhea, or infertility. Tumors secreting growth hormone may cause either acromegaly or gigantism. Adrenocorticotropic hormone (ACTH)–secreting adenomas cause Cushing's disease. About 15% of pituitary tumors secrete more than one hormone. Nonsecretory tumors may present with symptoms of hypopituitarism.

Acute hemorrhagic infarction of a PA may cause a dramatic syndrome of pituitary apoplexy, which includes severe headache, nausea, vomiting, and depressed consciousness. Ophthalmoplegia, visual and pupillary disturbances, and meningismus may be present. These symptoms are caused by direct pressure from the tumor and meningismus resulting from blood in the cerebrospinal fluid spaces. Pituitary apoplexy may evolve slowly over a period of 24–48 hours or may present with rapid progression to death.

Space-occupying lesions other than pituitary adenomas may sometimes expand the sella. Sellar enlargement may be due to carotid artery aneurysm, cyst of the pituitary gland, or intrasellar craniopharyngioma. Head CT or MRI with contrast are usually sufficient to define the pathology in the intrasellar or suprasellar regions. Conventional skull x-rays define the contours of the sella turcica and may show enlargement, erosion, or calcification of this region. Angiography is sometimes required when aneurysm or vascular malformation is suspected. PAs are generally isointense on T1 weighted MR images and moderately hyperintense on T2 weighted images, and show a variable degree of contrast enhancement.

The scope of endocrinologic testing in patients with newly diagnosed PAs is dependent on the clinical findings and patient's age. In addition to routine chemistries, electrolytes, and thyroid function tests, all patients should have prolactin levels checked. Other useful tests may include growth hormone (GH), insulin-like growth factor 1 (IGF-1), cortisol, testosterone, estrogen, follicle-stimulating hormone (FSH), and luteinizing hormone (LH) levels.

Therapy for pituitary adenomas includes medical and surgical interventions. Prolactinomas are the most common hypersecreting pituitary tumors and may be successfully treated with a dopamine agonist bromocriptine. It reduces the prolactin levels in most patients and in approximately 90% of patients marked reduction of the tumor size may be achieved. If tumor reduction is not sufficient, surgery should be performed. Somatostatin analog octreotide may reduce the growth hormone level and reduce tumor size of adenomas that secrete growth hormone, but these tumors usually require surgical treatment. ACTH-producing tumors can be treated surgically by transsphenoidal approach. Patients with nonsecretory adenomas presenting with signs of a mass lesion should be treated surgically. Although most patients can be treated by a transsphenoidal approach, craniotomy may be required. Total resection is often not possible because of invasion of surrounding structures, and postoperative irradiation may be required. Complications of surgery are usually minimal but may include hypopituitarism, transient or permanent diabetes insipidus, spinal fluid rhinorrhea, permanent visual loss, oculomotor palsy, and meningitis.

The present patient underwent craniotomy with subtotal resection of the pituitary tumor and also received radiation therapy. She also underwent a ventriculoperitoneal shunt placement to treat the hydrocephalus. The pathologic studies confirmed the diagnosis of a pituitary adenoma. Immunocytochemical studies were negative for ACTH, GH, LH, TSH, and prolactin with few small foci of cells with mild FSH positivity. Postoperatively the patient developed hypopituitarism and required replacement treatment with levothyroxine and hydrocortisone.

Clinical Pearls

1. Patients with pituitary tumors may present with symptoms of hormonal disturbance or neurologic deficits caused by compression of adjacent structures such as the optic chiasm.

2. Bitemporal hemianopia localizes lesions to the optic chiasm.

3. Prolactin-hypersecreting tumors may be successfully treated with the dopamine receptor agonist bromocriptine.

4. Most pituitary tumors that require surgical treatment can be resected through a transsphenoidal approach.

5. Total resection of large pituitary macroadenomas may not be possible and postoperative radiation therapy should be considered.

REFERENCES

1. Andrews DW: Pituitary adenomas. Curr Opin Oncol 1997; 9:55–60.
2. Kane LA, Leinung MC, Scheithauer BW, et al: Pituitary adenomas in childhood and adolescence. J Clin Endocrinol Metab 1994; 79:1135–1140.
3. Molitch ME: Approach to the incidentally discovered pituitary mass. Cancer Treat Res 1997; 89:73–90.
4. Weinstein J, Isaacs S, Shore D, et al: Diagnosis and management of pituitary tumors. Compr Ther 1997; 23:594–604.

PATIENT 51

A 49-year-old man with a 1-year history of fatigue, bilateral arm weakness, recurrent diplopia, and difficulty chewing

A 49-year-old man presented with a 1-year history of progressive difficulty chewing. He had also noticed recurrent episodes of diplopia, which initially bothered him only toward the end of the day, but then became constant. He complained of easy fatigability during any activities that required him to keep his arms above his head. He denied weakness in lower extremities, sensory disturbances, or difficulty with bladder or bowel function. He had a history of hypothyroidism treated with thyroid replacement, and adult-onset diabetes mellitus treated with insulin. He was not aware of any family members with similar symptoms.

Physical Examination: Vital signs: normal. Cardiac and chest: normal. Neck: supple, no bruits. Mental status and speech: normal. Cranial nerves: pupils equal, 3 mm in diameter, with normal reaction to light and accommodation; bilateral ptosis (left > right) that worsened with sustained effort to keep his eyes open; bilateral weakness (left > right) of eye adduction, worsened by sustained effort to look upward, which induced diplopia; mild jaw weakness; no other cranial nerve abnormalities. Motor examination: minimal proximal weakness in the upper extremities with significant increase of weakness after brief exercise. Sensory examination: normal. Muscle stretch reflexes: normal. Plantar reflexes: flexor. Coordination and gait: normal.

Stop and Consider: What is the significance of fluctuating weakness that worsens with effort?

Laboratory Findings: CBC, chemistry panel, electrolytes, TSH, ESR: normal. Hemoglobin A_1C: 7.1% (normal 4.3–6.1%). Acetylcholine receptor (ACHR) binding and modulating antibodies: negative. Anti-striational muscle antibodies: negative. Antinuclear antibodies: negative. Nerve conduction study (NCS): normal latencies and normal amplitudes of motor and sensory responses, normal sensory and motor conduction velocities. Repetitive nerve stimulation (RNS) test at low (2 Hz) stimulation frequency: see figure. Needle electromyography: normal. Chest CT: normal.

Question: What is the physiologic significance of the RNS findings and how do they relate to this patient's symptoms?

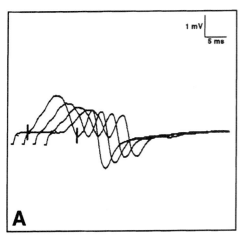 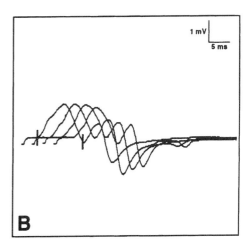

2 Hz repetitive nerve stimulation (RNS) test. Stimulation of the facial nerve, recording over the nasalis muscle. *A,* At rest. *B,* After maximal voluntary exercise for 10 seconds.

Diagnosis: Myasthenia gravis

Discussion: The patient's fluctuating symptoms, worsened by exercise or effort, and particularly the pronounced fluctuating ocular weakness, were typical for myasthenia gravis (MG). The mild proximal weakness in the upper extremities, worsened by exercise, was also typical of MG. The absence of ACHR antibodies is not an unusual finding, because 20–30% of patients with diffuse MG and up to 50% of patients with ocular MG have no detectable ACHR antibodies. Cranial neuropathies secondary to diabetes or botulism, which also may produce ocular and bulbar weakness, were unlikely. The RNS showed a significant decrement (35%) with low (2 Hz) frequency of stimulation (panel *A*) and repair of the decrement after 10 seconds of maximal voluntary exercise (panel *B*) (post-exercise facilitation), which was followed 2 minutes later by worsening of the decrement (post-exercise exhaustion), consistent with the diagnosis of MG. Lack of any significant increment of the compound muscle action potential (CMAP) amplitude after exercise pointed away from conditions caused by a presynaptic neuromuscular transmission defect, such as Lambert-Eaton myasthenic syndrome (LEMS) or botulism.

MG is a disorder of neuromuscular transmission caused by an autoimmune response against the acetylcholine receptor (ACHR), a postsynaptic element of the neuromuscular junction. The diagnosis of MG is typically made on the basis of clinical findings, electrodiagnostic studies, pharmacologic testing (edrophonium test), and laboratory testing for ACHR antibodies.

The most characteristic clinical feature of MG is fluctuating weakness of voluntary muscles that is exacerbated by exercise and improves with rest. The weakness, fatigue, and other symptoms frequently progress in the course of the day. Ocular weakness (manifesting as diplopia or ptosis) or bulbar weakness (manifesting as dysphagia, dysarthria, or weakness of mastication) are the most common initial complaints. Approximately 80% of patients have ocular involvement after 1 month from onset of symptoms. Most patients develop more generalized weakness within 1 year from the onset, but in approximately 20% of patients the weakness remains limited to ocular muscles.

The differential diagnosis of MG should include other conditions affecting the neuromuscular transmission. Botulism or LEMS can be usually excluded on the basis of distinct clinical features, characteristic electrodiagnostic findings, which typically show a marked increase in the CMAP amplitude after brief intense exercise or incremental

response on high-frequency (20–50 Hz) RNS test, and laboratory tests. Progressive ophthalmoplegia may be a feature of several mitochondrial disorders but the weakness in these disorders is not fluctuating, as is the case in ophthalmoplegia caused by hypothyroidism. Ptosis, facial, and limb weakness are common in many myopathies and sometimes may cause diagnostic difficulties, but weakness in muscle diseases is typically fixed and characteristic fluctuation with exercise is not appreciated. It is not uncommon that patients presenting with bulbar symptoms are initially thought to have a brain stem stroke or motor neuron disease.

Approximately 70–80% of patients with diffuse MG and 50–70% of patients with ocular MG have ACHR-binding antibodies. Rare patients (< 5%) who lack binding antibodies may have ACHR-modulating antibodies. Approximately 30% of patients with generalized MG have anti-striational antibodies, but in cases of MG associated with thymoma they are positive in 80% of cases.

Electrodiagnostic evaluation with the RNS test, if at least one distal and one proximal muscle are tested, is positive in 75% of generalized and less than 50% of ocular MG cases. Single-fiber electromyography (SFEMG), which is very sensitive for detection of a defect in neuromuscular transmission, is abnormal in 97–99% of patients. It is important to remember that both RNS and SFEMG are not specific for neuromuscular junction disorders and may be abnormal in both myopathic and neurogenic conditions. Tensilon (edrophonium) test is very helpful, especially in ocular MG, but should be placebo-controlled and double-blinded. Precautionary measures should be taken to avoid unnecessary complications. CT scan should be performed in all patients with MG to assess for the presence of thymoma.

Transient neonatal MG is observed in infants of mothers with MG as result of passive transplacental transfer of maternal ACHR antibodies. These babies may be floppy, hypotonic, have respiratory and feeding difficulties, but only about 15% have ocular abnormalities. In general, about 10–12% of babies born to mothers with MG develop this complication. Neonatal MG should be distinguished from different forms of congenital myasthenic syndromes, which are genetically determined conditions. Congenital myasthenic syndromes should always be considered in children and adults with seronegative MG. As in this case, there is increased prevalence of other autoimmune conditions in MG patients and their families, such as thyroid disease, systemic lupus erythematosus, rheumatoid arthritis, pernicious anemia, or polymyositis.

The goal of treatment in patients with MG is to improve weakness and induce remission with minimal side effects. The natural history of MG is variable and up to 20% of patients may achieve significant remission without any treatment. At the time of diagnosis patients should be educated and counseled about signs and symptoms of MG and different treatment modalities and their side effects. All medications that may interfere with neuromuscular transmission should be avoided.

Treatment of MG is usually initiated with cholinesterase inhibitors, such as pyridostigmine or neostigmine. These agents alone may provide symptomatic relief of weakness in many patients. Side effects caused by muscarinic receptor stimulation may be prevented or minimized by avoidance of unnecessary high doses or by anticholinergic preparations (e.g., atropine). Most frequent side effects include gastrointestinal symptoms, such as diarrhea or abdominal cramping, increased oral or bronchial secretions, and rarely bradycardia. Excessive treatment with high doses may produce additional weakness, frequently associated with increased oral and upper respiratory secretions, which is referred to as cholinergic crisis and may be life-threatening if not promptly recognized and treated. The dose should be adjusted individually, and once remission is achieved with other forms of therapy, these medications can be discontinued.

Thymectomy may produce long-term remissions in many patients and should be considered in most patients younger than 50–60 years with significant generalized MG. Severely weak patients should be pretreated prior to surgery with plasmapheresis or high-dose intravenous immunoglobulin. If possible, steroids should be avoided prior to thymectomy. After thymectomy, up to 30% of patients may have complete or near-complete remission of MG and do not need medications. Another 30% may improve but still need treatment with cholinesterase inhibitors or immunosuppressive drugs. The remaining patients do not improve with thymectomy; however, the beneficial effect of that procedure may not be observed in some patients until 1–2 years later. Median sternotomy with cervical exploration is the most frequently used technique that allows best visualization and removal of the thymic tissue. Thymectomy is usually not recommended in purely ocular MG. All patients who have MG associated with a thymoma, with rare exceptions (e.g. very old, debilitated patients), should have surgical treatment to remove the tumor. In some patients postsurgical radiation may be necessary.

Corticosteroids have been used successfully for many years in patients with MG and up to 70% may achieve remission or marked improvement. In some patients there may be transient worsening of weakness after initiation of steroids, which needs close monitoring. Once improvement is achieved, steroids should be gradually tapered down to a minimal dose that controls the symptoms without significant side effects. Monitoring for possible iatrogenic side effects is necessary and all prophylactic measures should be taken to avoid unnecessary complications, including osteoporosis, hypertension, or diabetes. Azathioprine is a relatively weak immunosuppressant but is frequently used as an adjuvant treatment to corticosteroids. Cyclosporine or cyclophosphamide are sometimes used but have significant side effects. Medications that may have teratogenic effects should be avoided in pregnancy.

Patients with myasthenic or cholinergic crisis should be admitted to the intensive care unit and elective endotracheal intubation may be necessary. Approximately 20% of patients develop myasthenic crisis with severe deterioration of respiratory function at least once in the course of the disease, which is most frequently precipitated by infection. Patients in myasthenic crisis are treated with plasmapheresis or high-dose intravenous immunoglobulin.

The present patient was initially treated with cholinesterase-blocking agents and later underwent thymectomy. Because of the persistence of diplopia and weakness, he was started on a combination of prednisone and azathioprine with marked improvement of limb muscle weakness and resolution of diplopia and dysphagia within a few weeks. He required close monitoring of glucose levels and his insulin dosages were adjusted frequently. One year after thymectomy he was asymptomatic with only minimal left ptosis and prednisone was reduced to 10 mg/day.

Clinical Pearls

1. Ocular or bulbar symptoms are the most common initial complaints in MG patients.

2. Most patients with MG can be diagnosed on the basis of clinical examination, electrodiagnostic studies, testing for ACHR antibodies, and pharmacologic testing (edrophonium test).

3. A chest CT scan should be performed in all patients with MG to assess for the presence of thymoma.

4. Thymectomy may be beneficial in patients with MG but the positive effects of this procedure may not be observed until several months to a year from the time of procedure.

5. Patient education about symptoms of MG and spectrum of side effects of their medications is a crucial element of effective and successful treatment.

6. Patients suspected of myasthenic or cholinergic crisis should be hospitalized and managed in intensive care units until their respiratory function is stable.

REFERENCES

1. Grob D, Arsura EL, Brunner MG, Namba T: The course of myasthenia gravis and therapies affecting outcome. Ann N Y Acad Sci 1987; 505:472–499.
2. Plauche WC: Myasthenia gravis in mothers and their newborns. Clin Obstet Gynecol 1991; 34:82–99.
3. Verma P, Oger J: Treatment of acquired autoimmune myasthenia gravis: A topic review. Can J Neurol Sci 1992; 19:360–375.
4. Howard JF Jr, Sanders DB, Massey JM: The electrodiagnosis of myasthenia gravis and the Lambert-Eaton myasthenic syndrome. Neurol Clin 1994; 12:305–330.
5. Massey JM: Treatment of acquired myasthenia gravis. Neurology 1997; 48 (Suppl 5):S46–S51.
6. Mayer SA: Intensive care of the myasthenic patient. Neurology 1997; 48(Suppl 5):S70–S75.

PATIENT 52

A 68-year-old man with acute headache, left-sided weakness, sensory neglect, and partial left visual field loss

A 68-year-old man with a history of coronary artery bypass surgery, aortic aneurysm repair, and prosthetic mitral valve implantation suffered an abrupt onset of headache, stiff neck, left-sided weakness and clumsiness, and unsteadiness of gait 5 days prior to presenting for evaluation. His wife observed that he was inattentive to events on his left side. He denied recent head or neck trauma, right body weakness or numbness, or difficulties with speech or swallowing. He had been treated with warfarin but did not remember the dose.

Physical Examination: Vital signs: pulse 68 and regular, blood pressure 112/78, temperature and respiratory rate normal. Neck: supple, no bruits, Cardiac: well-healed sternal scar, midsystolic click consistent with prosthetic mitral valve. Mental status, affect, speech, and language: normal. Cranial nerves: left inferior visual field loss; fundi, gaze, pupillary reflexes normal; facial musculature normal and symmetric; oral and pharyngeal structures midline. Motor examination: mild spasticity with grade 4 weakness of the left upper extremity. Sensory examination: left hemineglect, otherwise normal. Muscle stretch reflexes: increased (grade 3) in the left upper extremity, normal and symmetric in lower extremities. Coordination: mild incoordination of the left hand, otherwise normal. Plantar reflexes: flexor. Gait: decreased left arm swing, no gait ataxia. Romberg test: negative.

Stop and Consider: What is the time course and localization of his neurologic dysfunction?

Laboratory Findings: Head CT: see figure. CBC, platelets, chemistry panel, electrolytes, ESR: normal. Prothrombin time: 38 seconds (normal 11.5–13.5); International Normalized Ratio (INR): 6.1 (normal 0.9–1.1). Cerebral angiography: normal.

Question: What is the likely etiology of the abnormality observed on head CT?

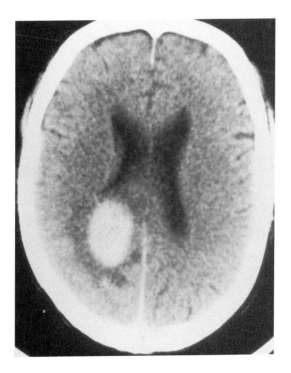

Diagnosis: Lobar intracerebral hemorrhage in the right parietal cortex

Discussion: The clinical presentation of acute, severe headache, neck stiffness, and focal symptoms suggested a subarachnoid hemorrhage. The presence of focal neurologic signs with left inferior homonymous visual field loss, mild left-sided weakness with long tract signs, and left hemineglect suggested an intracranial hemorrhage in the right frontoparietal cortex. The differential diagnosis included other processes that could present with an acute cortical dysfunction in that area, such as hemorrhagic or embolic infarction or hemorrhage into a neoplasm. The most important diagnostic step was a cranial CT, which showed a circumscribed acute intracerebral hemorrhage in the right parietal cortex. Because the cerebral angiography was normal and revealed no evidence of an aneurysm or an arteriovenous malformation, it was thought that the intracranial hemorrhage was related to excessive anticoagulation.

Intracerebral hemorrhage (ICH) represents approximately 10–20% of all vascular events in the brain. The most frequent cause of ICH is hypertension, and the typical locations of the hypertensive ICH are the internal capsule, putamen, caudate, thalamus, cerebellum, and pons. Other etiologies include trauma, vascular malformations, amyloid angiopathy, and coagulopathies. Amphetamine and cocaine abuse may also cause nonhypertensive ICH.

Lobar intracerebral hemorrhage accounts for as many as 30% of nontraumatic intracerebral hemorrhages, and may be associated with aneurysms, arteriovenous or venous malformations, cerebral amyloid angiopathy, hypertension, and hemorrhage into cerebral neoplasms. Bleeding diatheses, including hemorrhages associated with warfarin treatment, account for 30–40% of all lobar intracerebral hemorrhages and often occur in association with hypertension.

ICH is a relatively rare but well recognized complication of therapy with warfarin (warfarin derived its name from Wisconsin Alumni Research Foundation, in recognition of the discovery of the drug at the University of Wisconsin). The ICHs that develop as complication of anticoagulation frequently evolve more gradually and insidiously than in other types of cerebral hemorrhages and are more likely to be lobar in distribution then hypertensive hemorrhages.

The clinical presentation of ICH depends on the localization and the size of the hematoma. Occipital intracerebral hemorrhage typically presents with headache, visual difficulty at the onset, and visual field loss contralateral to the occipital hemorrhage. Motor signs are uncommon, but dysgraphia, dyslexia, and hemineglect may be observed when lesion extends into parietal cortex. In addition to headache, temporal lobe ICH in the dominant hemisphere may present with speech problems, confusion, difficulty in comprehension due to involvement of Wernicke's area, right-sided visual field deficits such as homonymous superior quadrantanopsia due to involvement of Meyer's loop, or the optic radiations in the temporal lobe. Frontal ICH is typically associated with headache, lethargy, contralateral arm weakness, mild leg weakness, minimal facial weakness, and, on occasion, expressive dysphasia due to involvement of Broca's area. Parietal hemorrhage presents with headache, drowsiness, contralateral hemisensory deficits and neglect, contralateral weakness when there is extension into the precentral gyrus, and contralateral homonymous inferior quadrantanopsia.

Patients with ICH as a complication of anticoagulation therapy or hematologic conditions require therapy to correct the bleeding tendency. Treatment with fresh frozen plasma and vitamin K should be considered, but needs to be carefully balanced against the risk of thrombotic or embolic events, especially in patients with artificial cardiac valves. All patients need careful monitoring in the intensive care unit. Follow-up CT scans should be obtained if there is any deterioration of neurologic status. Small ICHs usually have good recovery and most hemorrhages smaller than 3 cm do not need surgical drainage. Larger hematomas may require evacuation or ventriculostomy if there is intraventricular hemorrhage causing hydrocephalus.

The present patient was monitored in the intensive care unit and followed with frequent neurologic evaluations. Warfarin was held and he received an infusion of fresh frozen plasma. The INR was followed to avoid overcorrection, taking into account his prosthetic cardiac valve. Warfarin dose was adjusted to maintain the INR between 2.5 and 3.0. His treatment was monitored closely and at follow-up evaluation 6 months later his neurologic signs completely resolved. A follow-up head CT showed only a small area of encephalomalacia.

Clinical Pearls

1. Suspect intracranial hemorrhage in patients presenting with severe acute headache, with or without focal neurologic signs.

2. Causes of lobar intracerebral hemorrhages that occur without arterial hypertension include bleeding diatheses, vascular malformations, amyloid angiopathy, or hemorrhage within a primary or metastatic brain tumor.

3. Intracranial hemorrhage is a risk in patients receiving chronic anticoagulation therapy.

REFERENCES

1. Ropper AH, Davis KR: Lobar cerebral hemorrhages: Acute clinical syndromes in 26 cases. Ann Neurol 8:141–147, 1980.
2. Kase CS: Intracerebral hemorrhage: Non-hypertensive causes. Stroke 1986; 17:590–595.
3. Caplan L: Intracerebral hemorrhage revisited. Neurology 1988; 38:624–627.
4. Wilterdink JL, Feldmann E: Cerebral hemorrhage. Adv Neurol 1994; 64:13–23.
5. Molinari GF: Lobar hemorrhages: Where do they come from? How do they get there? Stroke 1993; 24:523–526.

PATIENT 53

A 63-year-old man with a subacute onset of back pain with bilateral leg weakness and numbness

A 63-year-old right-handed man presented with a 3-day history of severe, progressive low back pain with lower extremity weakness, numbness, and unsteady gait. There was no history of recent injuries or any other precipitating events. He denied any symptoms in upper extremities, headache, fever, chills, nausea, vomiting, shortness of breath, chest pain, or difficulty with bowel or bladder function, but complained of decreased appetite. Two years prior to this evaluation he underwent bilateral orchiectomy for treatment of adenocarcinoma of the prostate with pelvic lymph node metastases, followed by antiandrogenic treatment with flutamide. He had no prior history of significant back pain or any neurologic symptoms and his medical history was otherwise unremarkable.

Physical Examination: Vital signs: normal. Spine: tenderness over T7 and T8 spinal processes. Mental status and speech: normal. Cranial nerves: normal. Motor examination: normal muscle bulk and tone, bilateral grade +4 lower extremity weakness. Sensory examination: diminished sensation to pain and light touch below the level of T8 dermatome, marked loss of vibratory sensation and proprioception in bilateral lower extremities. Muscle stretch reflexes: normal in upper extremities, increased (grade 3) in lower extremities. Cremasteric reflex: normal. Anal sphincter tone: mildly decreased. Plantar reflexes: bilateral Babinski signs. Coordination: mild difficulty on heel-to-shin test. Gait: unsteady, marked difficulty on tandem gait test.

Stop and Consider: What anatomic structures are involved, and what is the most likely cause of this patient's neurologic deficit?

Laboratory Findings: MRI of the spine (noncontrast): see figure. CBC, chemistry panel including liver function tests, electrolytes: normal. ESR: normal. Prostate-specific antigen (PSA): 56.9 ng/ml (normal 0–2.8).

Question: What emergent therapy is required?

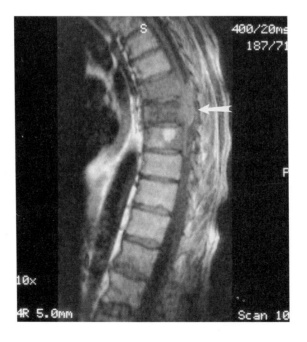

Diagnosis: Prostate cancer with spinal metastasis

Discussion: Acute onset of back pain and neurologic symptoms in a patient with a known history of cancer should immediately raise suspicion of spinal metastatic disease. The tenderness of the thoracic spine, signs of myelopathy, history of prostate cancer, and marked PSA elevation strongly indicated acute cord compression caused by an epidural metastatic process. Emergent diagnostic evaluation including imaging studies is required because severe irreversible neurologic deficit may develop very rapidly.

While metastatic epidural compression is overwhelmingly the likely diagnosis in this setting, carcinomatous meningitis may also produce spinal cord metastases causing cord compression or polyradiculopathy syndromes. Other considerations that are unlikely in this case are thoracic disc herniation, epidural hematoma (in patients who are anticoagulated), and epidural abscess in patients presenting with fever and back pain. Transverse myelitis and arteriovenous malformations of the spinal cord may also present with myelopathy and pain. Acute myelopathy from spinal cord infarction is usually not associated with severe back pain. The spine MRI study in this patient revealed tumor infiltration of the T7–T9 vertebral bodies with extension of the tumor into the epidural space and spinal cord compression (figure, arrow).

Epidural metastases are relatively frequent complication of disseminated neoplasms. The most common neoplasms causing epidural metastases include carcinomas of the lung, breast, prostate, and kidney, lymphoma, and sarcoma. Spinal cord compression occurs in approximately 7% of men with prostate cancer. The most frequent location of epidural metastases is thoracic spine (70% of cases), followed by lumbosacral (20%) and cervical spine regions (10%).

Pain is the initial complaint of more than 90% of patients with epidural metastases and usually precedes the development of other neurologic symptoms and signs by a few days to a few months, but may be followed by a rapidly developing severe neurologic deficit. The pain is often most severe in the local site of the involved vertebral body but frequently also has radicular features. It is sometimes worse in the supine position and some patients experience severe nocturnal pain.

Sensory symptoms are present in approximately 70% of patients with epidural metastases at the time of diagnosis, and many patients have a dermatomal sensory level. Weakness is present in approximately 80% of patients at the time of diagnosis and as many as 15% may be paraplegic. The progression of the neurologic dysfunction may be very rapid, and about 30% of patients become severely paraparetic within a week from the onset of weakness. The severity of the deficit at the time of diagnosis is the most important predictor of outcome. Symptoms of bowel or bladder dysfunction are frequent, and exist in up to 50% of patients at the time of presentation. Lumbosacral epidural metastases with involvement of conus medullaris and cauda equina present with flaccid paralysis and areflexia, and frequently cause sphincter involvement. Patients with cervical and thoracic epidural metastases may manifest with signs of a myelopathy, including spasticity and hyperreflexia.

Routine x-rays of the spinal column show bony invasion in more than 90% of patients at the time of the clinical presentation and therefore should be performed urgently in all patients with suspected spinal metastases. In addition to AP and lateral views, oblique views may be helpful. Radioisotope bone scan may show increased isotope uptake in the vertebrae before abnormalities are apparent in routine x-rays, but false-positive results are relatively common. MRI or CT-myelography are the most definitive diagnostic techniques for evaluation of epidural metastases and define the relation of metastases to the spinal cord and nerve roots. Lumbar puncture is not routinely performed if imaging studies demonstrate an epidural mass.

Because of the risk of rapid progression to irreversible neurologic dysfunction, treatment should be initiated rapidly. Dexamethasone at an initial dose of 100 mg IV followed by 24 mg IV every 6 hours should be administered. This dose can be gradually tapered once radiation is started or surgical decompression is performed. Radiation therapy is the treatment of choice for radiosensitive tumors. The optimal radiation dose that avoids radiation-induced myelopathy is often difficult to predict with certainty, but usually 30 Gy in 10 fractions is given. Surgical treatment with decompressive laminectomy or anterior vertebral body resection with stabilization is sometimes performed and may be considered if a primary neoplasm is not apparent and tissue diagnosis is required. Surgery should also be considered in patients who develop progressive myelopathy despite radiation. Once paraplegia has developed, surgery is usually of little value, and treatment with radiation in combination with corticosteroids should be considered. Chemotherapy may be helpful as adjuvant treatment for neoplasms that are known to be responsive. Prognosis for meaningful recovery from paraplegia in adults is poor, but

50% of pediatric patients may have good recovery with combination of surgery and radiation. Prognosis depends significantly on the histology of the tumor. Metastases from lung or renal cancer or melanoma are associated with poor prognosis even with aggressive treatment.

The present patient was immediately started on intravenous steroids, followed by radiation therapy the same day. Within 3 days his pain and leg weakness markedly improved and his sensory symptoms also resolved. Several weeks later he was able to ambulate with only mild, residual leg weakness.

Clinical Pearls

1. Patients with suspected epidural metastases require emergent evaluation because the neurologic deficit may progress very rapidly and be irreversible.

2. Most epidural metastases occur in the thoracic spine.

3. Spinal MRI is the most useful diagnostic test in patients with suspected epidural metastases.

4. The most important prognostic factor in acute epidural metastases is the severity of neurologic deficit at the time of diagnosis.

5. High-dose steroids and radiation therapy are treatments of choice for most patients with epidural metastases.

REFERENCES

1. Liskow A, Chang CH, DeSanctis P, et al: Epidural cord compression in association with genitourinary neoplasm. Cancer 1986; 58:949–954.
2. Berman CG, Clark RA: Diagnostic imaging in cancer. Prim Care 1992; 19:677–713.
3. Osborn JL, Getzenberg RH, Trump DL: Spinal cord compression in prostate cancer. J Neurooncol 1995; 23:135–147.
4. Gilbert RW, Kim JH, Posner JB: Epidural spinal cord compression from metastatic tumor: Diagnosis and treatment. Ann Neurol 3:40–51, 1978.
5. Klein SL, Sanford RA, Muhlbauer MS: Pediatric spinal epidural metastases. J Neurosurg 1991; 74:70–75.

PATIENT 54

A 15-year-old boy with visual impairment, mental retardation, and seizures

A 15-year-old boy with a history of global developmental delay, autistic behavior, visual impairment, and seizures since early childhood was brought to the clinic by his mother because of increased frequency of seizures. The boy experienced at least 15–20 seizures daily that were described as staring spells, sometimes associated with brief "eye jerking" and head nodding. The spells had a duration of 30 seconds–1 minute. He had experienced 2–3 generalized tonic-clonic seizures per year that began with head deviation to the left, followed by loss of consciousness, posturing of extremities, and later brief shaking of the arm, followed by confusion. He had been treated with ethosuximide, primidone, and clonazepam, which failed to control his seizures, and valproic acid, which appeared to control the generalized tonic-clonic seizures but did not reduce the staring spells. Metabolic testing to rule out inborn errors of metabolism did not reveal abnormalities. There was no family history of neurodegenerative disorders.

Physical Examination: Vital signs: normal. Head circumference 58 cm (98th percentile). Height: 161 cm (20th percentile). Skull: nontender. Neck: supple, no bruits. Skin, cardiac, chest, and abdomen: normal. Spine: no deformity, nontender, good range of motion. Mental status: uncooperative, with markedly decreased attention span, hyperactivity, and poor response to simple commands. Speech: limited spontaneous speech consisting of 2–3-word phrases. Cranial nerves: responds to visual threat symmetrically; pupils equal, 3 mm in diameter, sluggishly reactive to light; fundi: bilateral optic nerve hypoplasia and atrophy; facial expressions symmetric; the rest of cranial nerve examination unremarkable. Motor examination: muscle bulk, tone, and strength: normal; no tremor or dystonia. Sensory examination: localizing touch and pain stimuli. Muscle stretch reflexes: normal (grade 2). Plantar reflexes: flexor. Coordination and gait: normal.

Stop and Consider: Based on the available description, how would you classify this patient's seizures?

Laboratory Findings: CBC, chemistry panel, electrolytes: normal. Serum valproic acid: 72 μg/ml (normal 50–100 μg/ml). EEG: see figure, *left*. Brain MRI: see figure, *right*. Serum growth hormone, thyroid-stimulating hormone, follicle-stimulating hormone, luteinizing hormone, testosterone, and cortisol: normal.

Question: Are the EEG findings consistent with the staring spells? What abnormalities does the MRI show?

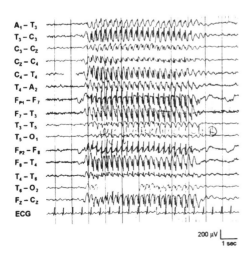
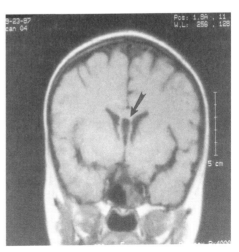

Diagnosis: Septo-optic dysplasia with a mixed seizure disorder (atypical absence seizures and generalized tonic-clonic seizures)

Discussion: The clinical description suggested a mixed seizure disorder with absence seizures and generalized tonic-clonic seizures. The EEG showed paroxysmal bursts of generalized 3-Hz spike and wave discharges, a pattern consistent with absence seizures. The bilateral hypoplastic, atrophic optic nerves suggested the possibility of septo-optic dysplasia. The brain MRI revealed a small optic chiasm, cavum septum pellucidum (figure on the right, arrow), and cavum velum interpositum, consistent with the diagnosis of septo-optic dysplasia. No suprasellar or parasellar mass lesions were observed. There was no convincing clinical or laboratory evidence of coexisting hypopituitarism.

Septo-optic dysplasia (SOD) is a developmental disorder associated with hypoplastic optic discs and abnormalities or absence of the septum pellucidum. In some patients there is coexisting hypopituitarism and dwarfism, and these cases are referred to as septo-optic-pituitary dysplasia. The hypopituitarism is usually related to hypothalamic dysfunction.

The main clinical feature of SOD is visual impairment. Patients with coexisting hypopituitarism may show progressive growth failure secondary to growth hormone deficiency, or other hormonal abnormalities such as hypothyroidism, corticotropin deficiency, diabetes insipidus, or hyperprolactinemia.

The visual impairment may vary from mild decrease of visual acuity to visual field defects or complete blindness. The optic nerves are usually small, hypoplastic, and sometimes with coexisting atrophy. The abnormalities are usually bilateral, but may be unilateral or markedly asymmetrical. The visual impairment is usually stable but may be slowly progressive. Depending on the extent of brain abnormalities patients may exhibit other neurologic abnormalities, including seizures, mental retardation, hemiparesis, or hearing impairment.

Cranial CT or MRI in SOD show spectrum of morphologic abnormalities involving the optic nerves, septum pellucidum, or pituitary gland. Schizencephaly, gray matter heterotopia, absence of corpus callosum, and other developmental abnormalities may also be noted. Although the absence of the septum pellucidum is common, a significant proportion of patients with optic atrophy and pituitary dysfunction may have a septum pellucidum that appears normal. Cavum septum pellucidum is a common incidental finding on MRI studies and may not be associated with neurologic deficits.

The pathogenesis of SOD is uncertain. Intrauterine exposure to toxic agents, viral infections, and maternal diabetes mellitus have been suggested as possible etiologic factors. In rare familial cases a genetic defect has been postulated. Treatment is symptomatic. Patients with hypopituitarism need appropriate replacement therapy. Patients with seizures are treated with anticonvulsants.

Valproic acid produced a good control of generalized tonic-clonic seizures in the present patient, but he continued to experience absence seizures. Lamotrigine was added to valproic acid and this combination markedly improved control of absence seizures.

Clinical Pearls

1. Hypoplastic optic nerves in a child with visual impairment suggest the possibility of septo-optic dysplasia.

2. Patients with septo-optic dysplasia may exhibit coexisting structural brain abnormalities on neuroimaging studies and may present with a wide spectrum of neurologic disabilities.

3. Hypothalamic dysfunction in septo-optic dysplasia may cause hypopituitarism.

4. Ethosuximide is the drug of choice for isolated absence seizures and valproic acid is usually a good choice for absence seizures associated with generalized tonic-clonic seizures.

REFERENCES

1. Hoyt WF, Kaplan SL, Grumbach MM, et al: Septo-optic dysplasia and pituitary dwarfism. Lancet 1970; 1:893–894.
2. Brook CG, Sanders MD, Hoare RD: Septo-optic dysplasia. BMJ 1972; 3:811–813.
3. Purdy F, Friend JC: Maternal factors in septo-optic dysplasia. J Pediatr 1979; 95:661.
4. Morishima A, Aranoff GS: Syndrome of septo-optic-pituitary dysplasia: The clinical spectrum. Brain Dev 1986; 8:233–239.
5. Barkovich AJ, Fram EK, Norman D: Septo-optic dysplasia: MR imaging. Radiology 1989; 171:189–192.
6. Bodensteiner JB, Schaefer GB: Wide cavum septum pellucidum: A marker of disturbed brain development. Pediatr Neurol 1990; 6:391–394.
7. Wales JK, Quarrell OW: Evidence for possible Mendelian inheritance of septo-optic dysplasia. Acta Paediatr 1996; 85:391–392.
8. Willnow S, Kiess W, Butenandt O, et al: Endocrine disorders in septo-optic dysplasia (De Morsier syndrome): Evaluation and follow-up of 18 patients. Eur J Pediatr 1996; 155:179–184.

PATIENT 55

A 59-year-old man with progressive proximal and distal weakness of arms and legs

A 59-year-old right-handed man presented with bilateral weakness of hand grip, which was slowly progressive for the last 2 years and markedly limited his ability to make a fist, especially with the right hand. He also complained of progressive leg weakness manifesting as difficulty lifting his feet from the ground while walking. He denied sensory disturbances, double vision, speech or swallowing difficulties, or excessive fatigue. His medical history was significant for obstructive sleep apnea, treated successfully with uvulopalatopharyngoplasty 10 years previously. There was no family history of neuromuscular diseases or consanguinity.

Physical Examination: Pulse 78, respirations 16, blood pressure 140/78. Skull and spine: normal. HEENT, cardiac, and chest: normal. Mental status: normal. Cranial nerves: normal. Motor examination: muscle tone normal, severe atrophy and grade 4 weakness of wrist flexors, brachioradialis, biceps, quadriceps, and anterior tibialis muscles bilaterally. Sensory examination: normal. Muscle stretch reflexes: normal except for markedly depressed knee reflexes bilaterally. Coordination: mildly compromised because of weakness. Gait: wide-based, with stepping pattern.

Stop and Consider: Are the findings consistent with weakness caused by an upper motor neuron lesion or a disorder affecting the motor unit?

Laboratory Findings: CBC, chemistry panel, electrolytes, ESR: normal, except for elevated creatine kinase (CK) level at 780 U/L (normal 0–250 U/L). Nerve conduction study (NCS): normal in both upper and the lower extremities. Needle EMG: fibrillation potentials, combination of short-duration low-amplitude and rare long-duration high-amplitude motor unit potentials (MUPs), and many polyphasic MUPs in the majority of muscles. Muscle biopsy: see figures (light microscopy, *left*, electron microscopy, *right*).

Question: What abnormalities were demonstrated on the muscle biopsy?

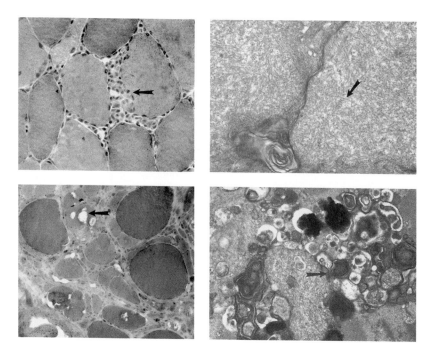

162

Diagnosis: Inclusion body myositis

Discussion: The pattern of slowly progressive weakness with prominent muscle atrophy and depressed reflexes suggested a motor unit disorder. The needle EMG findings and a markedly elevated CK level indicated a myopathy, which was confirmed by muscle biopsy. Histopathologic examination of the muscle specimen showed evidence of muscle degeneration, atrophy, and inflammatory changes with focal invasion of non-necrotic muscle fibers (figure on the left, top, arrow). It also showed numerous fibers with vacuoles rimmed by basophilic material (figure on the left, bottom, arrow), best observed in the modified Gomori trichrome section. Electron microscopy revealed numerous fibers containing filamentous inclusions (figure on the right, top, arrow) and autophagic vacuoles containing myeloid figures, membranous fragments, and debris (figure on the right, bottom, arrow), which are characteristic of inclusion body myositis (IBM).

IBM, polymyositis, and dermatomyositis are the most common types of inflammatory myopathy. Approximately one third of patients with inflammatory myopathy have IBM. Although children have been described with this disorder, the majority of patients are older than 50 years of age. Men are slightly more likely to be affected then women. IBM typically presents with painless, progressive weakness that predominates in proximal muscles. However, distal weakness is also present in as many as 50% of cases and may be as severe or more severe than the proximal weakness. In the lower extremities the knee extensors and hip flexors are preferentially affected and in most cases the knee reflexes are depressed after 5 years and absent after 10 years from disease onset. A footdrop is not an uncommon finding. In the upper extremities the biceps muscles are frequently weak, and most patients have a characteristic wasting of the wrist flexors, which are more severely affected than other forearm muscles. Many patients complain of dysphagia, which may be a presenting symptom, but otherwise muscles supplied by cranial nerves are not affected. CK is usually mildly elevated (5–10 times normal value) but in some patients CK levels may be normal.

EMG examination typically shows short-duration low-amplitude (myopathic) MUPs, but in many patients with IBM there are also abundant long-duration high-amplitude MUPs, which sometimes may suggest a "neurogenic" condition. The myopathic features predominate in most cases. Some patients may have an associated, usually mild, distal axonal polyneuropathy.

The muscle biopsy shows evidence of inflammatory myopathy with endomysial infiltrates and focal invasion of non-necrotic fibers by mononuclear cells, but the inflammatory changes may be very sparse. A characteristic but unspecific finding is presence of fibers containing autophagic vacuoles rimmed by basophilic material and small groups of atrophic fibers. Eosinophilic inclusions are seen in a minority of patients. Amyloid deposits on Congo red stain have been demonstrated in vacuolated muscle fibers in many sporadic IBM cases. Electron microscopy reveals large autophagic vacuoles and filamentous inclusions of 15–20 nm in diameter.

The differential diagnosis should include motor neuron disease, especially when lower motor neuron signs predominate. In some patients differentiation from polymyositis can be difficult if the rimmed vacuoles are sparse. Predominantly motor polyneuropathies can be differentiated on the basis of nerve conduction studies. Familial IBM may histologically resemble sporadic IBM, but usually little or no inflammation on muscle biopsy is observed. Most cases of familial IBM likely represent a form of genetically determined myopathy.

The etiology and pathogenesis of IBM are unclear. It has been postulated that the abundant vacuoles and inclusions may be secondary to myonuclear matrix degeneration and that inflammatory reaction may be just an epiphenomenon of the myodegenerative process. The observation that IBM patients, in contrast to polymyositis or dermatomyositis, do not respond to immunosuppressive treatment would support that notion.

There is no convincing evidence that any therapeutic interventions are effective. Transient improvement with corticosteroids or high-dose intravenous immunoglobulin have been reported, but the course of IBM is slowly progressive.

The present patient received supportive physical therapy and was fitted with braces to prevent the bilateral footdrop. His condition has been gradually progressive.

Clinical Pearls

1. Although most myopathies are characterized by proximal weakness, distal weakness is a common finding in IBM.
2. IBM is the most common form of acquired myopathy in elderly patients.
3. Characteristic light microscopy findings of IBM are endomysial inflammatory changes with invasion of non-necrotic muscle fibers, groups of atrophic fibers, rimmed vacuoles, and eosinophilic inclusions.
4. The EMG finding of a mixture of "myopathic" and "neurogenic" motor unit potentials should always raise the suspicion of a diagnosis of IBM.
5. Currently there is no effective treatment for IBM.

REFERENCES

1. Lotz BP, Engel AG, Nishino N, et al: Inclusion body myositis: Observations in 40 patients. Brain 1989; 112:727–747.
2. Karpati G: Inclusion body myositis: Status 1997. The Neurologist 1997; 3:201–208.
3. Griggs RC, Askanas V, DiMauro S, et al: Inclusion body myositis and myopathies. Ann Neurol 1995; 38:705–713.
4. Massa R, Weller B, Karpati G, et al: Familial inclusion body myositis amongst Kurdish-Iranian Jews. Arch Neurol 1991; 48:519–522.

PATIENT 56

A 49-year-old man with medically intractable epilepsy

A 49-year-old right-handed man presented for evaluation of medically intractable epilepsy. At age 7, he suffered the first generalized tonic-clonic seizure following a brief febrile illness with gastrointestinal symptoms. He was then seizure-free until age 29, when he had another generalized tonic-clonic seizure. He continued to have stereotyped seizures at a frequency of about one per day, consisting of brief episodes of staring, poorly characterized feeling of "well-being," followed by motor automatisms and an approximately 30-second episode of uncontrollable laughter. There was no loss of consciousness, loss of bladder control, or tongue biting. After the seizure he usually felt depressed and tired. His medical history was otherwise unremarkable and there was no family history of seizures. The patient grew up in South America but later relocated to the U.S.

Physical Examination: Vital signs: normal. General examination, including head and spine: normal. Mental status, speech, cranial nerves, motor, and sensory examinations: normal. Muscle stretch reflexes: grade 2 and symmetric. Plantar reflexes: flexor. Coordination and gait: normal.

Stop and Consider: How would you classify this patient's seizure type using the international seizure classification?

Laboratory Findings: CBC, chemistry panel, electrolytes, calcium, magnesium: normal. Noncontrast cranial head CT scan: see figure. Brain MRI: confirmed the presence of the lesion observed on head CT and showed a mild ring enhancement of the surrounding brain parenchyma after gadolinium contrast injection; no abnormality in the hippocampal region. Cerebral angiogram: normal. Positron emission tomography (PET): focal, severe hypometabolism associated with the lesion demonstrated on CT, otherwise normal. Interictal EEG: focal sharp waves and delta wave slowing in the posterior right temporal region. Prolonged video-EEG monitoring: two episodes with inappropriate laughing were associated with a run of well-developed spike-wave complexes recorded from an electrode in the right foramen ovale, but the electrographic onset was not captured.

Clinical Course: The patient underwent lesionectomy with excision of the calcified lesion and surrounded gliotic tissue, guided by intraoperative electrocorticographic recordings. Pathologic examination: a calcified remnant of a parasite surrounded by a layer of gliosis.

Question: What is the likely etiology of the intracerebral lesion?

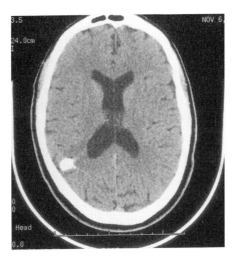

Diagnosis: Partial seizures caused by cerebral cysticercosis

Discussion: The clinical presentation of this patient's seizures was consistent with partial epilepsy. The head CT (figure) and MRI showed a calcified lesion in the posterior temporal-parietal region. The relationship of that lesion to the patient's seizures was initially unclear, and he underwent evaluation to determine if the structural lesion was associated with an epileptic focus. The intraoperative electrocorticography revealed a focus of epileptiform activity in the cortical area around the calcified lesion, which was resected with surrounding epileptogenic tissue. The pathologic examination revealed calcified remnants of a cysticercus.

Cysticercosis is the most frequent parasitic CNS infection in humans. It develops when humans are the intermediate host of *Taenia solium*. In more than 90% of patients the infection develops after ingestion of food or water contaminated by *Taenia solium* ova. In the stomach the ova release oncospheres that penetrate the stomach and intestinal mucosa, and may spread to brain, skeletal muscle, and other organs via hematogenous dissemination. In the brain they may be located in the parenchyma, meninges, ependyma, or in the ventricular system. The living cysts cause minimal inflammatory reaction, but after a few years the cysts may degenerate and calcify. The leaking walls of the degenerating cysts may induce a severe inflammatory reaction that is usually associated with neurologic symptoms. Cysticercosis-associated vasculitis may lead to focal brain ischemia caused by vascular occlusions.

The neurologic presentation depends on the anatomic site, developmental stage of the cyst, the number of parasites, patient's age, and the immune responses of the host. Seizures may be generalized or focal, and are the most common manifestations of neurocysticercosis. Symptoms related to an increase in the intracranial pressure are also relatively frequent and some patients may present with mental status changes. Focal neurologic signs are present in approximately 10% of cases. Chronic meningitis may develop in about 5% of patients and may be associated with development of communicating hydrocephalus. Cysts in the third or fourth ventricles may obstruct the CSF flow and cause an obstructive hydrocephalus. The spinal form of cysticercosis is rare.

Neurocysticercosis should be included in differential diagnosis of new-onset seizures or other neurologic symptoms, especially in persons coming from endemic areas. Cranial CT or MRI with contrast usually demonstrate the focal cerebral lesions, hydrocephalus, or inflammation of meninges. Depending on the biologic stage of the infection, there may be variable degree of edema surrounding the cysts, calcification, and contrast enhancement. However, the lesion must be differentiated from lesions of different etiologies such as tumors, arteriovenous malformations, tuberculomas, or other infectious or parasitic conditions, e.g., schistosomiasis. Cerebrospinal fluid examination is usually normal, but may show mild elevation of protein content or mild pleocytosis, sometimes with decreased glucose levels. In some patients there may be eosinophilia in the CSF. Anti-cysticercus antibodies in the CSF or serum may provide support for the suspected diagnosis of neurocysticercosis.

Most patients have a very good prognosis and up to 15% are asymptomatic. Many patients develop relatively severe neurologic symptoms during the stage of cyst degeneration, usually secondary to inflammatory reaction in the area of the cyst. Massive infestation with cysticercosis is rare.

Most symptomatic patients are treated with praziquantel or albendazole. Treatment in some patients may be accompanied by transient headaches, mental status changes, or other neurologic symptoms after initiation of medical treatment, which is usually related to the release of the cysticercus antigen to the surrounding brain and reactive inflammatory response. Corticosteroids may minimize the inflammation and edema caused by dying cysticerci. Patients with very few lesions and minimal symptoms may initially be followed with serial imaging studies without cystidal therapy, since many cysts may spontaneously disappear. However, if the cysts persist, treatment should be initiated and may diminish the risk of secondary epilepsy. Patients with inactive lesions should not be treated. MRI with contrast distinguishes between inactive and active lesions by showing significant edema and contrast enhancement. Anticonvulsants are usually effective for seizure control. Surgical treatment includes lesionectomy for medically intractable seizures, and should ventricular shunting in patients with obstructive hydrocephalus.

Avoidance of ova-contaminated water or food in the endemic areas is the most important means of preventing neurocysticercosis. Affected patients and families should have stool examination for presence of tapeworms and should be treated because of risk of reinfection.

The present patient had a very successful outcome after resective brain surgery and became seizure-free. His anticonvulsants were tapered without recurrence of seizures.

Clinical Pearls

1. Consider neurocysticercosis in the differential diagnosis of patients with a seizure disorder and evidence of calcified lesions on cranial CT or MRI, especially in patients from endemic areas for cysticercosis.

2. There is a wide spectrum of neurologic and psychiatric presentations in patients with neurocysticercosis depending on number, developmental stage, and location of the parasites. The clinical course also depends on patient's age and host immune responses.

3. Many cases of brain cysticercosis have a benign course and may not need pharmacologic treatment, but in patients with acute brain infection whose lesions do not improve on serial imaging studies, cystidal therapy is recommended and may diminish the risk of intractable epilepsy or other neurologic sequelae.

4. Surgical treatment can be successful in some patients with medically intractable seizures if an epileptic focus can be localized and surgery can be performed safely without significant morbidity.

REFERENCES

1. Lawson JR, Gemmell MA: Hydatidosis and cysticercosis: The dynamics of transmission. Adv Parasitol 1983; 22:261–308.
2. Vazquez V, Sotelo J: The course of seizures after treatment for cerebral cysticercosis. N Engl J Med 1992; 327:696–701.
3. Del Brutto OH, Sotelo J, Roman GC: Therapy for neurocysticercosis: A reappraisal. Clin Infect Dis 1993; 17:730–735.
4. Davis LE, Kornfeld M: Neurocysticercosis: Neurologic, pathogenic, diagnostic, and therapeutic aspects. Eur Neurol 1991; 31:229–240.

PATIENT 57

A 76-year-old man with recurrent brain hemorrhages

A 76-year-old male nursing home resident was admitted after he had been found obtunded with a right hemiparesis. Four years prior to admission he suffered abrupt onset of left hemiparesis caused by an intracerebral hemorrhage in the right frontal lobe. At that time his cerebral angiogram was normal for age and an extensive evaluation for possible coagulopathy was negative. One year later he again became abruptly obtunded in association with worsening of left-sided weakness and sensory deficit as a result of a right parietal hemorrhage that extended into the right lateral ventricle. He had a relatively good recovery, became alert and cooperative, but was left with cognitive impairments and mild left-sided weakness. He was treated with a ventriculo-peritoneal shunt for hydrocephalus secondary to intracerebral hemorrhages, but the shunt produced no further improvement of his cognitive status. He had a history of hypertension well controlled with diuretics and no previous episodes of head trauma.

Physical Examination: Vital signs: pulse 80 and regular, blood pressure 140/70, respirations and temperature: normal. Skin, neck, cardiac, chest, and abdomen: normal. Mental status and speech: severely obtunded, purposeful movements to painful stimuli on left hemibody, otherwise unresponsive. Cranial nerves: normal fundi and pupillary reflexes; visual fields: no response to threat; left gaze preference; weakness of right lower facial muscles, oral and pharyngeal structures midline. Motor examination: muscle bulk normal, marked spasticity in all extremities but worse on the left side; withdrawal movements of the left extremities to pain stimuli; no movement of the right extremities. Muscle stretch reflexes: increased (grade 3) in left extremities, pathologically increased (grade 4) in right upper and lower extremities; brisk (grade 3) jaw jerk. Plantar reflexes: bilateral Babinski signs. Coordination and gait: untestable.

Stop and Consider: What is the localization of the new neurologic dysfunction?

Laboratory Findings: Head CT: see figure, *left*. CBC, platelet count, PT, PTT, chemistry panel, ESR: normal.

Clinical Course: The patient's condition did not improve and he was discharged to a nursing home and died 2 months later. Brain autopsy: gross pathology specimen (see figure, *right*). Histopathologic examination: presence of congophillic material with birefringence in the polarized light within the arterial blood vessel walls.

Question: Is the localization of the hematoma typical for a hypertensive hemorrhage? What is the relationship of the recurrent lobar hemorrhages and the pathologic findings?

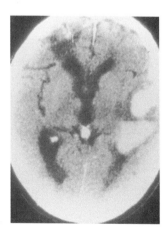 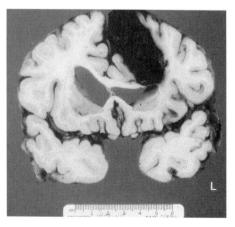

Diagnosis: Recurrent intracerebral hemorrhages associated with cerebral amyloid angiopathy

Discussion: The clinical presentation of this patient, with acute obtundation, right hemiparesis, and bilateral corticospinal tract signs raises the possibility of numerous CNS conditions, but with a prior history of recurrent intracerebral hemorrhages another hemorrhagic stroke should be considered. This presentation is also consistent with an ischemic stroke, hemorrhage within a neoplasm, or possible traumatic cerebral hematoma. Brain abscess and encephalitis are less likely. The differential diagnosis should be influenced by history of the recurrent nature of this patient's intracerebral lobar hemorrhages, which suggests cerebral amyloid angiopathy, but bleeding diatheses, including iatrogenic coagulation abnormalities, should also be considered.

Head CT showed two areas of an intracerebral hemorrhage within the left cerebral hemisphere (figure, *left*), encephalomalacia in the right frontal cortex, and moderately enlarged lateral ventricles. Cerebral angiography performed during his prior admission was unremarkable and showed no evidence of a vascular malformation or vasculitis. The lobar localization of the hemorrhage was not typical for a hypertensive bleed. Brain autopsy showed evidence of new subarachnoid blood over the bifrontal region, recent bifrontal intracerebral hemorrhages, and hemosiderin-stained cystic changes in multiple areas, suggestive of previous hemorrhages. The largest lesion, after the most recent hemorrhage, was in the left hemisphere (figure, *right*). Histopathologic studies demonstrated significant amyloid deposits in blood vessel walls, which suggested that recurrent intracranial hemorrhages were most likely caused by amyloid angiopathy. Microscopy showed extensive neurofibrillary tangles, senile plaques, and reduction in the number of large neurons in the cerebral cortex.

Etiologies of nontraumatic intracerebral hemorrhage include hypertension (40–60% of cases), amyloid angiopathy (5–20%), iatrogenic hemorrhages related to anticoagulation or thrombolytic therapy (5–10%), hemorrhage related to cerebral neoplasms (5–10%), hemorrhages caused by amphetamine or cocaine abuse (5%), and hemorrhages associated with aneurysms or arteriovenous malformations (5%). Occasionally no specific etiology for an intracerebral hemorrhage can be determined.

Cerebral amyloid angiopathy is an important cause of lobar intracerebral hemorrhage in the elderly, and is probably the most common cause of recurrent lobar hemorrhage in that age group. Amyloid infiltrates are found in the media and adventitia of the cerebral microvasculature and vessels affected by cerebral amyloid angiopathy frequently bridge leptomeninges and the superficial areas of cerebral cortex, which may explain the tendency for lobar hemorrhage in these patients. Affected vascular channels frequently show a distinctive "double barrel" lumen, and the blood vessels may undergo fibrinoid degeneration or necrosis, either with or without microaneurysmal formation.

Clinical and pathologic conditions associated with cerebral amyloid angiopathy include sporadic and familial recurrent hemorrhages, degenerative dementia of the Alzheimer's type, Down syndrome, CNS vasculitis, cerebral microinfarctions, and leukoencephalopathy. Amyloid angiopathy has also been observed in association with late postradiation CNS necrosis, spongiform encephalopathy, angiopathic changes within arteriovenous malformations, or Lewy body disease.

Hemorrhages caused by cerebral amyloid angiopathy have no clear sex preponderance and may be associated with hypertension in up to 30% of cases. Frontal and parietal lobes are the most common locations of hemorrhages secondary to amyloid angiopathy. Dementia occurs in as many as 40% of cases, and autopsy findings consistent with degeneration of the Alzheimer's type are found in more than 40% of cases. While cerebral amyloid angiopathy is an important cause of lobar cerebral hemorrhage, severe cerebral amyloid angiopathic changes may be present without cerebral hemorrhage, and may also be observed in patients with cerebral infarction. When cerebral amyloid angiopathy is severe and accompanied by fibrinoid necrotic changes of the blood vessels, the association between cerebral amyloid angiopathy and cerebral hemorrhage is particularly common.

In the present patient, the pattern and localization of recurrent hemorrhages was typical of amyloid angiopathy but the definitive diagnosis required histopathologic confirmation.

Clinical Pearls

1. Cerebral amyloid angiopathy is a frequent cause of nontraumatic primary cerebral hemorrhages, particularly in individuals who are normotensive and elderly.

2. Patients with cerebral amyloid angiopathy may have coexisting microscopic features typical of Alzheimer's disease and dementia.

3. Some forms of amyloid angiopathy may be familial.

4. Intracerebral hemorrhage in cerebral amyloid angiopathy most frequently affects frontal and parietal lobes.

REFERENCES

1. Vinters HV: Cerebral amyloid angiopathy: A critical review. Stroke 1987; 18:311–324.
2. Hendricks HT, Franke CL, Theunissen PH: Cerebral amyloid angiopathy: Diagnosis by MRI and brain biopsy. Neurology 1990; 40:1308–1310.
3. Feldmann E. Tornabene J: Diagnosis and treatment of amyloid angiopathy. Clin Geriatr Med 1991; 7:617–630.
4. Vonsattel JP, Myers RH, Hedley-Whyte ET, et al: Cerebral amyloid angiopathy without and with cerebral hemorrhages: Comparative histologic study. Ann Neurol 1991; 30:637–649.
5. Rosenberg RN: A causal role for amyloid and Alzheimer's disease: The end of the beginning. Neurology 1993; 43:851–856.
6. Molinari GF: Lobar hemorrhages: Where do they come from? How do they get there? Stroke 1993; 24:523–526.

PATIENT 58

A 42-year-old woman with a 2-day history of bilateral leg numbness, weakness, and urinary retention

A 42-year-old woman presented with a 2-day history of intense upper abdominal pain and bilateral lower extremity numbness and tingling. One day after the onset of the sensory symptoms she developed progressive leg weakness and difficulty walking. On the day of admission she developed urinary retention. She denied fever, headache, vomiting, nausea, or any other systemic or neurologic symptoms. She had no significant medical history except for an upper respiratory illness approximately 2 weeks prior to admission. There was no history of recent trauma.

Physical Examination: Vital signs: normal. HEENT, cardiac, chest, abdomen: normal. Spine: nontender, no deformity. Mental status and speech: normal. Cranial nerves: normal. Motor examination: muscle bulk normal; muscle tone: normal in upper extremities, mildly decreased in lower extremities; strength: normal in upper extremities, bilateral lower extremity weakness (grade 3 on the right and grade 4 on the left). Sensory examination: diminished sensation to pain, temperature and light touch below T8–T9 dermatomal level, decreased proprioception and vibration in lower extremities; positive Romberg test. Muscle stretch reflexes: normal in upper extremities, brisk knee reflexes (grade 3), ankle reflexes pathologically increased (grade 4) with sustained ankle clonus. Plantar reflexes: bilateral Babinski signs. Coordination: normal in upper extremities, marked difficulty on heel-to-shin test bilaterally. Gait: unable to walk without assistance.

Stop and Consider: What is the anatomic localization of the lesion? What conditions should be considered in the differential diagnosis of this patient?

Laboratory Findings: MRI of the thoracic spine: see figure. CBC, ESR, PT, PTT, electrolytes, chemistry including liver function tests: normal. ANA, rheumatoid factor, VDRL: negative. Urinalysis: normal. CSF analysis: nucleated cells 6/μl (83% lymphocytes, 17% macrophages), red blood cells 9/μl, protein 38 mg/dl (normal 15–45), glucose 80 mg/dl (serum glucose 110 mg/dl), myelin basic protein: 5.60 ng/ml (normal 0.0–1.0), IgG index: 0.5 (normal 0.3–0.7), no oligoclonal bands. CSF Lyme titer: negative. CSF cultures and cytology: negative. Brain MRI, chest x-ray, thoracic, abdominal, and pelvic CT: normal.

Question: What is the likely etiology of the abnormality demonstrated on the spinal MRI?

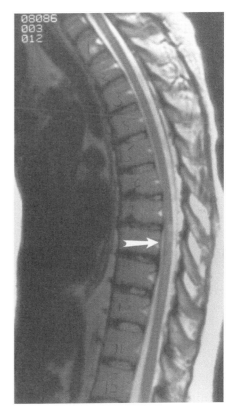

Diagnosis: Transverse myelitis

Discussion: This patient presented with a subacute neurologic deficit that was characterized by bilateral involvement of motor and sensory pathways and autonomic dysfunction in a pattern typical of a myelopathy. The sensory level and the type of a motor deficit indicated a lesion in the thoracic cord. In the differential diagnosis consideration should be given primarily to conditions that may present as acute or subacute myelopathy, such as spinal cord compression due to primary or metastatic neoplasm, epidural hematoma, abscess, intervertebral disc herniation, vascular lesions such as aortic dissection or arteriovenous malformations, demyelinating conditions, such as postinfectious transverse myelitis, or multiple sclerosis.

Spine MRI showed abnormally high signal intensity on the T2 weighted images within the thoracic cord from T7 through T10 vertebral levels (figure, arrow). There was no significant cord enlargement or contrast enhancement. Taking into account the MRI findings, the pattern and evolution of the neurologic deficit, antecedent viral infection, and otherwise unremarkable extensive diagnostic studies, the diagnosis of postinfectious transverse myelitis was most likely.

Transverse myelitis is an acute, inflammatory, primarily demyelinating condition affecting the spinal cord. The etiology and pathogenesis of this condition are poorly understood. In about 30% of cases there is evidence of preceding or underlying viral infection and these cases are typically referred to as postinfectious or parainfectious transverse myelitis. In most cases, however, there is no antecedent event and no underlying disease is identified and these cases are typically classified as idiopathic.

Acute myelopathy may also develop in association with a variety of systemic conditions. Transverse myelitis has been reported in association with toxic exposures (e.g., heroin), after radiation treatment, or in association with connective tissue diseases, most commonly systemic lupus erythematosus, and may develop as an exacerbation or initial presentation of multiple sclerosis.

Numerous viral infections have been reported in association with transverse myelitis, including influenza, adenovirus, mumps, measles, rubella, herpes simplex, herpes zoster, or cytomegalovirus. Myelopathy may also develop in association with retroviral infections, such as HTLV-1 and HIV, as well as in the course of *Mycoplasma pneumoniae* or spirochetal infections, such as Lyme disease or syphilis. Cases following vaccinations are very rare.

The pathophysiology of myelitis associated with viral infections is uncertain. Several mechanisms

have been postulated, including possible direct viral invasion of the spinal cord parenchyma or autoimmune mechanisms with cross-reactivity between viral and myelin-related antigens. Some pathologic alterations may be caused by spinal cord ischemia secondary to vasculitis triggered by viral infection. The lesions of the cord in idiopathic or postinfectious transverse myelitis are typically more severe than cases that develop in the course of or as initial manifestation of multiple sclerosis, because in addition to demyelination there is frequently evidence of severe axonal loss.

Symptoms of transverse myelitis may evolve from onset to maximum neurologic deficit within a few hours to a few weeks, but typically they progress from a few days to a week. The most frequent initial symptoms are paresthesias. Severe, localized back pain is common. Sensory symptoms are typically followed by leg weakness and dysautonomia causing sphincter dysfunction. Some patients may develop dysesthetic, dermatomal pain. The weakness is initially associated with hypotonia and hyporeflexia, but spasticity and hyperreflexia usually develop within a few days. If cervical cord is affected, spastic quadriparesis may develop, and in cases with conus medullaris involvement severe flaccid paraparesis with sphincter incontinence is characteristic. Transverse myelitis typically affects the whole cord in cross-section, but it may be asymmetric and lead to different patterns of sensory and motor deficits, including Brown-Séquard syndrome.

Most patients with idiopathic or postinfectious transverse myelitis have a monophasic condition with signs of recovery visible within a few weeks from the onset of symptoms, but recovery may be very slow and is often incomplete. About 30% of patients have good outcome, with complete or near-complete resolution of the deficit. Patients who acutely develop severe and persistent motor deficit and sphincter incontinence usually have worse prognosis than patients with a more subacute course.

Spinal MRI is the most useful initial diagnostic test in patients with transverse myelitis. It also helps to rule out alternative diagnoses, especially compressive lesions that need emergent interventions. MRI typically shows increased signal intensity on T2 weighted images, which may spread within multiple segments. The changes may not be observed on the initial MRI, and it should be repeated in a few days unless an alternative diagnosis is made. There is usually a variable degree of contrast enhancement after gadolinium administration. The CSF examination may show elevated CSF protein content and a mild degree of pleocytosis. In necrotizing encephalomyelitis, red cells and polymorphonuclear cells may be present. Brain MRI should be obtained to evaluate possible coexisting demyelinating process in the brain. If severe axonal injury is present, electromyography may show signs of denervation in the limb muscles within 2–3 weeks from the onset.

Patients with transverse myelitis are commonly treated with intravenous corticosteroids. It is most important to identify and treat any possible underlying systemic conditions. Physical therapy should be initiated as soon as possible to prevent secondary complications. Spasticity can be managed with antispasticity medications. Many patients require prolonged management of sphincter incontinence. Neuropathic pain may be severe and may require narcotic analgesics.

The present patient was treated with intravenous steroids followed by a tapering regimen of oral prednisone. Physical therapy was initiated on the first day of hospitalization. Within 3 days significant improvement of lower extremity strength was observed, and she was able to walk short distances using a walker. Her sensory deficit also markedly improved. She required intermittent catheterization for several weeks but within 3 months she had near-complete recovery with minimal motor and sensory deficit, and used a cane mostly for safety of ambulation.

Clinical Pearls

1. In about 30% of cases of transverse myelitis there is evidence of antecedent viral infection, but most cases are idiopathic.

2. Most cases of transverse myelitis affect the thoracic spine.

3. MRI of the spinal cord is the most useful diagnostic test in transverse myelitis. If the initial MRI is negative, it should be repeated within a few days.

4. Treatment with intravenous corticosteroids should be considered in patients with transverse myelitis.

5. Acute transverse myelitis with rapidly progressing severe motor and sensory deficit and sphincter incontinence is frequently associated with poor outcome.

REFERENCES

1. Berman M, Feldman S, Alter M, et al: Acute transverse myelitis: Incidence and etiologic considerations. Neurology 1981; 31:966–971.
2. Dunne K, Hopkins IJ, Shield LK: Acute transverse myelopathy in childhood. Dev Med Child Neurol 1986; 28:198–204.
3. Misra UK, Kalita J, Kumar S: A clinical, MRI and neurophysiologic study of acute transverse myelitis. J Neurol Sci 1996; 138:150–156.
4. al Deeb SM, Yaqub BA, Bruyn GW, et al: Acute transverse myelitis: A localized form of postinfectious encephalomyelitis. Brain 1997; 120:1115–1122.

PATIENT 59

A 70-year-old man with a 3-month history of weight loss and left leg pain, weakness, and numbness

A 70-year-old man presented with pain, numbness, and weakness in his left leg that started about 3 months prior to his neurologic evaluation. He first became aware of numbness in the sole of his left foot, and shortly afterward developed weakness of his left calf muscles. The weakness progressed to severe impairment of left foot plantar flexion and dorsiflexion that interfered with ambulation. During the following 3 months he lost 30 pounds. He denied weakness or sensory disturbances in the upper extremities or in the right leg, visual symptoms, dysphagia, dizziness, and bowel or bladder problems. There was no history of headaches, fever, chills, or skin rashes. He had a history of childhood asthma, but no history of diabetes mellitus, heart disease, or malignancy. His mother had myasthenia gravis but there was no history of neuromuscular disorder in siblings or relatives. He denied alcohol or drug abuse.

Physical Examination: Pulse 90, blood pressure 110/68. Cardiac, chest, abdomen: normal. Skin: clean, mild distal edema around ankles. Neck: supple, no bruits, no adenopathy. Mental status and speech: normal. Cranial nerves: normal. Motor examination: severe atrophy and weakness of left gastrocnemius (grade 2), atrophy of the intrinsic foot muscles, relatively mild atrophy and weakness (grade +4) of the left anterior tibialis, and peroneus longus and brevis muscles. Sensory examination: decreased light pain and touch over the sole and the lateral aspect of the left foot. Muscle stretch reflexes: normal except for absent left ankle reflex. Coordination normal. Gait: impaired, with limping secondary to left leg weakness.

Stop and Consider: What is the time course and localization of this patient's neurologic deficit?

Laboratory Findings: CBC, chemistry panel with liver and renal function tests, electrolytes: normal. ESR: 95 mm/hr (normal 0–25). Urinalysis: normal. Creatinine clearance: normal. ANA, ANCA, anti-extractable nuclear antigen antibodies (ENA), C_3, C_4, CH_{50}, serum and urine electrophoresis: normal. CSF: normal. Hepatitis A to C virus serology, HIV antibodies, VDRL: negative. Urine toxicology screen: negative. Chest, left ankle, and foot x-rays, CT of chest and abdomen, bone scan: normal. NCS: markedly diminished amplitudes of the left tibial and peroneal CMAPs with borderline slowing of tibial and peroneal conduction velocities, absent left sural nerve response. Needle EMG: fibrillation potentials, decreased motor unit recruitment, and mild increase in polyphasic MUPs in the left gastrocnemius, anterior tibialis, and peroneus longus muscles; proximal lower extremity muscles and lumbar paraspinal muscles: normal. Left sural nerve biopsy: see figure.

Question: What abnormality was observed in the nerve biopsy?

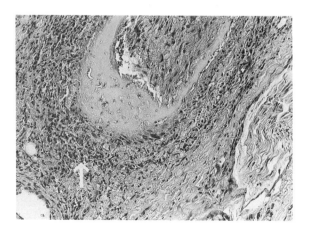

Diagnosis: Peripheral nervous system vasculitis

Discussion: This patient presented with weakness and sensory loss in a pattern indicative of left tibial, peroneal, and sural nerve dysfunction, which was suggestive of mononeuropathy multiplex but it may also be observed in some cases of sciatic neuropathy or lumbosacral plexopathy. The electrodiagnostic studies showed severe axonal injury in the distribution of the left peroneal, tibial, and sural nerves. Lack of paraspinal muscle involvement pointed away from possible radiculopathy. The markedly elevated ESR and weight loss immediately raised suspicion of a systemic process, such as vasculitis involving peripheral nerves. The sural nerve biopsy confirmed the diagnosis of suspected vasculitis and showed evidence of severe axonal loss and intense inflammatory cell infiltration around perineurial blood vessels, with mononuclear cells extending into the arterial blood vessel walls (figure, arrow). Secondary thrombosis in the vascular lumen was also observed. There was no evidence of other organ system involvement, which suggested that the vasculitis was confined primarily to the peripheral nervous system (PNS).

Several different types of vasculitis can involve the peripheral nerves. The most common systemic necrotizing vasculitis is polyarteritis nodosa (PAN), which produces neuropathy in 50–75% of patients. Other forms of systemic necrotizing vasculitis that may involve PNS include Churg-Strauss syndrome, Wegener's granulomatosis, and vasculitis associated with connective tissue diseases such as rheumatoid arthritis, systemic lupus erythematosus, or Sjögren's syndrome. The systemic necrotizing vasculitides affect the small- and medium-size arteries with frequent involvement of other organs. In classic PAN, renal, hepatic, and skin involvement are common. The pulmonary circulation is usually not affected in PAN but in Churg-Strauss syndrome pulmonary blood vessel involvement is typical, and is frequently associated with eosinophilia and asthma. Wegener's granulomatosis is a granulomatous vasculitis involving the respiratory system and also causing glomerulonephritis. Peripheral nerve involvement has also been reported in giant-cell arteritis, and may manifest as syndromes of temporal arteritis or polymyalgia rheumatica. The clinical and pathologic features of vasculitis syndromes may overlap.

Hypersensitivity vasculitides caused by reactions to certain drugs (e.g., cocaine, amphetamines, penicillin), infectious processes of different etiologies, and malignancies usually involve small vessels, including capillaries, arterioles, and veins. Skin involvement in that group is typical. In some reports 30% of patients with necrotizing vasculitis have evidence of exposure to hepatitis B, as documented by positive antibody titers.

Vasculitis confined to the PNS has been recognized with increasing frequency. It appears to be the third most common cause of vasculitic neuropathy, after PAN and rheumatoid vasculitis. The etiology of this syndrome is uncertain but it has been postulated that the isolated PNS vasculitis may represent a restricted form of PAN. In some histopathologic studies, 80% of patients with isolated PNS vasculitis had evidence of vasculitis or other inflammatory changes in muscle biopsies, which suggests the possibility of subclinical involvement of other organs.

Vasculitis of the peripheral nervous system presents most commonly as mononeuritis multiplex. This term refers to discrete lesions involving two or more nerves. Some patients may present with a symmetric distal polyneuropathy, polyradiculoneuropathy, and brachial or lumbosacral plexopathies. The presentation of mononeuritis multiplex is typically acute and most patients also have features of other organ system involvement.

Evaluation of patients with PNS vasculitis requires search for possible involvement of other organ systems. Laboratory studies should include complete blood count, ESR, C-reactive protein, complement levels, renal and liver function tests, urinalysis, hepatitis antigens, VDRL, ANA, ENA, ANCA, and cryoglobulins.

The NCS/EMG is the most helpful test to classify the type of peripheral nerve involvement and typically shows evidence of mononeuritis multiplex with severe axonal damage. All cases of suspected peripheral nerve vasculitis should be confirmed by pathologic studies to demonstrate evidence of the vasculitic process. The typical pathologic abnormality is transmural inflammatory cell infiltration with fibrinoid necrosis. In some cases the changes may be very focal, and inflammatory infiltrate or the vessel wall necrosis may be missed in a limited biopsy specimen. The sensitivity of pathologic studies is markedly increased if the nerve biopsy is combined with a muscle biopsy. The diagnostic yield of combined peripheral nerve and muscle biopsies is approximately 80%, compared to 55% with nerve biopsy alone.

Peripheral neuropathy associated with systemic necrotizing vasculitis is usually treated with a combination of corticosteroids and cytotoxic agents such as cyclophosphamide. Neuropathies associated with hypersensitivity vasculitis are treated by elimination of the inciting agent or drug or treatment of underlying infection, but most patients still need some form of immunosuppressive treatment. Treatment of isolated PNS vasculitis is controversial. Most physicians initiate treatment with corticosteroids alone but if the condition does not improve a cytotoxic agent is often added. The dosage and duration of treatment depend on the clinical response. Once the condition has improved, an attempt to taper or reduce the immunosuppressive drugs should be considered. Relapses may require higher doses of corticosteroids or cyclophosphamide. The 3-year survival rate in patients with systemic narcotizing vasculitis is approximately 50%, but patients with nonsystemic PNS vasculitis have a better prognosis and some may have excellent recovery with full resolution or only minimal residual neurologic deficit. Physical therapy and pain management are important aspects of treatment. Patients should be carefully monitored for any side effects of corticosteroids or cytotoxic agents to avoid iatrogenic complications.

The present patient was treated with prednisone alone, and responded extremely well with nearly complete resolution of his neurologic deficit within 6 months.

Clinical Pearls

1. Suspect vasculitis in a patient who presents with a clinical picture of mononeuritis multiplex.

2. Patients with PNS vasculitis can present with different patterns of peripheral nerve involvement, including mononeuropathy multiplex, symmetric distal polyneuropathies, cranial neuropathies, brachial or lumbosacral plexopathies, or peripheral mononeuropathies.

3. Combined muscle and nerve biopsy markedly increases the diagnostic yield in patients with suspected PNS vasculitis as compared to nerve biopsy alone.

4. The diagnosis of PNS vasculitis usually depends on analysis of clinical findings, electrodiagnostic studies, and histologic features from nerve or muscle biopsy.

5. Patients with necrotizing vasculitis require immunosuppressive treatment with corticosteroids, frequently in combination with cytotoxic agents such as cyclophosphamide.

REFERENCES

1. Hawke SH, Davies L, Pamphlett R, et al: Vasculitic neuropathy: A clinical and pathological study. Brain 1991; 114:2175–2190.
2. Kissel JT: Vasculitis of the peripheral nervous system. Semin Neurol 1994; 14:361–369.
3. Davies L, Spies JM, Pollard JD, et al: Vasculitis confined to peripheral nerves. Brain 1996; 119:1441–1448.
4. Said G, Lacroix-Ciaudo C, Fujimura H, et al: The peripheral neuropathy of necrotizing arteritis: A clinicopathological study. Ann Neurol 1998; 23:461–465.

PATIENT 60

A 76-year-old man with recurring episodes of right-sided weakness, numbness, and expressive speech difficulty

A 76-year-old man with a history of hypertension presented for evaluation of episodes of sudden onset of right upper and lower extremity weakness associated with difficulty speaking. He reported three similar episodes during the previous month, which all resolved completely within 10 minutes. During the episodes his right hand felt clumsy and the leg weakness caused difficulty walking. The weakness was accompanied by numbness or tingling in his right hand and leg, and by speech difficulty that he described as "unable to say what [he] wanted to say." He had no difficulty with comprehension or other neurologic complaints and his review of systems was noncontributory.

Physical Examination: Vital signs: pulse 72 and regular, respirations 16, blood pressure 177/74, afebrile. Cardiac: normal. Neck: no carotid bruits. Mental status, affect, speech, and language: normal. Cranial nerves: normal. Motor examination: normal muscle tone, bulk, and strength, no tremor. Sensory examination: normal. Muscle stretch reflexes: grade 2 and symmetric. Plantar reflexes: flexor. Coordination and gait: normal.

Stop and Consider: What is the time course and localization of this patient's neurologic dysfunction?

Laboratory Findings: CBC, ESR, platelets, PT, PTT, chemistry panel: normal. EKG: normal. Head MRI: normal. EEG: normal. Carotid Doppler/ultrasound: normal. Transthoracic and thransesophageal echocardiograms: normal. Magnetic resonance angiography (MRA) of the neck: normal. Head MRA: see figure.

Question: What abnormality can be seen in the head MRA?

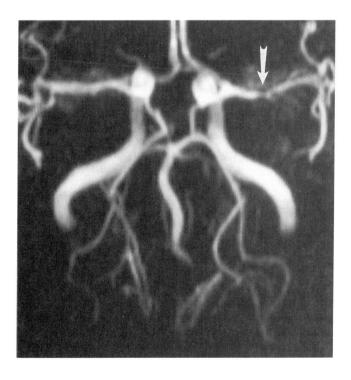

Diagnosis: Transient ischemic attacks associated with stenosis of the left middle cerebral artery

Discussion: The recurrent episodes of right-sided motor and sensory symptoms associated with dysphasia were suggestive of transient ischemic attacks (TIAs) affecting the left cerebral hemisphere in the distribution of the middle cerebral artery (MCA), but stenosis of the internal carotid artery (ICA) or common carotid artery (CCA) could also produce these neurologic symptoms. Transient monocular blindness (amaurosis fugax) is sometimes associated with ICA stenosis but is not encountered with isolated MCA stenosis. On rare occasions brain tumors, focal seizures, arteriovenous malformations, or subdural hematomas may present with recurrent episodes mimicking TIAs, but the symptoms experienced by this patient are almost always associated with transient ischemia caused by atherosclerosis affecting the carotid or middle cerebral arteries. An MRI of the brain showed no evidence of structural lesions. Carotid Doppler and ultrasound revealed no carotid artery stenosis. An MRA of head and neck was performed and demonstrated significant left middle cerebral artery stenosis (figure, arrow). This lesion was consistent with this patient's recurrent neurologic symptoms.

Intracranial stenosis of the major arterial vessels is increasingly recognized with improved resolution and availability of MRA. Patients who have ischemia in the MCA distribution may develop weakness, which is most severe in the face and upper extremity, with rather minor involvement of the contralateral lower extremity. Hemibody sensory loss, gaze preference toward the side of the lesion, visual or tactile neglect of the contralateral side, hemianopia, or upper quadrantanopsia may be observed. MCA-distribution ischemia in the dominant hemisphere may produce aphasia affecting comprehension or expression of speech.

Deep brain infarction in the MCA distribution is usually related to the occlusion of the main stem of the MCA, proximal to the lenticulostriate branches. In patients with good collateral flow, blood supply to the brain convexity may be preserved, but compromise of the blood supply to the deep branches of the MCA may produce severe hemiparesis that involves the arm and leg equally.

Patients with stem occlusion of the MCA without collateral flow to its cortical branches usually have a very severe motor and sensory deficit, hemianopia with conjugate gaze deviation to the side of infarction, and global aphasia in the dominant hemisphere lesions. Right hemispheric lesions of the main stem of the MCA may be associated with neglect or anosognosia, in addition to severe hemiparesis.

Patients with TIAs require a rapid evaluation to prevent brain infarctions and permanent neurologic deficits. Initial imaging studies should include urgent cranial CT or brain MRI, noninvasive vascular studies such as carotid Doppler and ultrasound and/or MRA of head and neck blood vessels, and cardiac evaluation with electrocardiogram and echocardiogram. Initial laboratory studies should include complete blood count, chemistries, ESR, and coagulation profiles. Conventional angiography may need to be performed in some cases to clarify the nature of underlying vascular pathology if MRA is not adequate.

Treatment considerations include surgical and/or medical therapy, depending on the nature, location, and severity of the specific mechanism underlying stroke or TIA. Both antiplatelet agents (e.g., aspirin) and warfarin have been used in treatment of patients with symptomatic stenosis of intracranial arteries. Extracranial–intracranial arterial bypass surgery for MCA occlusive disease was found to be of no significant benefit. Any underlying risk factors should be treated or modified.

The present patient developed another episode while waiting for the MRA and was promptly started on intravenous heparin. Warfarin therapy was initiated after the left MCA stenosis was identified. He suffered two more episodes while fully anticoagulated and a low-dose aspirin (81 mg) was added. He had no further ischemic events while taking both aspirin and warfarin.

Clinical Pearls

1. Transient ischemic attacks caused by middle cerebral artery stenosis are frequently indistinguishable from ischemic attacks secondary to internal carotid artery stenosis.

2. Magnetic resonance angiography is indicated in patients with transient ischemic attacks and may demonstrate stenosis of intracranial arteries.

3. Antiplatelet agents or warfarin may be beneficial in patients with symptomatic stenosis of major intracranial arteries.

REFERENCES

1. Caplan L, Babikian C, Helgason C, et al: Occlusive disease of the middle cerebral artery. Neurology 1985; 35:975–982.

2. Bogusslavsky J, Barnett HJ, Fox AJ, et al: EC/IC Bypass Study Group: Atherosclerotic disease of the middle cerebral artery. Stroke 1986; 17:1112–1120.

3. Chimowitz MI, Kokkinos J, Strong J, et al: The warfarin-aspirin symptomatic intracranial disease study. Neurology 1995; 45:1488–1493.

PATIENT 61

A 32-year-old man with low back pain radiating to left leg and foot

A 32-year-old man presented with a 4-week history of low back pain that developed following an accident at work. After a 10-foot fall from a truck, he immediately noted sharp low back pain that radiated into his left leg and foot and was accompanied by a tingling sensation in the same areas. X-rays of the lumbosacral spine were negative. His family physician prescribed bed rest, pain relievers, and muscle relaxants, without any significant improvement. The pain was constant, and was aggravated by coughing, sneezing, or bending, and limited his ambulation. He denied any bowel or bladder symptoms. His medical history was unremarkable and there was no prior history of back pain.

Physical Examination: Vital signs: normal. General exam: normal. Spine: muscle spasm and tenderness in the left lumbar paraspinal muscles. Straight leg raising test: positive on the left at 30°. Mental status, speech, and cranial nerves: normal. Motor examination: muscle bulk and tone normal; strength normal except for mild weakness (grade +4) of left foot plantar flexion. Sensory examination: diminished sensation to light touch and pain over the lateral aspect and the bottom of the left foot; vibratory sensation and proprioception: normal. Muscle stretch reflexes: grade 2 throughout except for absent left Achilles tendon reflex. Gait: slightly flexed, difficulty to bear weight on the left leg.

Stop and Consider: What is the localization of this patient's symptoms and signs, and what is the likely etiology?

Laboratory Findings: MRI of the lumbosacral spine: see figure. Nerve conduction studies: normal except for prolonged left H-reflex. Needle electromyography: fibrillation potentials and slight decrease of motor unit recruitment in the left medial gastrocnemius, gluteus maximus, and lumbosacral paraspinal muscles.

Question: Does the neurologic deficit in this patient correspond to the MRI and electromyographic abnormalities?

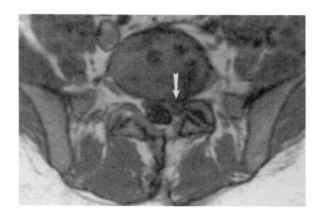

Diagnosis: Left S1 radiculopathy secondary to L5–S1 intervertebral disc herniation

Discussion: The pattern of pain, with radiation from lower back to the distal lower extremity ("sciatica"), was suggestive of lumbosacral radiculopathy. The distribution of sensory and motor deficits and absence of the left ankle jerk indicated a lesion of the left S1 nerve root, which was confirmed by the spinal MRI demonstrating compression of the left S1 nerve root by a herniated L5–S1 intervertebral disc (figure, arrow). The electromyographic findings confirmed the diagnosis by showing denervation changes in the left S1 myotome.

The most frequent sites of disc herniations in the lumbosacral spine are the L4–L5 and L5–S1 vertebral interspaces, with compression of the L5 or S1 nerve roots, respectively. Herniations at L3–L4 and L2–L3 levels are much less frequent. Severe low back pain is present in more than 90% of patients with lumbosacral radiculopathies. It may be constant or episodic and typically is aggravated by coughing, sneezing, or straining. In S1 radiculopathy the pain typically radiates to the posterolateral thigh, posterolateral leg, and lateral foot and small toe, and frequently is associated with paresthesias or sensory loss in the same distribution. Weakness may be observed in the gastrocnemius, gluteus maximus, and plantar flexors of the foot. The Achilles tendon reflex is lost or depressed. In L5 radiculopathy the pain and sensory disturbance affect the posterolateral thigh, lateral leg, dorsum of foot, and great toe. Significant weakness may be observed in anterior tibialis, peroneus longus and brevis, extensor hallucis longus, gluteus medius, and tensor fasciae latae muscles. Patients with large central disc herniations may develop cauda equina syndrome with flaccid paralysis and bladder and bowel dysfunction. Individuals with severe sciatica frequently walk with a slightly flexed posture and avoid weight bearing on the affected leg. There may be tenderness and muscle spasm in the ipsilateral paraspinal muscles. The straight leg raising test is regarded as positive if 60° elevation reproduces the pain, but is nonspecific for radiculopathy.

Although compressive radiculopathy producing severe pain (sciatica) is most frequently caused by intervertebral disc herniation or degenerative osteoarthritic changes, other conditions, including spinal fractures, neoplasms (especially epidural metastases), epidural hematoma, or abscess may be associated with spinal root compressions and require emergent evaluation if suspected. Noncompressive radiculopathies, such as Guillain-Barré syndrome, cytomegalovirus-associated radiculitis, vasculitis, or diabetes mellitus, may also develop in the course of inflammatory or infectious processes. Numerous nonspinal conditions, including abdominal or thoracic aortic aneurysms, kidney infections, nephrolithiasis, pancreatitis, peptic ulcer, and other abdominal or pelvic processes, may also present with severe low back pain and need to be excluded. Patients with spinal stenosis and neurogenic claudication may need to be differentiated from patients with vascular claudication.

The initial evaluation of a patient with acute low back pain should focus on detection of potentially serious spinal and systemic conditions that may require emergent evaluation. Imaging studies are not necessary in most patients on initial evaluation, unless neurologic deficits or risk factors for serious underlying disease are present. Plain x-rays of the lumbar spine are rarely useful in acute sciatica unless fractures, subluxations, neoplastic, or infectious processes are suspected. Computed tomography provides excellent imaging of the bony abnormalities within the spine, but for good visualization of nerve roots it should include contrast myelography. MRI is most useful and very sensitive for evaluation of patients with lumbar radiculopathies and suspected disc herniations but should be carefully correlated with clinical signs, because disc protrusions and herniations are common in asymptomatic individuals. Contrast-enhanced MRI may be necessary in some patients when tumor, infection, or arachnoiditis are suspected, but is not required routinely. Electrodiagnostic studies (nerve conduction study and needle electromyography) may be helpful to provide supportive evidence of specific root involvement, to obtain evidence about more widespread radiculopathies or to evaluate the severity of axonal degeneration and consider alternative diagnoses.

The choice of therapeutic options in patients with lumbosacral radiculopathies should be influenced by the fact that approximately 50% of patients with sciatica recover within 2 weeks, and 70% within 6 weeks. In patients treated with decompressive surgery, no difference in outcome has been observed at 4 and 10 years after surgery compared to patients treated with conservative methods, although a better outcome may be observed in the surgical group after 1 year.

Bed rest in patients with severe sciatica may initially be beneficial, but prolonged immobilization may be counterproductive. Patients should be treated with analgesics such as nonsteroidal anti-inflammatory agents, but in some cases a brief course of opioids may be necessary. Muscle relaxants are also frequently used but their efficacy is uncertain. Lumbar traction and lumbar bracing have not been found to be of any significant benefit. Once the acute pain is improved, patients should begin physical therapy, including stretching and strengthening exercises. Patients should be educated to avoid postures and activities that aggravate symptoms, and weight reduction may be recommended.

Emergent decompressive surgery is indicated in patients with the cauda equina syndrome. Patients who develop progressive motor deficits are also candidates for surgery. Patients who suffer intractable pain and severe activity limitation after at least 4 weeks of conservative therapy may be considered for surgical treatment if there is corroborative evidence of root compression on imaging studies.

The present patient was treated with physical therapy for 6 weeks but was unable to return to work because of persistent pain and paresthesias in his left lower extremity. He subsequently underwent laminectomy and discectomy, and within 4 weeks had a complete recovery.

Clinical Pearls

1. Initial evaluation of a patient with acute low back pain should be focused on exclusion of serious thoracic, abdominal, pelvic, and spinal conditions that may require emergent treatment.

2. Spinal MRI and electrodiagnostic studies supplement the clinical evaluation of patients with radiculopathies but should not be performed routinely.

3. Most patients with lumbosacral radiculopathies can be successfully treated with conservative methods.

4. Patients with acute intervertebral disc herniation causing a cauda equina syndrome should undergo an emergent decompressive surgery.

REFERENCES
1. Long DM: Failed back surgery syndrome. Neurosurg Clin North Am 1991; 2:899–919.
2. Long DM: Decision making in lumbar disc disease. Clin Neurosurg 1992; 39:36–51.
3. Malanga GA, Nadler SF: Nonoperative treatment of low back pain. Mayo Clin Proc 1999; 74:1135–1148.
4. Weber H: Lumbar disc herniation: A controlled, prospective study with ten years of observation. Spine 1983; 8:131–140.

PATIENT 62

A 39-year-old man with a sudden onset of weakness, numbness, and pain in the right lower extremity

A 39-year-old man woke up with pain in the right buttock and thigh area. The same day he developed marked difficulty walking, his right knee frequently buckled, and he fell a few times. He also had tingling and numbness in the right anterior thigh and the medial side of the right leg. He had no weakness or numbness in other extremities. He denied any bowel or bladder problems, headache, double vision, or difficulty swallowing. Two weeks previously he was started on warfarin for right leg deep vein thrombosis (DVT) complicated by pulmonary emboli. A diagnostic evaluation for the cause of the DVT was unrevealing. He had no history of diabetes, malignancy, or recent trauma.

Physical Examination: Vital signs: normal. Cardiac: normal. Extremities: distal pulses normal, no skin discoloration, edema, or tenderness. Spine: nontender. Straight leg raising test: negative. Mental status, speech, cranial nerves: normal. Motor examination: normal muscle bulk and tone, severe weakness of right knee extension (grade 3), mild weakness of right hip flexion (grade –5). Sensory examination: mildly diminished sensation to touch, light pain, and temperature on the anterior thigh and medial side of the right leg below the knee. Muscle stretch reflexes: absent right knee reflex, otherwise normal. Plantar reflexes: flexor. Gait: marked difficulty walking secondary to right lower extremity weakness, unable to arise from deep chair. Coordination: normal.

Stop and Consider: What is the time course and localization of the lesion producing this pattern of weakness and sensory deficit?

Laboratory Findings: CBC, chemistry panel: normal. Prothrombin time: International Normalized Ratio (INR) 2.5 (0.9–1.1). MRI of the pelvis (fast spin-echo T2 image): see figure. Nerve conduction study: markedly decreased amplitude of the right femoral compound muscle action potential (CMAP) with mildly prolonged femoral nerve latency, absent right saphenous nerve response. Needle electromyography performed 2 weeks after the onset of weakness: fibrillation potentials and markedly reduced motor unit recruitment in the right vastus lateralis and rectus femoris muscles and mildly decreased recruitment pattern in the right iliopsoas muscle; other lower extremity muscles and lumbar paraspinal muscles: normal.

Question: What is the likely etiology of the neurologic deficit?

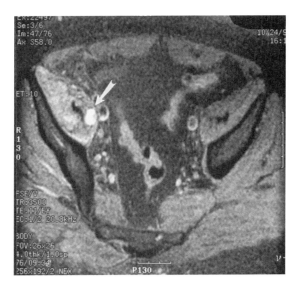

Diagnosis: Right femoral neuropathy secondary to iatrogenic hematoma within the iliopsoas muscle

Discussion: The neurologic deficit of this patient was indicative of femoral neuropathy. The lesion was very proximal, because in addition to knee extension weakness, the patient also had some weakness of the hip flexion. The distal sensory deficit on the right medial leg was consistent with saphenous neuropathy, which is the most distal sensory branch of the femoral nerve. Other L3–L4-innervated muscles, especially the thigh adductors (innervated by the obturator nerve), were not affected. The localization of abnormalities by clinical exam suggested an isolated femoral neuropathy rather than lumbar radiculopathy, lumbosacral plexopathy, or polyneuropathy. The pelvic MRI showed a hematoma with surrounding edema in the iliacus muscle (figure, arrow) and another hematoma in the psoas muscle. This hemorrhage caused compression of the femoral nerve and was most likely related to the patient's warfarin treatment. Electrodiagnostic studies confirmed femoral neuropathy with both demyelinating and axonal changes.

Patients with femoral neuropathy develop different degrees of weakness and atrophy of the quadriceps muscle. They frequently complain that the knee buckles when walking and experience difficulty climbing stairs or arising from chairs. Patients with complete quadriceps paralysis may be unable to walk without assistance. With very proximal lesions, at the site where the femoral nerve emerges from the lumbar plexus structures, patients also may have hip flexion weakness caused by involvement of the fibers to the iliopsoas muscle. Therefore, examination of the hip flexion may help to determine the site of the nerve lesion on purely clinical grounds. The ipsilateral knee reflex is diminished or absent and the sensory deficit usually affects the anterior thigh (anterior cutaneous branches of the femoral nerve) and medial calf (saphenous nerve). Severe pain sometimes observed at the onset of symptoms is not unusual, and the character and localization of the pain may depend on the underlying cause.

Femoral neuropathy may develop as result of trauma to the groin, upper thigh, or pelvic area, or with injuries associated with excessive extension or flexion of the hip. Femoral nerve may be damaged by pelvic malignancies or abscesses in the retroperitoneal area. Patients who undergo surgical procedures may develop femoral neuropathy because of intraoperative compression or traction forces. The lithotomy position itself is associated with an increased risk of perioperative femoral neuropathy. Isolated femoral neuropathy is also possible in the spectrum of diabetic amyotrophy, although most patients with that pathology have evidence of more diffuse plexus, nerve root, or other peripheral nerve involvement. Ischemia of the nerve is thought to play a role in development of diabetic amyotrophy and in femoral neuropathy that develops in the course of vasculitis. Hemorrhage following catheterization of the femoral artery may cause hematoma in the groin with secondary femoral neuropathy. Idiopathic femoral neuropathy is rare, but may develop in the course of parainfectious lumbosacral plexopathy. Femoral neuropathy may also develop secondary to radiation therapy in the groin or pelvic area.

Patients with bleeding disorders or anticoagulation treatment may develop femoral neuropathy from retroperitoneal hematoma. The hemorrhage within the iliacus or psoas muscles makes the femoral nerve vulnerable to compression, because it runs in the pelvis between these two muscles. Differential diagnosis should include L4 or L3 radiculopathy and lumbar plexus injury. The clinical examination of the motor and sensory deficit usually allows correct localization of the lesion, but electrodiagnostic studies are helpful to exclude radiculopathy or plexopathy and help to determine whether the lesion is predominantly axonal or demyelinating, which has implications for prognosis.

Large hematomas may require acute surgical exploration to decompress the nerve, but most patients can be followed conservatively and gradually recover from the neurologic deficit. Some degree of residual deficit is not unusual. Demyelinating lesions usually have more rapid and complete recovery than neuropathies with severe axonal loss. Some patients may benefit from long leg and knee braces to assist in ambulation and should also receive physical therapy.

The present patient required anticoagulation because of a recent life-threatening pulmonary embolus. Anticoagulation with warfarin was continued with close follow-up. He received physical therapy and within 10 months had a full neurologic recovery.

Clinical Pearls

1. Retroperitoneal hematoma should be considered in a patient who develops severe leg weakness and back pain in the course of anticoagulation treatment.

2. Femoral neuropathy caused by retroperitoneal hematomas typically improves with conservative treatment, but large hematomas may need surgical evacuation.

3. Femoral neuropathy is common in diabetic patients and is part of the clinical spectrum of diabetic amyotrophy.

4. Electrodiagnostic studies are helpful in evaluation of patients with femoral neuropathy and can rule out lumbar plexus involvement or lumbar radiculopathy.

REFERENCES

1. al Hakim M, Katirji B: Femoral neuropathy induced by the lithotomy position: A report of 5 cases with a review of literature. Muscle Nerve 1993; 16:891–895.
2. Kuntzer T, van Melle G, Regli F: Clinical and prognostic features in unilateral femoral neuropathies. Muscle Nerve 1997; 20:205–211.
3. Nobel W, Marks SC Jr, Kubik S: The anatomical basis for femoral nerve palsy following iliacus hematoma. J Neurosurg 1980; 52:533–540.
4. Young MR, Norris JW: Femoral neuropathy during anticoagulation therapy. Neurology 1976; 26:1173–1175.

PATIENT 63

A 49-year-old man with progressive mental status changes following heart transplantation

A 49-year-old man presented with signs of progressive cardiac failure 4 weeks after heart transplantation for idiopathic cardiomyopathy. His endocardial biopsy showed acute, severe transplant rejection, but despite intensive treatment of organ rejection, his cardiovascular status worsened. He experienced episodes of ventricular tachycardia and bradycardia, which required cardiopulmonary resuscitation. He did not appear to have any significant neurologic sequelae following resuscitation, but 2 days later became progressively confused, restless, and lethargic. Systemic complications included acute renal failure treated with hemodialysis, hepatic insufficiency, and respiratory insufficiency requiring mechanical ventilation. He suffered two generalized tonic-clonic seizures that were controlled with intravenous phenytoin. His medical history was also positive for right hemispheric "watershed" infarction with slight residual left hemiparesis. Medications included methylprednisolone, cyclosporin A, muromonab-CD3, azathioprine, phenytoin, broad-spectrum antibiotics, dobutamine, and dopamine.

Physical Examination: Vital signs: afebrile, pulse 82, blood pressure 114/54. Intubated, mechanically ventilated. Neck: supple, no bruits. Chest: lungs clear to auscultation. Cardiac: rhythm and rate regular, distant heart sounds. Abdomen: normal; moderate pitting edema in lower extremities. Mental status: lethargic but easily arousable, able to follow simple commands while intubated. Cranial nerves: pupils equal with normal reaction to light, visual fields full to threat, normal gaze, corneal reflexes preserved and symmetric, facial movements symmetric; funduscopic examination: normal. Motor examination: muscle bulk mildly diminished in lower extremities, muscle tone normal, strength grade +4 in all four extremities; mild pronator drift on the left. Sensory examination: normal to light touch, pain, and vibratory stimuli. Muscle stretch reflexes: grade 1 throughout and symmetric. Plantar reflexes: flexor. Coordination and gait: unable to test.

Stop and Consider: What etiologies should be considered as possible causes of this patient's diffuse cortical dysfunction and encephalopathy?

Laboratory Findings: Hemoglobin 8.5 g/dl (13.6–16.8), hematocrit 24% (40–50), WBC 8,300/μl (3,500–8,500), platelets 70,000/μl (160,000–370,00), PT: INR 1.2 (0.9–1.1), Na^+ 138 mmol/L (135–144), K^+ 5.3 mmol/L (3.5–4.8), Cl^- 102 mmol/L (97–106), HCO_3^- 20 mmol/L (22–32), NH_4^+ 48 mmol/L (0–40), calcium 7.8 mg/dl (8.5–10.2), albumin 2.3 g/dl (3.5–5.0) glucose 235 mg/dl, BUN 103 mg/dl (7–20), creatinine 4.8 mg/dl (0.6–1.3), GGT 485 U/L (0–85), AST 69 U/L (0–50), ALT 112 U/L (0–65), AP 245 U/L (35–130), LDH 488 U/L (90–200), total bilirubin 3.5 mg/dl (0–1.4). Arterial blood gases: pO_2 104 mmHg (80–90), O_2 saturation 96% (95–98), pH 7.40 (7.3–7.44), pCO_2 34 mmHg (34–46). Serum phenytoin: 14.7 μg/ml (10–20); cyclosporin A: 168 ng/ml. Cranial CT: old infarct in the right hemisphere between the middle cerebral artery and posterior cerebral artery watershed territories, no acute changes. EEG: see figure, next page.

Question: Are the EEG abnormalities consistent with the patient's clinical condition?

Diagnosis: Metabolic encephalopathy and seizures in a patient with acute cardiac transplant rejection and multiple metabolic disturbances

Discussion: This patient developed progressive mental status deterioration with features of delirium, lethargy, and seizures following acute heart transplant rejection complicated by cardiopulmonary failure. Systemic abnormalities contributing to encephalopathy included reduced cardiac output, renal and hepatic failure, and resulting metabolic disturbances. New focal brain abnormalities were not observed in the CT, and his mild left hemiparesis was a residual deficit from the prior right hemispheric infarct. The EEG demonstrated semirhythmic, bisynchronous slow activity consistent with bihemispheric dysfunction, and generalized sharp waves or sharp-contoured slow waves with triphasic features (arrows), as well as focal epileptiform discharges (arrowhead).

Acute toxic or metabolic encephalopathy may manifest as delirium, disorientation, inattention, restlessness, global cognitive impairment, or lethargy, and may evolve into coma if underlying abnormalities are not corrected. Neurologic examination usually reveals generalized, symmetric findings without focal abnormalities. When the neurologic examination reveals focal abnormality in addition to generalized impairment, structural brain lesions should be considered and excluded by imaging studies. In addition to metabolic disturbances, systemic and CNS infections, drug toxicity, or intoxication may contribute to encephalopathy. Seizures are common in critically ill patients with metabolic disturbances and may present as nonconvulsive status epilepticus. In critically ill patients, neuromuscular dysfunction produced by use of paralytic neuromuscular blocking agents and critical-illness polyneuropathy or myopathy may also contribute to neurologic abnormalities.

Laboratory studies should be obtained to define the systemic abnormalities and rapidly initiate correction or appropriate treatment. Typical laboratory studies include complete blood count, coagulopathy profile, electrolytes, glucose, liver and renal function tests, arterial blood gases, ammonia levels, and toxic drug screens of blood and urine. Blood cultures should be obtained if systemic infection is suspected. Other laboratory studies may be necessary depending on the clinical picture.

Neuroimaging studies should be obtained in all cases with focal abnormalities or asymmetric findings to exclude structural lesions. Lumbar puncture should be performed if meningitis or encephalitis are suspected. EEG should be obtained to look for focal dysfunction and to follow progression or improvement of the encephalopathy. The EEG may show findings consistent with toxic-metabolic etiologies, such as triphasic waves, but may also reveal epileptiform discharges including nonconvulsive seizures, which sometimes may be difficult to recognize clinically and have relatively high incidence in critically ill patients.

Neurologic complications related to cardiac transplantation are the major cause of morbidity and mortality in transplant recipients. In some early reports up to 54% patients suffered neurologic complications after heart transplantation, with hypoxic or metabolic encephalopathy, cerebral infarction or

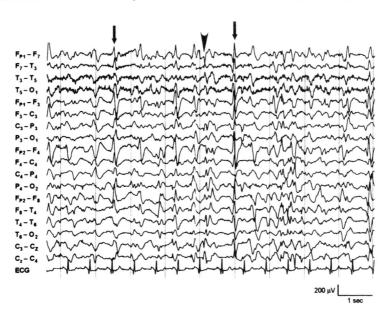

200 µV
1 sec

hemorrhage, and seizures being most frequent. Improvement in perioperative monitoring and treatment of cardiac rejection have markedly reduced the incidence of cerebral infarction in cardiac transplant patients.

Encephalopathy has been reported in one series in 12% of patients following heart transplantation and has multiple etiologies, including hypoxic brain injury, renal or hepatic failure, sepsis, or intracranial infection. Acute delirium and sometimes delusions and hallucinations have been reported immediately in the postoperative period but are usually transient.

The development of encephalopathy more than a few weeks after initiation of immunosuppression should suggest the possibility of CNS infections, including viral, fungal, and bacterial processes. Immunosuppressive drugs such as cyclosporin A or tacrolimus may be neurotoxic, and with higher blood levels may cause severe encephalopathy.

The present patient continued to deteriorate despite aggressive treatment of the heart transplant rejection and metabolic abnormalities. He later developed sepsis and meningitis and, despite all therapeutic efforts, expired due to multiorgan failure.

Clinical Pearls

1. Neurologic complications including delirium are common after organ transplantation.

2. Immunosuppressive drugs may be neurotoxic and cause acute encephalopathy.

3. EEG is very useful in evaluation of critically ill patients who develop acute mental status changes. It may reveal electrophysiologic abnormalities suggestive of toxic or metabolic encephalopathy, epileptiform discharges, or nonconvulsive seizures.

4. Rapid recognition and aggressive treatment of underlying metabolic abnormalities determine the outcome of critically ill patients who develop acute metabolic encephalopathy.

REFERENCES

1. Britt RH, Enzmann DR, Remington JS: Intracranial infection in cardiac transplant recipients. Ann Neurol 1981; 9:107–119.
2. Furlan AJ, Sila CA, Chimowitz MI, et al: Neurologic complications related to cardiac surgery. Neurol Clin 1992; 10:145–166.
3. Hotson JR, Enzmann DR: Neurologic complications of cardiac transplantation Neurol Clin 1988; 6:349–365.

PATIENT 64

A 20-year-old man with high-arched feet and progressive weakness and numbness of all four extremities

A 20-year-old man presented for evaluation of weakness and numbness in all extremities and progressive difficulty walking. In early childhood he developed unsteady gait and underwent two corrective orthopedic procedures for bilateral clubfoot deformities. He subsequently developed progressive distal weakness in lower extremities followed by weakness and atrophy in the hands and forearm muscles. By age 14 he required bilateral leg braces because of footdrop and experienced severe bilateral numbness, tingling, and electric shock-like sensation in his legs and feet. He denied any problems with bowel or bladder functions, visual or hearing symptoms, or difficulty swallowing. His father reported difficulty walking since adolescence and had a clubfoot deformity, but never lost the ability to ambulate independently.

Physical Examination: Vital signs: normal. Head and spine: normal. Mental status and speech: normal. Cranial nerves: normal. Motor examination: severe, bilateral foot deformities with high arches (pes cavus) and extensive scars secondary to orthopedic procedures (see figure); severe atrophy of distal muscles in upper and lower extremities; complete bilateral footdrop with no ability to dorsiflex the foot (strength grade 0), grade 2 bilateral plantar flexion weakness, proximal lower extremity muscle strength grade 4; upper extremity strength grade 4 distally and +4 proximally. Sensory examination: severe sensory loss in glove-and-stocking distribution to all modalities. Muscle stretch reflexes: absent throughout. Coordination: mild difficulty on heel-to-shin and finger-to-nose movements secondary to weakness. Gait: steppage pattern secondary to footdrop.

Stop and Consider: What is the anatomic localization for this patient's progressive extremity weakness and sensory dysfunction and what is the significance of the pes cavus? What diagnostic tests would be most useful in evaluation?

Laboratory Findings: CBC and chemistries: normal. Nerve conduction study (NCS): absent sensory and motor responses in lower extremities; marked slowing of motor and sensory conduction velocities in upper extremities with ulnar motor conduction velocity 22 m/s (normal: > 51) and median motor conduction velocity 26 m/s (normal: > 48); diminished amplitudes of sensory and motor responses in ulnar and median nerves. Needle electromyography (EMG): fibrillation potentials and long-duration, high-amplitude motor unit potentials with markedly decreased recruitment in distal upper and lower extremity muscles. Blood DNA analysis: duplication of chromosome 17p11.2–12 region containing the *PMP22* gene.

Question: What diagnosis was suggested by the clinical findings and the electrodiagnostic studies, and was confirmed by DNA analysis?

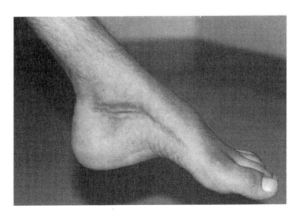

Diagnosis: Charcot-Marie-Tooth disease type 1A

Discussion: The neurologic deficit in this patient, with severe distal muscle atrophy, weakness, sensory loss in all four extremities, and areflexia was consistent with peripheral neuropathy. The presence of bilateral pes cavus and the family history of weakness and foot deformities suggested the possibility of a hereditary polyneuropathy. The severe slowing of conduction velocities on NCS in the setting of these clinical findings was consistent with Charcot-Marie-Tooth disease (CMT) type 1, also known as the demyelinating form of CMT. The DNA study confirmed the diagnosis by showing duplication in the *PMP22* gene locus on chromosome 17, the most frequent mutation associated with CMT disease type 1.

CMT, also known as hereditary motor and sensory neuropathy (HMSN), traditionally has been divided into CMT type 1 (CMT1), characterized by demyelination, and CMT type 2 (CMT2), characterized predominantly by axonal degeneration. Hereditary neuropathies demonstrate both clinical and genetic heterogeneity and classification has been based on clinical features, electrodiagnostic studies, inheritance patterns, and, in some cases, pathologic findings from nerve biopsy. DNA testing is currently available for several subtypes of CMT and has markedly improved the accuracy of diagnosis and classification. The most common inheritance pattern in CMT is autosomal dominant. The X-linked dominant form of CMT is also relatively common. Autosomal recessive forms of CMT are rare, and some cases present as *de novo* mutations.

CMT1 and CMT2 have similar clinical features, but there is considerable variability in the severity of the phenotype, even among the members of the same family. The disease typically manifests in the first or second decade of life and is slowly progressive. Patients develop progressive muscle weakness and atrophy that typically starts with distal muscles of lower extremities and affects the peroneal muscle group most severely. In addition to motor involvement, there is progressive distal sensory loss in characteristic glove-and-stocking distribution. Muscle stretch reflexes are markedly depressed and with disease progression are eventually lost in most patients. Foot deformities, including pes cavus (high-arched foot) and "hammer" toes, are very common. Patients with CMT1 frequently have markedly hypertrophic peripheral nerves that can be detected by palpation during examination. Mild cases of CMT1 and CMT2 may have minimal deficit or be asymptomatic; some cases may manifest only as foot deformities.

Electrodiagnostic studies in patients with CMT1 typically show severe, symmetric slowing of conduction velocities, which is consistent with a demyelinating pathologic process. Prior to introduction of DNA testing, the diagnosis of CMT1 was based on the typical clinical features accompanied by motor conduction velocity below 38 m/s in the upper extremity nerves. Pathologically, CMT1 is characterized by prominent demyelinating and remyelinating changes, with onion bulb formations in nerve biopsies. In CMT2 electrodiagnostic studies typically show evidence of primarily axonal process, with decreased amplitudes of motor and sensory responses and normal or mildly decreased conduction velocities. Axonal degeneration is the dominant pathologic abnormality in CMT2. In some cases "overlapping" electrodiagnostic and pathologic features of CMT1 and CMT2 are observed.

Several different mutations have been identified in CMT1 patients. In the majority of patients (CMT1A) there is a duplication in the 17p11.2–12 chromosomal region that contains the peripheral myelin protein 22 (*PMP22*) gene. Rare patients with CMT may have a point mutation in the *PMP22* gene. Patients with CMT1B have a mutation in the *P0* protein gene on chromosome 1 and represent approximately 5% of patients with CMT1. About 6% of CMT1 cases are caused by mutation on chromosome X in the connexin 32 gene, with a dominant inheritance pattern. In this form males are usually severely affected, whereas females may be mildly affected and sometimes asymptomatic. Rare patients with CMT1 may have a mutation in the early growth response 2 (*EGR2*) gene on chromosome 10. There is a significant number of families with CMT1 in whom a gene mutation has not been identified

Patients with very-early-onset, markedly delayed developmental milestones, severe motor and sensory deficit, severe foot deformities, and severe slowing of motor nerve conduction velocities (usually to less than 10 m/s) have been referred to as Dejerine-Sottas disease or HMSN type 3. Most of these patients have *de novo* mutations in the *PMP22*, *P0*, or *EGR2* genes; therefore, it appears to be a severe form of CMT type 1.

Patients with hereditary neuropathy with liability to pressure palsies (HNPP), also known as tomaculous neuropathy, typically present with focal neuropathies affecting different peripheral nerves, but many patients with HNPP have more diffuse demyelinating changes on electrodiagnostic studies. Most patients with HNPP have a 1.5-Mb deletion in the locus containing the *PMP22* gene (which is duplicated in CMT1A).

Several loci have been identified in families with the CMT2 (axonal form) by genetic linkage studies, but the specific genes have not been identified. There are no DNA diagnostic tests available at the present time to assist clinicians in diagnostic evaluation of patients who appear to have CMT2.

With availability of genetic testing, noninvasive accurate diagnosis of many patients with CMT is now possible and nerve biopsies are rarely necessary. In a patient with a CMT phenotype and demyelinating changes on NCS, the test for duplication of the locus containing the *PMP22* gene should be performed first. If negative, testing for less common mutations associated with CMT1 should be considered. Linkage studies may be useful in evaluation of families with CMT2.

Currently there is no effective treatment for CMT. Genetic counseling should be offered to patients and their families. Physical and occupational therapy should be directed toward maintaining function and symptom control and prevention of contractures and other musculoskeletal complications. Ankle-foot orthoses can improve ambulation. Corrective orthopedic procedures can be considered for severe foot deformities. Patients should avoid potentially neurotoxic medications. The CMT is a slowly progressive disease that is frequently associated with severe disability, but patients rarely become wheelchair-dependent.

Clinical Pearls

1. Hereditary neuropathy such as Charcot-Marie-Tooth (CMT) disease should be suspected in patients with early-onset, progressive polyneuropathy and associated foot deformities.

2. The peroneal muscle group is most severely affected in CMT disease.

3. CMT type 1 is characterized by primarily demyelinating changes and in CMT type 2 the dominant pathologic alteration is axonal degeneration.

4. CMT type 1 and type 2 can be distinguished in most cases on the basis of nerve conduction studies.

5. Duplication of the locus containing the *PMP22* gene in the 17p11.2–12 chromosomal region is the most frequent mutation in CMT1.

6. Phenotypes of CMT disease are variable; some individuals may have only slight foot deformities as the sole manifestation of the disorder.

REFERENCES

1. Harding AE, Thomas PK: The clinical features of hereditary motor and sensory neuropathy type I and II. Brain 1980; 103: 259–280.
2. Pareyson D: Charcot-Marie-Tooth disease and related neuropathies: Molecular basis for distinction and diagnosis. Muscle Nerve 1999; 22:1498–1509.
3. Vance JM, Baker D, Yamaoka LH, et al: Localization of Charcot-Marie-Tooth disease type 1A (CMT 1A) to chromosome 17p11.2. Genomics 1991; 9:623–628.

PATIENT 65

A 38-year-old woman with left arm and shoulder pain and skin rash

A 38-year-old woman developed severe pain in the left shoulder and left arm that increased in severity within 2 days after onset. She described the pain as burning, sharp, and stabbing, with radiation to the 4th and 5th digits of the left hand. A few days after the onset of pain she developed a vesicular rash in the left upper back (see figure), which later spread to the medial aspect of the left upper extremity. The severity of the pain continued to increase in association with the spread of the rash. A diagnosis of herpes zoster infection was established and she was treated with intravenous acyclovir. Her pain was well controlled with intravenous morphine and lidocaine. The rash subsequently resolved, but she continued to experience severe shoulder pain, numbness of the 4th and 5th digits of her left hand, and weakness of left hand grip. Six weeks after resolution of the rash she returned to the neurology clinic complaining of severe, intractable pain in the left upper extremity. Her medical history was significant for Hodgkin's lymphoma treated with radiation and chemotherapy 2 years prior to the development of the rash and pain, but oncologic evaluation indicated that the Hodgkin's disease appeared to be in complete remission.

Physical Examination: Vital signs: normal. Skin: patchy hyperpigmentation in the areas of previous rash. Mental status, speech, and cranial nerves: normal. Motor examination: atrophy of the left hand muscles, weakness (grade 3) of thenar, hypothenar, and interosseous muscles on the left. Sensory examination: diminished sensation to light touch, vibration, pin prick, and temperature in the left medial forearm and hand including 4th and 5th digits; dysesthesias were reported in response to light touch; hyperalgesia in the whole left upper extremity was evoked by pin prick. Muscle stretch reflexes: normal (grade 2). Coordination and gait: normal.

Stop and Consider: What is the neuroanatomic localization of the lesion causing the weakness and sensory deficit in this patient?

Laboratory Findings: CBC, chemistry panel: normal. ESR 27 mm/hr (normal 0–25). Nerve conduction study: diminished amplitudes of left ulnar and median compound muscle action potentials, normal conduction velocities. Needle electromyography: fibrillation potentials and decreased motor unit recruitment in the C8 and T1 nerve root innervated muscles in the left upper extremity, spontaneous activity in the left cervical paraspinal muscles. Cervical spine MRI: normal. Chest x-ray: normal.

Question: What is the cause of this patient's persistent pain?

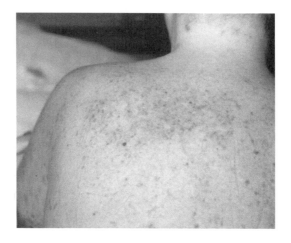

Diagnosis: Postherpetic neuralgia and left C8 and T1 radiculopathies secondary to herpes zoster infection

Discussion: A dermatomal rash associated with severe radiating pain is typical of herpes zoster virus (HZV) infection. In this patient the motor and sensory deficits in the left upper extremity were consistent with a C8/T1 radiculopathy, and corresponded with the dermatomal distribution of the rash (which probably also involved the T2 dermatome). A similar neurologic deficit may be encountered in lesions of the lower trunk of the brachial plexus, but electromyography confirmed a radiculopathy by showing denervation in the cervical paraspinal muscles in addition to the C8/T1 myotome in the left upper extremity. Although the neurologic deficit appeared to be related to HZV infection, a cervical spine MRI was obtained to assess for a possible compressive lesion. The persistence of pain for 6 weeks after resolution of the skin rash was consistent with postherpetic neuralgia.

After initial systemic infection (chickenpox), varicella zoster virus persists for life in the sensory ganglia. Reactivation of the virus causes zoster infection, which typically manifests as dermatomal rash (commonly referred to as "shingles"). The rash most frequently occurs in the thoracic region but can occur in any region of the neural axis. Neurologic syndromes of HZV infection may include myelitis, encephalitis, aseptic meningitis, vasculitis, ischemic stroke secondary to thrombotic cerebral vasculopathy, ascending polyradiculitis, multiple cranial neuropathies such as herpes zoster ophthalmicus, or Ramsay-Hunt syndrome (involvement of the 8th nerve ganglia and the geniculate ganglion of the 7th nerve), or radiculopathies with significant motor deficit. In patients who develop neurologic complications without typical skin rash (zoster sine herpete), examination of the CSF with PCR analysis for HZV DNA may be helpful to confirm the diagnosis.

Postherpetic neuralgia (PHN) is unfortunately the most frequent long-term neurologic complication of HZV infection. The skin rash itself is usually very painful and is often associated with dysesthetic sensory disturbance. In most cases, the pain gradually diminishes in intensity as the rash clears, but a number of patients continue to experience pain after the resolution of the rash. PHN is usually defined as persistence of pain for longer than 1 month after resolution of skin rash. It is characterized by severe pain with burning, lancinating features, frequently associated with allodynia and variable sensory alterations involving multiple modalities in the skin dermatome affected by zoster infection. The incidence of postherpetic neuralgia is low in younger patients (less than 40 years old), but the risk of this complication dramatically increases in elderly patients, and may be as high as 75% in patients older than 70. Some patients may show local signs of autonomic dysfunction. The affected skin areas may develop hyperpigmentation or excessive scarring.

Pathologic studies of PHN show axonal loss and areas of demyelination in sensory nerve roots, but similar changes are also observed in patients who do not develop PHN. Ongoing inflammation has been postulated as one of the possible mechanisms of PHN based on the observation that in some patients persistence of HZV DNA in mononuclear cells has been demonstrated for months to years after resolution of the skin rash. It has also been postulated that pain and allodynia can be caused by alterations in the peripheral and central nervous systems that result in dysfunctional central processing of sensory information.

Treatment with antiviral drugs such as acyclovir, valacyclovir, or famciclovir does not appear to prevent the eventual development of PHN, but may relieve the pain during the acute infection and may minimize the scar tissue formation. Corticosteroids have been used for many years and may ameliorate pain in acute infection but do not prevent development of PHN. Tricyclic antidepressants (e.g., amitriptyline or desipramine) have been found effective in alleviating the neuralgic symptoms and should be initiated early in the course of HZV infection. Satisfactory results and reduction in pain may be achieved in as many as 60–70% of patients. Nonsteroidal anti-inflammatory drugs or anticonvulsants such as carbamazepine have not been particularly effective, but recently patients treated with the anticonvulsant gabapentin have reported improvement. Topical analgesics such as capsaicin cream usually have a modest effect. In some patients treatment with opioids should be considered, although this form of therapy should be used as a last resort.

The present patient did not respond to tricyclic antidepressants, but partial improvement was observed with gabapentin. She reported satisfactory pain control with a small dose of extended-release morphine. Physical and occupational therapy were started after satisfactory pain control was achieved. Her sensory and motor deficits fully recovered within 3 months and she was able to return to work.

Clinical Pearls

1. Herpes zoster infection is diagnosed on the basis of a dermatomal vesicular skin rash and neuralgic pain in the areas supplied by peripheral sensory nerves projecting to the affected dorsal root ganglia.

2. Some cases of herpes zoster may never demonstrate a skin rash (zoster sine herpete) or the rash may develop several days after the onset of pain or neurologic deficit.

3. Postherpetic neuralgia is defined as persistence of pain for more than 4 weeks after resolution of vesicular eruption.

4. Age is the most important risk factor for development of postherpetic neuralgia, with incidence rising to 75% in patients older than 70.

5. Radiculopathies with motor deficit may develop in the course of herpes zoster infection.

6. Acyclovir should be given early in the course of herpes zoster infection.

7. Tricyclic antidepressants may markedly improve symptoms in patients with postherpetic neuralgia and should be considered early in the course of infection.

REFERENCES

1. Bowsher D: Acute herpes zoster and postherpetic neuralgia: Effects of acyclovir and outcome of treatment with amitriptyline. Br J Gen Pract 1992; 42:244–246.
2. Gilden DH, Kleinschmidt-DeMasters BK, LaGuardia JJ, et al: Neurologic complications of the reactivation of varicella zoster virus. N Engl J Med 2000; 342:635–645.
3. Liesegang TJ: Varicella zoster viral disease. Mayo Clin Proc 1999; 74:983–998.
4. Nurmikko T: Clinical features and pathophysiologic mechanisms of postherpetic neuralgia. Neurology 1995; 45(Suppl 8): S54–S55.
5. Watson CP: The treatment of postherpetic neuralgia. Neurology 1995; 45(Suppl 8):S58–S60.

PATIENT 66

A 26-year-old woman with recurrent ischemic strokes

A 26-year-old woman with a history of migraine presented to the emergency room after abrupt onset of right-sided weakness. She denied other neurologic symptoms, recent headache, or trauma. At age 22 she experienced abrupt onset of mild left-sided weakness associated with a right internal capsule infarct, but recovered completely after 3 months of rehabilitation. Despite extensive diagnostic evaluation an etiology for the infarct was not determined, and the only abnormality detected was a mild mitral valve prolapse. She was not taking any medications or oral contraceptives, and denied using alcohol, tobacco, or any drugs. Her medical and family history were unremarkable.

Physical Examination: Pulse 88 and regular; blood pressure 106/66; temperature and respiratory rate: normal. Neck, cardiac, chest, and abdomen: normal. Skin: mild livedo reticularis in both upper extremities. Skull and spine: normal. Mental status, affect, speech, and language: normal. Cranial nerves: pupils symmetric and reactive; normal fundi, visual fields, and gaze; mild right lower facial weakness with symmetric forehead movements, normal oral, pharyngeal, and tongue movements. Motor examination: normal muscle bulk; mild spasticity in both lower extremities; right hemiparesis with grade 4 strength in both arm and leg. Sensory examination: normal. Muscle stretch reflexes: increased (grade 3) but symmetric. Coordination: mildly decreased coordination of the right-sided extremities secondary to weakness. Plantar reflexes: bilateral Babinski signs. Gait: unsteady because of right hemiparesis.

Stop and Consider: What are the neuroanatomic structures that underlie this patient's deficits? What is the most likely cause of her abrupt-onset weakness?

Laboratory Findings: CBC, chemistry panel, electrolytes, ESR, ANA, PT, PTT: normal. Platelet count 108,000/μl (160,000–370,000). IgG anticardiolipin antibodies: 50 g/L (0–29); IgM and IgA anticardiolipin antibodies: normal. Kaolin clotting time test: abnormal. Head MRI: see figure. Intra-arterial four-vessel angiography: normal. Transthoracic and transesophageal echocardiography: normal, except for mild mitral valve prolapse and mild thickening of the mitral valve.

Question: Are the MRI abnormalities consistent with this patient's clinical findings? What is the significance of the elevated anticardiolipin antibodies?

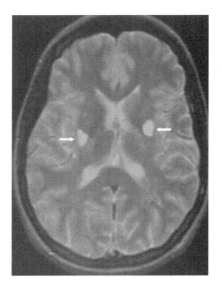

Diagnosis: Coagulopathy with recurrent ischemic strokes of the left and right subcortical regions involving internal capsules

Discussion: The neurologic examination revealed bilateral abnormalities of the corticospinal tracts, with the more severe and recent-onset deficit involving the left cerebral hemisphere. The pure motor deficit suggested a subcortical lesion. The acute presentation of the new deficit and the similar episode 4 years earlier were consistent with recurrent strokes. The head MRI showed deep ischemic lesions involving the posterior limbs of both right and left internal capsules (arrows). The laboratory evaluation revealed antiphospholipid antibodies, including high titers of anticardiolipin antibodies, and presence of the lupus anticoagulant indicated by the abnormal Kaolin clotting time test. The abnormalities were indicative of coagulopathy and are risk factors for ischemic stroke or transient ischemic attacks. The livedo reticularis, thrombocytopenia, history of migraine, and thickening of the mitral valve may also be associated with antiphospholipid antibodies, but there was no other evidence for systemic lupus erythematosus. The constellation of antiphospholipid antibodies, stroke, and livedo reticularis in the absence of other systemic disease is sometimes referred to as Sneddon's syndrome.

Antiphospholipid antibodies (anticardiolipin antibodies and lupus anticoagulants) are associated with an increased risk for venous and arterial thrombosis. In approximately 25% of patients with the antiphospholipid syndrome both anticardiolipin antibodies and lupus anticoagulant are present. Testing for both classes of antibodies is necessary if this syndrome is suspected. The frequency of antiphospholipid antibodies in patients with established diagnosis of systemic lupus erythematosus varies between 7–58%.

Strokes and transient ischemic attacks, involving both large and small arteries, or veins, have been described in persons with antiphospholipid antibody syndromes. Pathologic reports have demonstrated nonspecific microvascular platelet fibrin plugs in affected patients, suggesting ongoing thrombosis *in situ*. Additional cardiovascular manifestations, such as mitral valve thickening, often accompany antiphospholipid antibody syndrome and raise the possibility of cardioembolic events. Other systemic manifestations of the antiphospholipid antibody syndrome include livedo reticularis, recurrent miscarriages, migraine, and thrombocytopenia.

The proposed criteria for neurologic diagnosis of probable antiphospholipid antibody syndrome include: (1) age less than 55 years; (2) episodes of brain infarction, TIA, amaurosis fugax, retinal infarction, myelopathy, vascular dementia, or abnormal movements such as chorea; and (3) high levels of IgG anticardiolipin antibodies, presence of lupus anticoagulant, or both.

Management of patients with the antiphospholipid antibody syndrome is controversial and specific treatment is not available. Patients with minimal symptoms or a single transient ischemic event are often treated with an antiplatelet agent (such as aspirin), and those with more severe or recurring ischemic events are usually treated with chronic anticoagulation therapy.

The present patient was anticoagulated with warfarin (INR 2.5–3.0) and was followed closely because of the associated thrombocytopenia. She spent 2 months in the rehabilitation center, was fully independent when discharged, and had no additional recurrent ischemic cerebrovascular events. In addition, she has not manifested any rheumatologic problems.

Clinical Pearls

1. Antiphospholipid antibodies (both anticardiolipin antibodies and lupus anticoagulant) are associated with an increased risk of venous and arterial thrombosis, including ischemic stroke and transient ischemic attacks.

2. Approximately 25% of patients with the antiphospholipid antibody syndrome have both anticardiolipin antibodies and lupus anticoagulant. Testing for both classes of antibodies should be pursued if this syndrome is suspected.

3. Vascular dementia may be a consequence of recurrent strokes in patients with the antiphospholipid antibody syndrome.

4. Both antiplatelet agents and warfarin are used in management of patients with the antiphospholipid antibody syndrome, but the efficacy of these treatments is uncertain.

REFERENCES

1. Bick RL, Baker WF Jr: The antiphospholipid and thrombosis syndromes. Med Clin North Am 1994; 78:667–684.
2. Coull BM, Levine SR, Ray LB: The role of antiphospholipid antibodies in stroke. Neurol Clin 1992; 10:125–143.
3. Greaves M: Coagulation abnormalities and cerebral infarction. J Neurol Neurosurg Psychiatry 1993; 56:433–439.

PATIENT 67

A 57-year-old man with acute onset of headache, fever, chills, confusion, and restlessness

A 57-year-old man presented with a severe generalized headache, fever, chills, and malaise. The symptoms developed rapidly in one day and he became progressively irritable and drowsy. He had mild symptoms of an upper respiratory infection for about a week prior to the onset of headache. His medical history was significant for head trauma approximately 15 years ago that required surgical reconstruction of the frontal and maxillary bones, but was not associated with any neurologic sequelae. The patient was taking no medications and had no history of alcohol, tobacco, or drug abuse.

Physical Examination: Vital signs: pulse 102, respirations 22, blood pressure 140/80, rectal temperature 39.5°. HEENT: severe nuchal rigidity of the neck; positive Brudzinski's sign (passive flexion of the neck induced leg flexion), positive Kernig's sign (passive flexion of the neck induced pain in hamstrings). Cardiac, chest, abdomen, and skin: normal. Mental status: restless, confused, able to follow only one-step commands. Speech: minimal verbal output, very short, slurred phrases. Cranial nerves: pupils equal, round, reactive to light; funduscopic exam: no papilledema; otherwise normal. Motor examination: normal bulk, tone, symmetric movements of all four extremities, no evident weakness. Sensory examination: localized pain stimuli well. Muscle stretch reflexes: grade 3 throughout and symmetric. Plantar reflexes: flexor bilaterally. Coordination and gait: unable to test because of altered mental status.

Stop and Consider: What neurologic conditions should be considered in a patient with rapidly developing headache, fever, mental status changes, and signs of meningeal irritation?

Laboratory Findings: WBC count: 26,300/μl (53% segmented, 36% bands, 2% lymphocytes). ESR 17 mm/hr (0–25). Serum chemistries, electrolytes: normal. Arterial blood gases: normal. Chest x–ray: normal. Head CT scan: no midline shift, mass effect, hemorrhage, or hydrocephalus. Lumbar puncture: opening pressure 210 mmH$_2$O (65–195), glucose 16 mg/dl (40–80), protein 1,628 mg/dl (15–45); nucleated cell count: 30,000/μl (85% neutrophils, 2% lymphocytes, 13% macrophages). CSF Gram stain: abundant gram-positive cocci. CSF *Streptococcus pneumoniae* antigen: positive. CSF culture: penicillin-sensitive *Streptococcus pneumoniae*. Blood cultures: negative.

Question: What is the most appropriate treatment for this patient?

Diagnosis: Pneumococcal meningitis

Discussion: The presentation of this patient strongly suggested bacterial meningitis, although viral encephalitis, such as herpes encephalitis, or brain abscess may present with similar symptoms. Lumbar puncture confirmed the diagnosis by showing CSF abnormalities typical of bacterial meningitis and identified the causative microorganism.

Bacterial meningitis typically presents with headache, neck stiffness, fever, photophobia, and altered mental status. Patients may rapidly deteriorate into coma and develop focal neurologic signs and seizures. Prognosis depends on rapid recognition, determination of the cause of the infection, rapid institution of appropriate treatment with antibiotics, and management of complications. If untreated, 95% of patients with bacterial meningitis die, and delay in treatment may cause serious neurologic sequelae.

Lumbar puncture should be performed as soon as possible if meningitis is suspected. Neuroimaging studies (cranial CT) are often obtained prior to lumbar puncture in patients who may be at risk of brain herniation, especially those who present with focal neurologic signs, suggestive of asymmetric increase of intracranial pressure, patients who present with coma or rapidly deteriorating mental status, or in patients with papilledema. Appropriate broad-spectrum antibiotics should be started after obtaining CSF for laboratory studies. If lumbar puncture is delayed for cranial CT, blood cultures should be obtained and antibiotics started immediately. The most common causes of community-acquired bacterial meningitis in adults in the U.S. are *Streptococcus pneumoniae, Neisseria meningitidis*, and *Listeria monocytogenes. Staphylococcus aureus* is common in meningitis caused by head trauma or neurosurgical procedures.

The CSF in bacterial meningitis typically shows marked pleocytosis (50–10,000 cells or more per microliter) with neutrophillic predominance, elevated protein content, and often depressed glucose levels. In many cases microorganisms can be seen on the CSF Gram stain. In addition to CSF cultures, blood cultures should routinely be performed. Serologic tests for bacterial antigens may assist in rapid identification of the pathogenic organism. CSF tests for viral, fungal, or parasitic etiologies should be performed as suggested by the clinical presentation, underlying systemic conditions, and results of other laboratory studies.

The initial choice of antibiotic therapy is influenced by the patient's age, coexisting illnesses, and known bacterial antibiotic resistance in the community. When culture and sensitivity results are obtained antibiotics should be modified as appropriate, and are usually administered intravenously for 10–14 days. Typical initial treatment in adults with community-acquired meningitis includes ceftriaxone or cefotaxime, frequently with addition of vancomycin and rifampin for resistant streptococcal strains. In immunosuppressed or elderly patients ampicillin is frequently added to cover for *Listeria monocytogenes.* Nafcillin or oxacillin is used for staphylococcal meningitis, but if methicillin resistance is likely, vancomycin and rifampin should also be added.

Patients with acute bacterial meningitis are usually treated in the intensive care unit, with careful monitoring of vital signs and frequent neurologic evaluations. Appropriate management of fluid and electrolyte balance in patients at risk of increased intracranial pressure is most important. Signs of increased intracranial pressure usually subside rapidly with treatment, but if there is no improvement, patients should be evaluated with cranial CT or MRI to assess for hydrocephalus and severity of brain edema. Some patients may need treatment with hyperventilation and osmotic agents such as mannitol. Use of corticosteroids in adults with meningitis is controversial, but they have been reported to be beneficial in children with bacterial meningitis. Brain MRI and MR angiogram or venogram should be considered if focal neurologic signs are observed in order to rule out brain infarct, abscess, subdural empyema, vasculitis, or cerebral venous thrombosis.

The present patient initially received intravenous ceftriaxone and vancomycin, and penicillin was started after the Gram stain results were available. Because of severe obtundation he was electively intubated, but within 24 hours the fever subsided, his mental status markedly improved, and he was weaned from the ventilator. Ceftriaxone and vancomycin were discontinued after the results of CSF cultures were obtained and sensitivity to penicillin was confirmed. Intravenous penicillin was continued for 14 days and full recovery was confirmed on follow-up evaluation.

Clinical Pearls

1. Successful outcome of bacterial meningitis depends on rapid recognition and treatment with appropriate antibiotics.

2. Untreated meningitis is fatal in over 95% of cases; delay in treatment may be associated with serious permanent neurologic deficits.

3. The most frequent causes of community-acquired bacterial meningitis in adult U.S. population are *Streptococcus pneumoniae, Neisseria meningitidis*, and *Listeria monocytogenes*.

4. The initial choice of antibiotic treatment in bacterial meningitis depends on the patient's age, coexisting illnesses, and known bacterial antibiotic resistance in the community.

REFERENCES

1. Ashwal S: Neurologic evaluation of the patient with acute bacterial meningitis. Neurol Clin 1995; 13:549–577.
2. Davis LE: Acute bacterial meningitis. In: Johnson RT, Griffin JW (eds): Current Therapy in Neurologic Disease, 5th ed. St. Louis, Mosby, 1997, pp 120–127.
3. Quagliarello VJ, Scheld WM: Treatment of bacterial meningitis. N Engl J Med 1997; 336:708–716.

PATIENT 68

A 48-year-old woman with metastatic renal carcinoma and progressive bilateral leg weakness, numbness, and episodic urinary incontinence

A 48-year-old woman with a history of renal carcinoma presented with a 2-week history of progressive bilateral leg numbness and paresthesias, which gradually ascended to the mid-thoracic level. She experienced progressive problems with balance and needed a cane for walking. She also noted increased urinary frequency and urgency and was incontinent on several occasions. One year prior to the onset of symptoms she received radiation treatment to the T6–T10 spinal region for metastases to the T7 and T8 vertebrae. The total dose of radiation was 57 Gy, administered in 30 fractions over 27 days. She reported chronic low back pain that was unchanged over the last several years and denied any pain, numbness, or weakness in upper extremities, swallowing difficulty, or headache. Her medical history was otherwise unremarkable.

Physical Examination: Vital signs: normal. Cardiac, chest, abdomen: normal. Head and neck: normal. Spine: nontender, good range of motion. Mental status and speech: normal. Cranial nerves: normal. Motor examination: normal muscle bulk, upper extremity muscle tone and strength normal, bilateral grade 4 lower extremity weakness with significant spasticity. Sensory examination: able to distinguish hot from cold and sharp from dull over the legs and trunk, but identified the sensations as "different" at approximately T8 dermatome level; vibratory sensation and proprioception markedly diminished in both feet. Muscle stretch reflexes: normal in upper extremities, pathologically brisk in lower extremities (grade 4) with sustained ankle clonus. Plantar reflexes: bilateral Babinski signs. Coordination: normal in upper extremities, mild difficulty on heel-to-sheen test bilaterally. Gait: wide-based, unsteady.

Stop and Consider: What is the neuroanatomic localization of the neurologic deficit in this patient?

Laboratory Findings: CBC: normal. ESR: 11 mm/hr (normal 0–20). Alkaline phosphatase: 361 U/L (normal 35–130). MRI of the thoracic region: see figure (T1 weighted image after gadolinium contrast injection).

Question: What is the likely etiology of the spinal cord abnormality demonstrated on the spinal MRI?

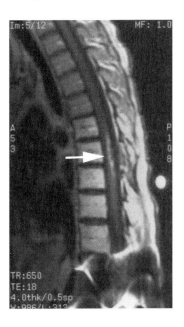

Diagnosis: Radiation-induced myelopathy

Discussion: This patient developed signs of progressive myelopathy with a sensory level localizing the spinal cord lesion to the T8 level 1 year after radiation to the spine. In a patient with metastatic cancer, epidural metastases causing cord compression should initially receive strong consideration, but the lack of significant back pain was unusual. Paraneoplastic myelopathy, epidural abscess or hematoma, transverse myelitis, or arteriovenous malformation should also be considered. The history of prior radiation therapy to the spine suggested that the myelopathy could be related to delayed effects of radiation on the spinal cord.

The MRI showed abnormal signal within the vertebral bodies of T6–T10 vertebrae consistent with postradiation bone marrow changes, but fractures and epidural metastases were not observed. There was diffusely abnormal signal within the spinal cord on T2 weighted images between T7–T10 vertebral levels. Abnormal enhancement was seen in the same cord region on T1 weighted images after gadolinium contrast administration (figure, arrow). The pattern of MRI abnormalities, with absence of mass effect, strongly suggested radiation-induced myelopathy.

Radiation-induced myelopathy may present within several months after treatment or as a delayed long-term complication. The most frequently observed is transient radiation-induced myelopathy, which occurs within 1–30 months after completion of radiation therapy, with the peak onset within 4–6 months. This syndrome is characterized predominantly by sensory disturbances, and paresthesias are the most frequently reported symptom. Many patients develop Lhermitte's sign, which refers to a sudden, electric shock–like sensation extending down the spine, induced by neck flexion. The majority of patients with this syndrome never develop any objective signs of myelopathy, and neuroimaging with spinal MRI typically is unremarkable. Most patients gradually improve within a few weeks to a year.

The syndrome of delayed radiation-induced myelopathy has bimodal incidence, with peaks at 12–14 months and 25–28 months. This syndrome may sometimes develop as long as 10 years after completion of radiation treatment. In the delayed syndrome sensory symptoms in the legs are followed by weakness and frequently urinary and bowel sphincter dysfunction. Some patients also complain of severe pain in lower extremities. The neurologic deficit may gradually evolve over the period of several months, and in most patients eventually reaches a plateau. In most cases the neurologic deficit is bilateral but a unilateral presentation, with a Brown-Séquard syndrome, may be observed. Radiation-induced injury may also produce prominent signs of lower motor neuron injury, with severe muscle atrophy, fasciculations, depressed reflexes, and signs of active and chronic neurogenic changes on electromyography. This syndrome is likely related to radiation-induced anterior horn cell degeneration.

Most patients who develop postradiation myelopathy receive incidental radiation to the spinal cord in the course of treatment of malignancies outside of the nervous system, especially for cancer of the lung, esophagus, and neoplasms of the head and neck. In cases of radiation-induced myelopathy after radiation treatment of a primary spinal cord tumor, it may be very difficult to distinguish whether neurologic deterioration is caused by radiation injury or by regrowth of the tumor.

MRI of the spine typically shows abnormally increased signal on T2 weighted images within the affected cord, and in some cases there may be cord enlargement due to cord edema. In most patients there is evidence of contrast enhancement that may have a streaky or ring-like pattern. Cerebrospinal fluid (CSF) examination may show mild elevation of the protein content or mild pleocytosis, but in most patients is normal.

Pathologic examination of the spinal cord in patients with delayed radiation-induced myelopathy typically shows areas of demyelination and axonal degeneration. In more severe cases there may be areas of necrosis. Some pathologic changes may also be secondary to ischemia caused by radiation-induced damage to the blood vessels.

The risk of radiation-induced myelopathy is higher in patients who receive higher total doses, higher daily fractions, have shorter total treatment duration, and have treatment administered to more extensive levels of the spinal cord. There is much variability in individual susceptibility to radiation-induced injury to the nervous system, but the incidence of postradiation myelopathy increases significantly in patients who receive a total dose of radiation to the region of the spinal cord above 5000 cGy, or daily fractions of 200 cGy or more. In patients who receive radiation doses less than these values, the risk of myelopathy is less than 5%. No effective treatment for radiation-induced myelopathy is available.

In the present patient the neurologic deficit eventually stabilized, but significant paraparesis remained. The spasticity improved with baclofen, and the back pain responded to oral morphine. She was able to walk short distances with a cane.

Clinical Pearls

1. Radiation-induced myelopathy may develop within months after radiation treatment or as late as 10 years after completion of the radiotherapy.

2. MRI is the best diagnostic test to evaluate patients with suspected radiation-induced myelopathy.

3. The risk of radiation-induced myelopathy may be reduced by avoidance of high total doses and administration of smaller daily fractions of radiation.

REFERENCES

1. Dropcho EJ: Neurologic complications of radiation therapy. In Biller J (ed): Iatrogenic Neurology. Boston, Butterworth-Heinemann, 1998, pp 461–483.
2. Goldwein JW: Radiation myelopathy: A review. Med Pediatr Oncol 1987; 15:89–95.
3. Schultheiss TE, Stephens LC, Peters LJ: Survival in radiation myelopathy. Int J Rad Oncol Biol Phys 1986; 12:1765–1769.
4. Yasui T, Yagura H, Komiyama M, et al: Significance of gadolinium-enhanced magnetic resonance imaging in differentiating spinal cord radiation myelopathy from tumor: Case report. J Neurosurg 1992; 77:628–631.

PATIENT 69

A 35-year-old woman with excessive daytime sleepiness

A 35-year-old woman who worked as a microelectronics technician was referred by her employer for evaluation of safety concerns related to excessive sleepiness at work. In high school she began experiencing episodes of suddenly falling asleep, which impaired her school performance. She ignored her tendency to excessive sleeping until she was nearly electrocuted when she fell asleep while working on oscilloscopes. She reported an episode of a sudden difficulty holding her head up after an argument with a friend, and another brief episode of sudden-onset leg weakness that produced difficulty walking and imbalance. Both episodes had a duration of about 1–2 minutes. She also reported several episodes of "paralysis" on awakening. The typical duration of her overnight sleep was 7–8 hours, and she used minimal amounts of caffeine, alcohol, or tobacco. The patient's father had a lifelong history of excessive sleepiness and frequent episodes of falling asleep at the dinner table. Her 13-year-old son was reported to have attention deficit disorder and excessive sleepiness at school where his teachers commented that he was frequently "daydreaming." The patient observed that her son could "sleep his life away" and often went back to sleep for 1–2 hours after breakfast. Her medical history was otherwise unremarkable.

Physical Examination: Vital signs: normal. General: normal. Mental status, speech, and cranial nerves: normal. Motor and sensory exam: normal. Muscle stretch reflexes: grade 2 and symmetric. Plantar reflexes: flexor. Coordination and gait: normal.

Stop and Consider: What are the possible causes of the excessive daytime sleepiness in this patient?

Laboratory Findings: CBC, chemistries: normal. Routine EEG: normal. Night-time sleep study (polysomnogram): normal. Multiple sleep latency test (MSLT): mean sleep latency 3.5 min. (normal > 10, borderline 5–10, abnormal < 5); sleep-onset rapid eye movement (REM) periods: 2 (normal < 2). Human leukocyte antigen (HLA) typing: DR2 negative; DQw1 positive. Both the patient's father and son underwent MSLT and were observed to have mean sleep latency of 4.5 and 4 minutes, respectively, and 2 sleep-onset REM periods.

Question: What is the diagnosis in this family based on the clinical presentation and results from multiple sleep latency tests?

Diagnosis: Narcolepsy, possibly with cataplexy and sleep paralysis

Discussion: Excessive daytime somnolence with "sleep attacks," episodes of probable cataplexy and sleep paralysis, and a strong family history of similar symptoms, should suggest narcolepsy. The MLST was markedly abnormal and confirmed pathologic daytime somnolence, indicated by abnormally short mean sleep latency and sleep-onset REM periods. The abnormal MSLT results in the patient's father and son were consistent with a familial disorder. She had no evidence of sleep apnea, systemic disease, or affective disorder, and her excessive daytime sleepiness was not explained by sleep deprivation.

Narcolepsy is characterized by excessive daytime sleepiness with sleep attacks and sleep-onset REM periods. Approximately 70–90% of patients with narcolepsy have cataplexy and many have episodes of sleep paralysis and hypnagogic hallucinations. Most patients with narcolepsy develop symptoms during the first or second decades of life, and the onset of symptoms can be very insidious. Excessive daytime sleepiness is the most common initial symptom and frequently precedes development of typical sleep attacks. In children, a decline in school performance may be the first noticeable manifestation of the disorder.

Patients with cataplexy experience sudden attacks of profound weakness and muscle hypotonia, which may last for a few seconds to a few minutes. Multiple attacks per day are not unusual. There is no loss of consciousness and respiratory or ocular muscles are not affected. Attacks of cataplexy are frequently precipitated by sudden positive or negative emotions. The extent of weakness and hypotonia in cataplectic attacks is variable. Some patients may experience attacks of complete paralysis; in other patients the attacks may be limited to a head drop, slumping into a chair, or feeling "weak." A significant proportion of narcoleptic patients with characteristic sleep attacks and abnormal sleep-onset REM periods do not have history of typical cataplexy and are typically referred to as monosymptomatic narcolepsy. Some of these patients may eventually develop typical cataplexy later in life.

Sleep paralysis occurs in many narcoleptic patients, and consists of episodes of inability to move at the onset of sleep or upon awakening, and may last up to a few minutes. Hypnagogic hallucinations typically occur in the sleep-wake transition and sometimes may occur during episodes of sleep paralysis.

Narcolepsy can sometimes be familial, and there is a strong association between narcolepsy and HLA haplotypes DR-15 (subtype of DR2) and DQB1*0602 (subtype of DQw1). Although the HLA association suggests a genetic predisposition, many individuals and families with narcolepsy do not have these HLA haplotypes and both DR-15 and DQB1*0602 antigens are common in general population. Narcolepsy has also been observed only in one of the monozygotic twins, which suggests that environmental factors may play a role in the development of this disorder. It is presumed that narcolepsy is a disorder involving abnormalities in monoaminergic or cholinergic systems and the generation of REM sleep.

In a patient with excessive daytime somnolence, conditions such as obstructive sleep apnea, structural CNS lesions involving hypothalamic area, chronic substance abuse, medication withdrawal, chronic sleep deprivation (sleep debt), and neuromuscular disorders such as myotonic dystrophy should be considered in addition to narcolepsy. The presence of cataplexy is the most helpful distinguishing clinical feature in patients suspected of having narcolepsy. Multiple sleep latency test is the most useful diagnostic study in evaluation of patients with suspected narcolepsy and shows abnormally short mean sleep latency and increased frequency of sleep-onset REM periods during daytime and night-time sleep episodes.

Narcolepsy is typically a lifelong disorder, and while completely effective treatment is rarely achieved, in approximately 75% of patients the symptoms can be markedly improved. Seep hygiene should be emphasized, and patients typically benefit from scheduled napping. Stimulants such as methylphenidate, modafinil, or amphetamines may be helpful. Cataplexy can be improved with imipramine or clomipramine.

The present patient was treated with several medications but continued to have sleep attacks and experienced treatment side effects. Eventually she had to stop working and received permanent disability.

Clinical Pearls

1. Cataplexy frequently accompanies narcolepsy, and in a patient with excessive day-time sleepiness and sleep attacks supports a clinical diagnosis of narcolepsy.

2. Multiple sleep latency test is the most useful diagnostic tool in evaluation of patients with suspected narcolepsy. It typically shows abnormally short mean sleep latency and increased frequency of sleep-onset REM periods.

3. Pharmacologic treatment is effective in as many as 75% of patients with narcolepsy, but complete control of symptoms is rarely achieved.

4. HLA haplotypes DR-15 and DQB1*0602 are strongly associated with narcolepsy, but are not specific as diagnostic tests.

REFERENCES

1. Aldrich MS: Diagnostic aspects of narcolepsy. Neurology 1998; 50(Suppl 1):S2–S7.
2. Bassetti C: Narcolepsy. Curr Treat Opt Neurol 1999; 1:291–297.
3. Neely S, Rosenberg R, Spire JP, et al: HLA antigens in narcolepsy. Neurology 1987; 37:1858–1860.

PATIENT 70

A 38-year-old woman with severe progressive dystonia

A 38-year-old woman was referred for evaluation of progressive problems with ambulation and dystonia. Her mother stated that at age 10–12 her daughter insidiously developed intermittent "twisting" motions in her hands and elbows. At about the same time she started exhibiting involuntary orofacial movements, and was noted to be "toe-walking." Her school performance deteriorated. Over the next decade she developed recurrent episodes of severe neck dystonia characterized by extreme forward neck flexion and spasms of the jaw muscles. Severe mandibular dystonia resulted in dental problems and she eventually became prematurely edentulous. She also developed tremors in both upper extremities that did not respond to carbidopa/levodopa. She had eating difficulties due to orofacial dystonia, and her speech was poorly intelligible. She was the product of a normal pregnancy and delivery, and her early childhood development was normal. There was no family history of a similar disorder. Her medical history was significant for a head trauma with brief loss of consciousness at age 3. At age 10 she experienced two generalized tonic-clonic seizures that were well controlled by Dilantin.

Physical Examination: Vital signs: normal. Head: normocephalic. Mental status: alert, awake, follows only very simple commands, poor attention span. Speech: severe dysarthria. Cranial nerves: pupils equal in size with normal reaction to light, visual fields normal to confrontation; funduscopic examination: normal, no pigmentary degeneration; normal gaze, severe, recurrent blepharoclonus, dystonic orofacial movements, hearing normal, oropharyngeal structures midline, no palatal myoclonus, bilateral hypertrophy of sternocleidomastoideus and trapezius muscles. Motor examination: diffusely diminished muscle bulk, rigidity; severe dystonic posturing in all four limbs with extreme flexion in elbows and wrists, frequent episodes of severe dystonia of axial muscles with extreme anterocollis (see figure, *left*); bilateral episodic low-frequency (3–5 Hz) resting tremor of hands and fingers. Sensation: difficult to evaluate because of poor cooperation but preserved to light pain, touch, and vibration. Muscle stretch reflexes: brisk throughout (grade 3). Plantar reflexes: bilateral Babinski signs. Coordination: unable to test because of severe dystonia. Gait: very unsteady, able to walk only with assistance.

Stop and Consider: What types of movement abnormalities are present in this patient and which systems and neuroanatomic pathways are involved?

Laboratory Findings: CBC, chemistries, liver function tests, electrolytes, thyroid function tests, ESR, ANA: normal. Serum ceruloplasmin and hexosaminidase A and urine copper levels: normal. Cranial CT: normal. Brain MRI (T2 weighted image): see figure, *right*. EEG: normal. Slitlamp examination: no Kayser-Fleischer rings.

Question: How would you classify this disorder and what is the significance of the abnormalities demonstrated on the brain MRI?

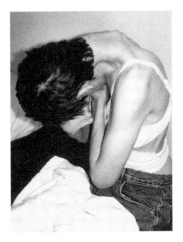 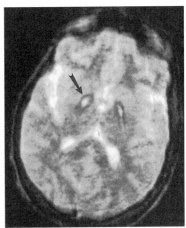

Diagnosis: Hallervorden-Spatz disease

Discussion: The clinical examination in this patient was characterized by severe dystonia affecting orofacial, limb, and axial muscles, rigidity, tremor, corticospinal tract signs, and intellectual impairment that apparently developed progressively after onset in late childhood. Her symptoms, signs, and the course of the disease were strongly suggestive of Hallervorden-Spatz disease. Wilson's disease may present with similar abnormalities, but was excluded by normal serum ceruloplasmin, normal urine copper levels, and normal slit-lamp examination.

MRI of the brain showed symmetric bilateral areas of increased signal surrounded by low signal in the area of globus pallidus on T2 weighted images (figure on the right, arrow). This appearance of the basal ganglia, sometimes referred to as "eyes of the tiger" sign, is usually related to iron deposits in the globus pallidus area and strongly supports the diagnosis of Hallervorden-Spatz disease. The MRI appearance, with characteristic abnormalities, varies from patient to patient and also depends on the stage of the disease.

Hallervorden-Spatz disease is a neurodegenerative condition characterized by abnormal iron metabolism in the brain. The symptoms typically start in the first decade of life and are relentlessly progressive. Patients with adult onset may have a relatively slower course of progression. Typical clinical features include prominent extrapyramidal signs with rigidity, dystonia, choreoathetosis, and tremor. Most patients also develop corticospinal signs with prominent spasticity, hyperreflexia, and Babinski signs. Severe dysarthria and dysphagia develop in most patients. Respiratory compromise may develop as a result of severe dystonic posturing. There is typically progressive cognitive decline and optic atrophy and retinitis pigmentosa are observed in some cases. Approximately 20% of patients with Hallervorden-Spatz disease may develop seizures. Most patients do not survive beyond early adulthood, but the clinical manifestations and the rate of progression vary from individual to individual. Most cases are sporadic, but familial cases also occur and suggest an autosomal recessive inheritance pattern.

Hallervorden-Spatz disease is characterized by large iron deposits in the globus pallidus and the pars reticulata of the substantia nigra, which at autopsy may produce a "rusty" appearance. Iron accumulation is observed in large astrocytes, microglial cells, neurons, and may also be observed extracellularly. Iron deposition is accompanied by neuromelanin accumulation, focal demyelination, axonal swelling, gliosis, and characteristic spheroid bodies, which may represent swollen axons. Abnormal cytosomes in circulating lymphocytes and sea-blue histiocytes in the bone marrow are present in some cases, and support the diagnosis.

The differential diagnosis of patients with suspected Hallervorden-Spatz disease should include other conditions that may be associated with severe dystonia and extrapyramidal signs, especially Wilson's disease that can be effectively treated. In some cases it may be difficult to distinguish Hallervorden-Spatz disease from Huntington's disease. Some childhood-onset cases may be difficult to differentiate from neuronal ceroid lipofuscinosis or gangliosidoses.

Therapeutic attempts to improve Hallervorden-Spatz disease with iron chelation treatment have been unsuccessful. Some patients may have transient improvement with levodopa. Spasticity may be treated with baclofen. Many patients eventually need gastrostomy placement.

The present patient had a relentlessly progressive course and severe dystonia did not improve with drug therapy. Botulinum toxin injections improved her severe anterocollis, but she eventually required gastrostomy, and was placed in a nursing home.

Clinical Pearls

1. Hallervorden-Spatz disease should be considered in the differential diagnosis of a patient with early onset of dystonia, pyramidal signs, and intellectual decline.

2. Hallervorden-Spatz disease is characterized by excessive iron deposition in the globus pallidus and pars reticulata of the substantia nigra.

3. Brain MRI in patients with Hallervorden-Spatz disease often shows symmetric abnormalities in the basal ganglia resulting from iron deposition, which have a characteristic appearance known as the "eyes of the tiger" sign.

4. Abnormal cytosomes in blood lymphocytes or sea-blue histiocytes in the bone marrow may be observed in some patients with Hallervorden-Spatz disease and support the diagnosis.

5. Some cases of Hallervorden-Spatz disease are familial and appear to show an autosomal recessive inheritance pattern.

REFERENCES

1. Sethi KD, Adams RJ, Loring DW, et al: Hallervorden-Spatz syndrome: Clinical and magnetic resonance imaging correlations. Ann Neurol 1988; 24:692–694.
2. Swaiman KF: Hallervorden-Spatz syndrome and brain iron metabolism. Arch Neurol 1991; 48:1285–1293.
3. Tanfani G, Mascalchi M, Dal Pozzo GC, et al: MRI imaging in case of Hallervorden-Spatz disease. J Comput Assist Tomogr 1987; 11:1057–1058.

PATIENT 71

**A 26-year-old-man with progressive weakness of both arms
and winging of shoulder blades**

A 26-year-old man presented with a 5-year history of gradually progressive weakness of both arms. During the past year he was unable to lift his arms above the head. His wife noted that his shoulder blades were "sticking out" when he attempted to raise his arms. He had no weakness of the hands or legs, difficulty walking, or any sensory symptoms. He denied neck or back pain, but had a history of bilateral shoulder dislocations. His medical history was otherwise unremarkable, and he denied any family history of similar symptoms.

Physical Examination: Vital signs: normal. Head: normocephalic, skull nontender. Neck: supple, no bruits. Spine: no deformity, nontender, good range of motion. Cardiac: normal. Mental status and speech: normal. Cranial nerves: mild facial weakness, especially in the orbicularis oris and orbicularis oculi muscles, otherwise normal. Motor: severe atrophy and weakness of bilateral trapezius, pectoralis, triceps, biceps and brachioradialis muscles, with relatively spared deltoids (see figure, *left*); unable to forward flex his arms more than 90°. Sensation: normal. Muscle stretch reflexes: depressed triceps reflexes (grade 1) bilaterally, otherwise normal. Plantar reflexes: flexor. Coordination and gait: normal. Screening neuromuscular examination of patient's mother and sister revealed that both had mild facial and shoulder girdle weakness, but not as severe as the proband.

Stop and Consider: What is the likely diagnosis in a patient presenting with this pattern of weakness and evidence of a similar condition in his mother and sister?

Laboratory Findings: Creatine kinase (CK): 749 U/L (normal 0–250). Nerve conduction study (NCS): normal. Needle electromyography (EMG): small, short-duration, polyphasisc motor unit potentials with a rapid recruitment in bilateral trapezius, supraspinatus, deltoid, biceps, triceps, and brachioradialis muscles. Muscle biopsy from the deltoid muscle: see figure, *right*.

Question: What other diagnostic test could be performed to confirm the diagnosis?

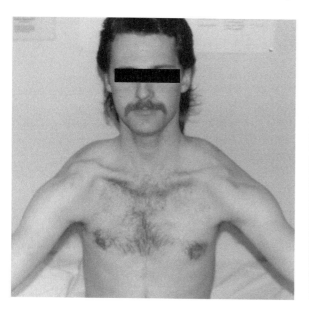
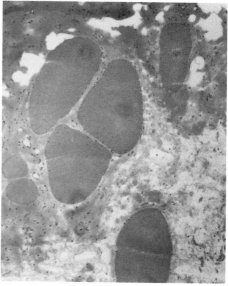

Diagnosis: Facioscapulohumeral muscular dystrophy

Discussion: The patient's painless weakness and muscle atrophy without sensory abnormalities, elevated CK, and myopathic changes on EMG strongly indicated a muscle disorder. The characteristic pattern of muscle atrophy and weakness, with involvement of facial and upper extremity muscles, and autosomal dominant inheritance pattern suggested by the abnormal neuromuscular examination of his mother and sister, were characteristic of facioscapulohumeral muscular dystrophy (FSHD). The muscle biopsy showed findings typical of a muscular dystrophy, with excessive variation in fiber sizes, fiber splitting, increase in the number of fibers with internal nuclei, and severe increase of endomysial and perimysial connective tissue elements (see figure, *right*). He subsequently underwent DNA testing that showed a deletion at chromosomal locus 4q35, confirming the diagnosis of FSHD.

FSHD is one of the most frequent forms of muscular dystrophy, with an approximate prevalence of 1 in 20,000–100,000 population. There is a very wide spectrum of clinical presentations in FSHD, with most patients developing some weakness by the second or third decade of life. Because this condition is relatively benign, patients typically develop weakness long before they finally seek medical attention. The initial weakness usually affects the facial muscles, such as orbicularis oris and orbicularis oculi. Many patients are unable to whistle and some degree of ptosis is present in most patients. The pattern of weakness is usually asymmetrical. Scapular fixators are typically severely affected and the scapular winging is usually most apparent on forward arm flexion. The scapula may ride into the substance of the trapezius muscle, giving a false "athletic" impression (figure, *left*). There is typically severe involvement of the pectoralis muscle. The deltoids are usually relatively spared, but triceps, biceps, and brachioradialis are usually severely affected. Lower extremities are minimally involved, but more weakness may develop with disease progression, which usually involves the anterior leg compartment with foot dorsiflexion weakness. Although some patients with disease progression may be severely disabled, most patients have a normal life span. Only rare patients become wheelchair-dependent. In contrast to several other forms of muscular dystrophies, symptomatic cardiac involvement in FSHD has not been well documented, but in a few patients with FSHD atrial dysrhythmias have been reported.

Some patients with FSHD develop high-frequency sensorineural hearing loss or retinal teleangiectasia and detachment (Coats' disease).

The CK is usually normal or mildly elevated (up to 5 times baseline). The EMG shows a myopathic pattern with focal distribution, but frequently demonstrates abnormalities in clinically unaffected muscles. Muscle biopsy typically shows nonspecific dystrophic features. An interesting feature is presence of endomysial and perimysial mononuclear cell infiltrates in some FSHD cases. The focality of the dystrophic process is frequently striking; biopsy from two different regions of the same muscle may show completely different findings, from advanced dystrophic changes to completely normal muscle histology, within a few inches. This underscores the importance of careful selection of the site of muscle biopsy in patients with myopathies. In a patient with typical clinical findings and chromosome 4q35 deletion, muscle biopsy or EMG is not necessary.

The gene responsible for FSHD has been mapped to 4q35 chromosomal locus, and the inheritance pattern is autosomal dominant. Approximately 90% of individuals with FSHD have this deletion and based on current data it appears that its identification is more than 90% specific for FSHD. How this DNA abnormality leads to development of muscular dystrophy is unclear. The disease severity appears to be related to the size of the deletion in the FSHD region; the largest deletions are usually associated with a congenital form of FSHD. Mental retardation and epilepsy may also be associated with very large deletions. As many as 10% of patients with clinical features of FSHD do not map to 4q35 locus. Genetic testing with DNA analysis for the typical 4q35 deletion is currently available.

At the present time there is no effective treatment of FSHD. The beta-2 agonist albuterol has recently been advocated for patients with FSHD and may have a modest effect on improvement of muscle mass and possibly also strength. Treatment is focused on prevention of secondary complications. In carefully selected patients, a surgical procedure to stabilize the scapula by fixing it to the rib cage may be considered.

The present patient had mild progression of weakness over the past 2 years and was unable to continue his current employment. Genetic counseling was provided to his family. He currently participates in a vocational rehabilitation program.

Clinical Pearls

1. In most patients with FSHD the diagnosis can be made on the basis of the characteristic pattern of atrophy and weakness, and evidence of an autosomal dominant inheritance pattern.

2. Genetic testing for chromosome 4q35 deletion is currently available and is positive in approximately 90% of patients with FSHD.

3. Because of the wide spectrum of phenotypic abnormalities in FSHD, DNA testing should be considered to confirm the diagnosis, especially in patients with subtle abnormalities.

4. DNA testing can identify possible family members in preclinical stages of the disease, and genetic counseling should be provided to all families with FSHD.

REFERENCES

1. Padberg GW, Frants RR, Brouwer OF, et al: Facioscapulohumeral muscular dystrophy in the Dutch population. Muscle Nerve 1995; 2:S81–S84.
2. van Deutekom JC, Wijmenga C, van Tienhoven EA, et al: FSHD-associated DNA rearrangements are due to deletions of integral copies of 3.2 kb tandemly repeated unit. Hum Mol Genet 1993; 2:2037–2042.
3. Woelfel A, Cascio W, Smith SW: Cerebral embolization in two young patients with facioscapulohumeral muscular dystrophy and atrial dysrhythmias. Am Heart J 1989; 118:632–633.
4. Wijmenga C, Hewitt JE, Sandkuijl LA, et al: Chromosome 4q DNA rearrangements associated with facioscapulohumeral muscular dystrophy. Nat Genet 1992; 2:26–30.

PATIENT 72

A 39-year-old man with progressive lower extremity pain and weakness

A 39-year-old man presented with a 5-week history of back pain and progressive weakness of lower extremities. The weakness began insidiously 2 days after the onset the back pain, initially causing some difficulty climbing stairs and rising from chairs, but over the next 5 weeks progressed to the point that he was unable to walk unassisted. His back pain radiated to the legs and was associated with numbness and tingling in both feet. He denied any upper extremity or facial weakness, dysphagia, respiratory problems, difficulty with bowel and bladder function, fever, or chills. A diagnosis of AIDS had been established 4 months prior to the onset the back pain and leg weakness, when he presented with fatigue, anorexia, and weight loss. His medications included zidovudine (AZT), lamivudine, azithromycin, and trimethoprim/sulfamethoxazole.

Physical Examination: Vital signs: afebrile, pulse 100, respirations 16, blood pressure 124/74. HEENT, chest, cardiac, abdomen: normal. Mental status and speech: normal. Cranial nerves: normal. Motor examination: muscle bulk and tone normal; mild upper extremity weakness (grade +4); lower extremity strength grade 3 bilaterally in multiple muscle groups. Sensory examination: severe loss of sensation to light touch, pain, and vibration in glove-and-stocking distribution; mild impairment of proprioception in the toes. Muscle stretch reflexes: grade 1 in upper extremities, areflexia in lower extremities. Plantar reflexes: flexor. Coordination: mildly diminished rapid alternating movements and fine motor skills in both upper extremities, marked difficulty on heel-to-sheen test secondary to weakness. Gait: unable to walk unassisted.

Stop and Consider: What is the time course and localization of the weakness and sensory loss in this patient? What types of neurologic complications may develop in the course of HIV infection?

Laboratory Findings: Lumbosacral spine MRI: see figure (T1 weighted image with gadolinium contrast). WBC 2,400/μl (3,500–8,500), CD4 cell count 23/μl (500–1300), CD4:CD8 ratio 0.3 (1.2–3.7), AST 76 U/L (0–40). ESR, BUN, creatinine, creatine kinase, electrolytes: normal. Cytomegalovirus (CMV) titers: negative. CSF studies: 1 nucleated cell/μl; glucose: 52 mg/dl (40–80), protein 110 mg/dl (15–45). CSF CMV culture: negative. Nerve conduction study (NCS): diffuse slowing of motor and sensory conduction velocities, prolonged distal motor and sensory latencies, mild decrease of tibial and peroneal compound muscle action potentials, absent bilateral sural nerve action poten-

tials. Needle electromyography (EMG): rare fibrillation potentials and decreased motor unit recruitment diffusely in bilateral lower extremity muscles, lumbar paraspinal muscles, and distal muscles in upper extremities.

Question: What is the most likely diagnosis in this patient? Are the electrodiagnostic abnormalities consistent with the results of the MRI and CSF examinations?

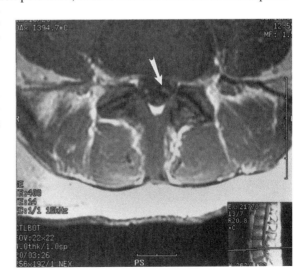

Diagnosis: HIV-associated subacute inflammatory demyelinating and axonal polyradiculoneuropathy

Discussion: The pattern of neurologic deficit suggested severe motor and sensory polyneuropathy. Spinal MRI, obtained because of severe back pain, showed marked contrast enhancement of lumbosacral nerve roots (arrow) and no evidence of compressive lesions. In a patient with AIDS and these neurologic and MRI findings, one should strongly consider the diagnosis of CMV-associated radiculitis, but CMV titers and cultures were negative, and the electrodiagnostic studies showed severe, diffuse, predominantly demyelinating polyradiculoneuropathy. The clinical presentation and electrodiagnostic abnormalities were consistent with an acute inflammatory demyelinating polyneuropathy, also known as Guillain-Barré syndrome (GBS), although the progression of weakness was longer (subacute) than in typical cases of GBS, in which the nadir of weakness is usually reached between 2–4 weeks from onset. Increased CSF protein content with normal cell count was also supportive of that diagnosis. The severe back pain was likely secondary to inflammatory changes in the spinal nerve roots, and is common in GBS. Normal creatine kinase level pointed away from possible HIV-associated polymyositis.

Numerous neurologic complications involving both central and peripheral nervous systems may develop in HIV-infected patients. These complications may be related to direct HIV infection of the nervous system, opportunistic infections, medication toxicity, or autoimmune pathogenesis. Distinct types of peripheral neuropathies may develop at different stages of HIV infection. Acute, subacute, or chronic inflammatory demyelinating polyneuropahties (AIDP, SIDP, CIDP) typically develop during early stages of HIV infection and may precede seroconversion. Clinically these cases are indistinguishable from non-HIV-related cases of AIDP or CIDP. Electrodiagnostic studies typically show evidence of a primarily demyelinating process with severe slowing of conduction velocities, but in some patients there is evidence of coexisting axonal loss. CSF examination may show significant pleocytosis, in addition to elevated protein content. The etiology of this syndrome appears to be autoimmune and is most likely triggered by HIV infection.

Treatment of HIV-associated demyelinating polyneuropathies is similar to non-HIV-related cases and includes plasmapheresis and high-dose intravenous immunoglobulin (IVIG). Some HIV-infected patients with CIDP have been successfully treated with corticosteroids, but it has to be carefully balanced with the possible risks in immunocompromised patients.

Distal symmetric axonal polyneuropathy typically occurs in advanced stages of HIV infection and is the most common form of HIV-associated polyneuropathy. It has been observed in as many as 30% of patients with AIDS. Most of these patients have evidence of opportunistic infections. It is characterized by severe dysesthetic pain, which starts in distal aspects of lower extremities and gradually spreads proximally. In addition to pain, there is usually severe sensory loss to all modalities in glove-and-stocking distribution. The weakness is usually less severe than the sensory symptoms, but may worsen with progression of polyneuropathy. Electrodiagnostic studies show evidence of sensory and motor axonopathy, with decreased sensory and motor evoked potentials, normal or mildly decreased conduction velocities, and denervation signs on the EMG. Pathologic studies in this form of polyneuropathy show severe axonal loss of both myelinated and nonmyelinated fibers. The etiology of this polyneuropathy is unknown but is probably multifactorial, with several underlying mechanisms, including direct HIV infection of the peripheral nervous system, coexisting opportunistic infections including CMV, and medication neurotoxicity. Laboratory studies to evaluate for other potentially treatable causes of polyneuropathy should be undertaken in this patient population. Pain control is an important aspect of management of this type of neuropathy.

Lumbosacral polyradiculopathy associated with CMV infection typically presents with severe back pain radiating to lower extremities, weakness, and sensory loss, which may rapidly progress to severe paraparesis with sphincter involvement. EMG usually demonstrates severe denervation in the limb and paraspinal muscles. Cerebrospinal fluid (CSF) examination typically shows high nucleated cell count (frequently > 1000 cells/µl), elevated protein, and reduced glucose levels. CSF viral cultures are usually positive for CMV, but PCR analysis for CMV allows more rapid diagnosis. Lumbosacral spine MRI in CMV radiculitis usually shows prominent contrast enhancement of cauda equina. Nerve root enhancement may also be observed in AIDP or CIDP without CMV infection and in neoplastic conditions affecting the nerve roots. Patients with CMV-related polyradiculitis are typically treated with intravenous gancyclovir or foscarnet.

The pattern of mononeuropathy multiplex, sometimes associated with vasculitis, and of different forms of focal mononeuropathies including cranial neuropathies, may also develop in the course of HIV infection. In HIV-infected patients who present with diffuse weakness without significant sensory symptoms, one should consider HIV-associated polymyosis or AZT-induced toxic myopathy. These patients frequently have elevated levels of creatine kinase, but muscle biopsy should be obtained if HIV-associated polymyositis is suspected.

The present patient was treated with a course of IVIG. Within a few days he showed a remarkable improvement of strength and was able to walk with the help of a cane. Four weeks later his weakness worsened again, but improved with another course of IVIG. After a second course of IVIG he had sustained improvement and he was able to return to work within 2 months.

Clinical Pearls

1. Distinct neuropathic syndromes may develop at different stages of HIV infection.

2. Acute and chronic inflammatory demyelinating polyneuropathies typically develop in early stages of HIV infection and may precede HIV seroconversion.

3. A characteristic feature of HIV-associated inflammatory demyelinating polyneuropathies is significant pleocytosis in the CSF.

4. Cytomegalovirus polyradiculitis should be suspected in AIDS patients who develop severe back pain with weakness and sensory deficit in lower extremities.

5. Both inflammatory demyelinating polyneuropathies and CMV radiculitis may be associated with prominent nerve root enhancement on spinal MRI.

6. Plasmapheresis and IVIG may be useful in management of HIV-associated inflammatory demyelinating polyneuropathies.

REFERENCES

1. Bacellar H, Munoz A, Miller EN, et al: Temporal trends in the incidence of HIV-1-related neurologic diseases: Multicenter AIDS Cohort Study, 1985–1992. Neurology 1994; 44:1892–1900.
2. Barohn RJ, Gronseth GS, LeForce BR, et al: Peripheral nervous system involvement in a large cohort of human immunodeficiency virus–infected individuals. Arch Neurol 1993; 50:167–171.
3. Miller RG, Parry GJ, Pfaeffl W, et al: The spectrum of peripheral neuropathy associated with ARC and AIDS. Muscle Nerve 1988; 11:857–863.
4. Simpson DM, Tagliati M: Neurologic manifestations of HIV infection. Ann Intern Med 1995; 121:769–785.
5. Tagliati M, Grinnell J, Godbold J, Simpson DM: Peripheral nerve function in HIV infection: Clinical, electrophysiologic, and laboratory findings. Arch Neurol 1999; 56:84–89.

PATIENT 73

A 43-year-old man with insidious onset of weakness and clumsiness in the right upper extremity

A 43-year-old man presented with a 6-month history of progressive weakness and clumsiness of the right upper extremity. Initially he noted difficulty with activities requiring dexterity, but later developed weakness of the right hand that made it difficult to hold an object. He also complained of progressive fatigue, frequent cramping in the legs, and muscle twitching on his chest. He had several episodes of coughing while eating. He denied headache, nausea, difficulty with memory, vision, hearing, or bowel and bladder problems. His medical history was otherwise unremarkable and there was no family history of neurologic disease.

Physical Examination: Vital signs: normal. Head and spine: normal. Mental status: normal. Speech: dysarthric. Cranial nerves: fasciculations and mild atrophy of the tongue. Motor examination: atrophy of the intrinsic muscles in the right hand, diffuse fasciculations in all extremities and pectoralis muscles; spasticity in all extremities; right upper extremity strength grade 3 distally and grade 4 proximally, grade +4 strength in the left upper extremity and bilateral lower extremities. Sensory examination: normal. Muscle stretch reflexes: hyperactive (grade 4) in all extremities; hyperactive jaw reflex (grade 4). Plantar reflexes: bilateral Babinski signs. Coordination: mild incoordination and decrease of fine motor skills in the right upper extremity secondary to weakness. Gait: decreased right arm swing, difficulty with tandem gait. Romberg test: negative.

Stop and Consider: What is the time course and localization of this patient's neurologic abnormalities?

Laboratory Findings: CBC, chemistries, electrolytes, creatine kinase, ESR, thyroid function tests, B_{12}, serum and urine electrophoresis, anti–GM1 ganglioside antibodies: normal. Urine heavy metal screen: normal. Nerve conduction studies (NCS): normal, except for mildly decreased amplitude of the right ulnar nerve compound muscle action potential (CMAP). Needle electromyography (EMG): diffuse fibrillation potentials and large, prolonged, and polyphasic motor unit potentials, with markedly reduced recruitment in all extremities, tongue, and paraspinal muscles in the cervical, thoracic, and lumbar regions. MRI of the brain and cervical spine: normal.

Question: What is the most likely diagnosis in a patient with these neurologic symptoms and electromyographic abnormalities?

Diagnosis: Amyotrophic lateral sclerosis

Discussion: The neurologic examination in this patient showed multifocal upper and lower motor neuron signs. With these neurologic findings and lack of any sensory, autonomic, or systemic abnormalities, motor neuron disease (amyotrophic lateral sclerosis) is the most likely diagnosis. This clinical diagnosis was supported by EMG that showed diffuse active and chronic denervation changes in all extremities, paraspinal muscles, and bulbar musculature, indicating widespread anterior horn cell and brain stem motor neuron involvement. Compressive lesions were excluded by the normal MRI of the brain and cervical spine. Laboratory tests did not reveal any underlying systemic illnesses.

Amyotrophic lateral sclerosis (motor neuron disease), known in the U.S. as Lou Gehrig's disease, is a neurodegenerative condition affecting the motor neurons of the cerebral cortex, brain stem, and spinal cord. The disease is characterized by relentless progression of weakness and atrophy of limb, axial, and bulbar muscles, usually leading to death within 3–5 years from the onset of symptoms. The etiology of ALS is unknown. About 10% of ALS cases are familial, and about 20% of the familial cases are associated with a mutation in the copper/zinc superoxide dismutase (*SOD1*) gene on chromosome 21, and are transmitted as an autosomal dominant trait. Deficiencies of this enzyme may predispose to neurotoxicity by free radicals.

The diagnosis of ALS is based on signs of upper and lower motor neuron dysfunction without signs of sensory or any other system involvement. There are a number of clinical variants of motor neuron disease. Cases that present with lower motor neuron signs are sometimes referred to as progressive muscular atrophy, but most of these patients eventually develop upper motor neuron signs and evolve into typical ALS. Rare cases present with upper motor neuron signs and never develop lower motor neuron signs and are referred to as progressive lateral sclerosis.

The diagnosis of ALS is usually unambiguous when the disease is advanced, but may be uncertain in the early stages, when the motor abnormalities are limited. ALS typically begins with focal weakness in one of the limbs or bulbar muscles, but with time there is progression to other body regions. Rare patients may present with exertional dyspnea secondary to denervation in the diaphragm or intercostal muscles as the only initial complaint. Severe cramps may develop at any stage of the disease, but are common in early stages. Fasciculations are very common and indicate lower motor neuron

involvement. The disease progresses relentlessly to severe paralysis of all limbs and bulbar muscles. A pseudobulbar syndrome with emotional lability may be observed in patients with degeneration of the corticobulbar motor tracts. Extraocular muscles are remarkably spared.

When the disease begins in the lower extremities, patients may initially complain of tripping and falls. Some develop footdrop and may be suspected of having a peroneal neuropathy or L5 radiculopathy. Patients with upper extremity onset may initially complain of difficulty with activities requiring normal dexterity and fine motor skills and later complain of difficulty holding objects. Patients who present with weakness and atrophy of hand muscles are often suspected to have ulnar or median neuropathies, cervical radiculopathy, or brachial plexopathy before the spread of upper and lower motor neuron signs to other regions is appreciated. Patients may also present exclusively with bulbar symptoms, such as dysphagia or dysarthria. Because of diagnostic difficulties in early stages of ALS, patients are frequently classified as suspected, possible, probable, or definite ALS based on the presence and distribution of upper and lower motor neuron signs and results of diagnostic studies.

Electrodiagnostic studies (NCS and needle EMG) can confirm the lower motor neuron involvement and rule out other conditions that may mimic ALS, such as multifocal motor neuropathy with conduction blocks, chronic inflammatory demyelinating polyneuropathy, radiculopathies, or plexopathies. The EMG may show widespread denervation changes in clinically affected and unaffected muscles.

MRI of the brain should be performed in patients with bulbar onset and MRI of the spine is obtained in most patients presenting with limb onset to exclude compressive lesions. Patients who present with upper motor neuron signs caudal to lower motor signs should be evaluated to exclude structural lesions affecting cervical cord or brain stem. For example, a patient with cervical spondylosis may have wasting and fasciculations in the upper extremities, and spasticity, brisk reflexes, and Babinski signs in lower extremities.

Laboratory studies in patients with suspected ALS should be focused on exclusion of conditions that may be associated with dysfunction of motor neurons and may mimic ALS. Motor neuron dysfunction has been observed in association with some systemic conditions such as lymphoma, monoclonal gammopathy, thyroid disorders, hyperparathyroidism, HTLV-1 or HIV infections, heavy metal toxicity, or high titers of anti-GM$_1$ ganglioside antibodies. Mild elevation of creatine kinase is not unusual in ALS, but muscle biopsy may be required in some patients suspected of ALS if creatine kinase is elevated in order to rule out a myopathy. DNA testing for *SOD1* mutation should be offered to patients in suspected familial cases.

There is no effective treatment of ALS. Management is focused on supportive and symptomatic measures to maximize function and minimize discomfort. Special attention should be paid to nutritional status, as many patients with dysphagia require gastrostomy to maintain nutritional intake. Communication devices should be provided when necessary. Cramps may be treated with quinine or phenytoin, and baclofen may relieve spasticity. Anticholinergic medications may reduce oral secretions. Patients with progressive respiratory difficulties may be assisted with respiratory support such as BiPAP. Riluzole, a glutamate release inhibitor, is currently the only FDA-approved medication for ALS, and appears to modestly slow disease progression.

The present patient was started on riluzole and received supportive physical therapy. Spasticity responded partially to baclofen treatment, but his condition has been relentlessly progressive. He underwent gastrostomy, and received ventilatory support with BiPAP at night.

Clinical Pearls

1. Amyotrophic lateral sclerosis is clinically characterized by presence of upper and lower motor signs and absence of any other system involvement.

2. Nerve conduction studies and needle electromyography should be performed in all patients with suspected motor neuron disease. Electrodiagnostic evaluation may reveal evidence of muscle denervation in clinically unaffected muscles, and helps in ruling out alternative diagnoses.

3. MRI of the brain and the spinal cord should be considered in patients suspected of motor neuron disease to rule out focal lesions that may mimic ALS.

4. Mild elevation of creatine kinase is not unusual in ALS. Muscle biopsy to rule out myopathy may be considered in some patients when signs of upper motor neuron involvement are absent.

5. Glutamate release inhibitor riluzole modestly slows disease progression, which usually leads to death within 3–5 years.

REFERENCES

1. Bensimon G, Lacomblez L, Meininger V: A controlled trial of riluzole in amyotrophic lateral sclerosis. ALS/Riluzole Study Group. N Engl J Med 1994; 330:585–591.
2. Rosen DR, Siddique T, Patterson D, et al: Mutations in Cu/Zn superoxide dismutase gene are associated with familial amyotrophic lateral sclerosis. Nature 1993; 362:59–62.
3. Subcommittee on Motor Neuron Diseases/Amyotrophic Lateral Sclerosis of the World Federation of Neurology Research Group on Neuromuscular Diseases: El Escorial World Federation of Neurology criteria for the diagnosis of amyotrophic lateral sclerosis. J Neurol Sci 1994; 124(Suppl):96–107.
4. Tandan R, Bradley WG: Amyotrophic lateral sclerosis: Part 1. Clinical features, pathology and ethical issues in management. Ann Neurol 1985; 18:271–280.

PATIENT 74

A 35-year-old woman with a 3-week history of painless, progressive leg weakness

A 35-year-old woman presented with a 3-week history of gradually progressive weakness of both lower extremities. Initially she noted difficulty walking and getting up from the sitting position. This gradually worsened and she began falling frequently. There was no pain or sensory disturbance, and she denied bladder or bowel dysfunction, upper extremity symptoms, diplopia, dysphagia, headache, and speech or cognitive problems. There was no history of trauma, unusual physical activity, or recent infection. Her medical history was significant for schizophrenia, treated with clozaril. Her family history was noncontributory.

Physical Examination: Vital signs: afebrile, pulse 96, respirations 16, blood pressure 122/75. HEENT, chest, heart, abdomen: normal. Spine: nontender, no deformity. Mental status and speech: normal. Cranial nerves: normal. Motor examination: normal bulk, tone, and strength in the upper extremities; grade 3 weakness in the right lower extremity and grade 4 weakness in the left lower extremity; bilateral lower extremity spasticity. Sensory examination: light touch, pain, and temperature sensation diminished below the T11 dermatome; vibratory sensation and proprioception diminished in both feet. Muscle stretch reflexes: grade 2 in upper extremities, pathologically brisk bilateral knee and Achilles tendon reflexes (grade 4), with bilateral ankle clonus. Plantar reflexes: bilateral Babinski signs. Coordination: normal in upper extremities; diminished in lower extremities secondary to weakness. Gait: unable to walk without support.

Stop and Consider: What is the likely anatomic location of the neurologic dysfunction in this patient?

Laboratory Findings: CBC, chemistry panel, ESR, electrolytes: normal. MRI of the thoracic spine: see figure.

Question: What kind of lesion is demonstrated on the thoracic MRI?

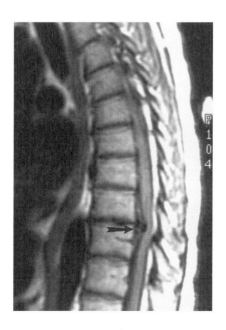

Diagnosis: Myelopathy caused by T9–T10 intervertebral disc herniation

Discussion: The clinical presentation of this patient with weakness, hyperreflexia, bilateral Babinski signs, and T11 level sensory changes was highly suggestive of myelopathy affecting lower thoracic cord. The differential diagnosis should include causes of myelopathy such as primary or metastatic tumors within the spinal canal, vascular lesions, transverse myelitis, or infectious conditions, including abscess. Thoracic disc herniation, although rare compared to lumbar or cervical disc disease, should also be included in the differential diagnosis. There was no history of trauma or significant pain in this patient, but traumatic cord compression was also considered. The MRI of the thoracic spine showed T9–T10 intervertebral disc herniation causing anterior thoracic cord compression with posterior displacement. The MRI findings were consistent with the neurologic deficit.

Thoracic disc herniation (TDH) is regarded as rare but has been increasingly diagnosed with widespread availability of MRI imaging. It is estimated that less than 1% of disc herniations occur in the thoracic spine and most of them occur at the lower (T8–T12) thoracic levels. Approximately 80% of TDHs occur between the third and fifth decade of life and equally affect males and females. Thoracic herniations are usually single, but multiple disc herniations may occur and there may not be a significant history of identifiable trauma or sudden strain.

Pain is the most common initial symptom and is present in about 50% cases of TDH. It is most severe in the midline, but may be unilateral or bilateral and have radicular features. Some patients with TDH are initially thought to have intercostal neuralgia or herpes zoster infection. In the upper thoracic region disc herniation may produce pain radiating into the upper extremities. In some cases, the pain may suggest a gallbladder disease, other abdominal conditions, or pain of cardiac origin.

Patients with T11–T12 herniations may have pain radiating to the groin or lower extremities. Sensory symptoms are the second most frequent initial manifestation. Patients may complain of numbness, paresthesias, or dysesthesias in lower extremities. In some cases Lhermitte's sign may be the presenting feature. About one third of patients report weakness as the initial symptom. The motor deficit typically evolves very slowly, but an acute-onset, rapidly progressing flaccid paraplegia can occur. Symptoms of urinary bladder dysfunction may accompany a progressing myelopathy, but are rarely an initial manifestation.

The diagnosis of a thoracic disc herniation is usually confirmed by spinal MRI or CT-myelography. Patients with mild, nonprogressive symptoms may be treated conservatively with physical therapy, immobilization in a brace, and anti-inflammatory drugs. Up to 75% of the patients treated conservatively improve or have complete recovery. Surgical treatment should be considered in patients with intractable pain or signs of myelopathy. There is controversy regarding the choice of surgical procedures, which include decompression of the thoracic cord by an anterior transthoracic approach or a posterolateral (costotransversectomy or transpedicular) approach. Posterior approach with laminectomy has been associated with poor outcome in many cases.

In the present patient the absence of pain was rather unusual. She underwent anterior transthoracic spinal cord decompression with T9–T10 discectomy. Postoperatively the patient showed a remarkable recovery. Strength in both lower extremities markedly improved and she was able to walk comfortably without any support within 3 weeks. A follow-up neurologic examination 2 months after spinal cord decompression revealed only mild weakness of the right lower extremity (grade +4) and no other signs of myelopathy.

Clinical Pearls

1. Thoracic disc herniation can cause severe myelopathy that may not be associated with pain.

2. Pain caused by thoracic disc herniation may mimic intra-abdominal or intrathoracic pathology, such as cholecystitis or myocardial ischemia.

3. Most thoracic disc herniations occur in the lower thoracic spine.

4. The diagnosis of a thoracic disc herniation can be confirmed by MRI and CT-myelography.

5. Surgical decompression by anterior transthoracic or posterolateral approach rather than laminectomy should be performed when disc herniation produces myelopathy.

REFERENCES

1. Arce CA, Dohrman GJ: Herniated thoracic disks. Neurol Clin 1985; 3:383–392.
2. Bohlman HH, Zdeblick TA: Anterior excision of herniated thoracic discs. J Bone Joint Surg 1988; 7A:1038–1047.
3. Brown CW, Deffer PAJ, Akmakjian J, et al: The natural history of thoracic disc herniation. Spine 1992; 17(Suppl 6):S97–S102.
4. Simpson MJ, Silveri CP, Simeone FA, et al: Thoracic disk herniation: Reevaluation of the posterior approach using a modified costotransversectomy. Spine 1993; 18:1872–1877.

PATIENT 75

A 48-year-old man with recurrent right-sided weakness and numbness

A 48-year-old man experienced several episodes of transient right-sided weakness and numbness during a 3-week period. The episodes were unprovoked, had an abrupt onset, lasted less than 10 minutes, and typically involved weakness and numbness of the right face, arm, or leg, and slurred speech. Two days prior to admission he again experienced the abrupt onset of weakness and numbness of the right face, arm, and leg, which persisted and resulted in hospital admission. He denied headache, nausea, vertigo, difficulty with bowel and bladder functions, memory problems, or any left-sided symptoms. His medical history was significant for hypertension treated with diuretics. He was a heavy smoker, but denied alcohol or substance abuse. His family history was noncontributory.

Physical Examination: Pulse 80 and regular; blood pressure 168/92; respirations and temperature: normal. Skin, cardiac, chest, and abdomen: normal. Neck: loud left carotid bruit. Mental status: normal. Speech: dysarthric. Cranial nerves: pupils equal, with normal pupillary reflexes; funduscopic examination: normal; vision, visual fields, and gaze: normal; moderate weakness of the lower facial musculature on the right; oral and pharyngeal structures: midline. Motor examination: muscle bulk normal, spasticity of right upper extremity, grade 4 right-sided weakness affecting equally arm and leg, no tremor. Sensory examination: mildly decreased sensation to light touch, pain, and vibration on right side of the body. Muscle stretch reflexes: mildly increased (grade 3) on the right, normal (grade 2) on the left. Plantar reflexes: extensor on the right; flexor on the left. Coordination: mildly diminished in the right hand and right foot secondary to weakness. Gait: circumductive on the right.

Stop and Consider: What is the time course and neuroanatomic localization of the symptoms and signs in this patient?

Laboratory Findings: Head CT: see figure, *left.* CBC, platelets, coagulation profile, chemistry panel, electrolytes, arterial blood gases: normal except for a total serum cholesterol level of 296 mg/dl (desirable < 200, borderline 200–239). EKG: normal sinus rhythm, mild left ventricular hypertrophy. Chest x-ray: mild cardiomegaly. Intra-arterial carotid angiography: selected image of the left internal carotid artery: see figure, *right.*

Question: What is the likely etiology of the neurologic deficit based on the head CT and angiography findings?

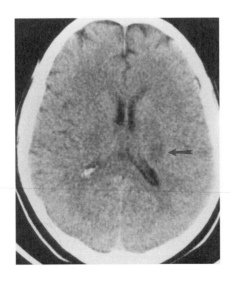 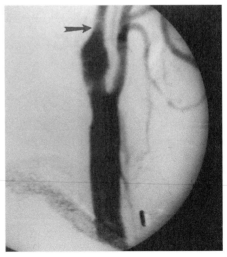

Diagnosis: Subcortical ischemic stroke in the left cerebral hemisphere, preceded by transient ischemic attacks, caused by artery-to-artery embolization from an atherosclerotic lesion of the left internal carotid artery

Discussion: The clinical presentation of this patient, with recurring episodes of right-sided weakness and numbness, followed by persistent right-sided hemiparesis, numbness, and dysarthria, is consistent with transient ischemic attacks (TIAs) culminating in brain infarction in the left cerebral hemisphere. The pattern of the neurologic deficit suggests involvement of the corticospinal tract in the subcortical region, most likely in the posterior limb of the left internal capsule. Right-sided sensory loss involving the face, arm, and leg suggests involvement of the thalamus or the thalamocortical fibers in the left cerebral hemisphere.

Ischemic stroke was the most likely cause of the neurologic deficit, but the differential diagnosis should also include an acute hemorrhagic stroke. The possibility of an epidural or a subdural hematoma or an unusual presentation of a malignant brain tumor or a brain abscess, while not likely, deserve some consideration.

The head CT scan confirmed an ischemic lesion in the subcortical region of the left cerebral hemisphere, involving the posterior limb of the left internal capsule (figure on the left, arrow). The left internal carotid artery angiogram showed stenosis (figure on the right, arrow), irregularity, and atherosclerotic nidus that suggested the possibility of artery-to-artery embolization from the carotid lesion to distal intracranial arteries. The cerebral angiography also showed evidence of an acute intraluminal thrombus occluding the left anterior choroidal artery at its origin from the intracranial portion of the left internal carotid artery. He had several risk factors for stroke, including arterial hypertension, tobacco smoking, elevated cholesterol, left ventricular hypertrophy, and recurrent TIAs.

Ischemic stroke may have several underlying mechanisms. In approximately 15% of cases there is severe large-vessel atherothrombosis with high-grade stenosis or occlusion of the ipsilateral extracranial or intracranial feeding vessel. About 15–20% have less severe large-vessel atherothrombosis, which predisposes to artery-to-artery embolization ipsilaterally to distal intracranial vessels. Approximately 15–30% of ischemic strokes are cardioembolic. About 15% patients have small deep ("lacunar") infarcts usually secondary to occlusive small-vessel disease, and 15–30% cases are indeterminate in regards to a specific cause.

TIAs are defined as abrupt-onset episodes of neurologic deficit consistent with a vascular distribution, which are of less than 24-hour duration, although majority of TIAs resolve within an hour. Vascular risk factors predispose to TIAs and strokes, and as many as 40% of patients with ischemic strokes have premonitory TIAs. TIAs typically occur before 25–50% of atherothrombotic, large-vessel ischemic strokes, but only before 11–30% of cardioembolic strokes and 11–14% of small, deep strokes. The clinical manifestations depend on the site of the lesion and the adequacy of collateral circulation.

All patients with symptoms of brain ischemia (TIA or completed stroke) should be rapidly evaluated. Once the diagnosis has been established, attention should be given to whether the patient may be a candidate for thrombolytic therapy. Patients who present within 3 hours from the onset of symptoms and have no contraindications are potential candidates for thrombolytic therapy with recombinant tissue plasminogen activator (rt-PA).

The initial diagnostic studies should include head CT, EKG, chest x-ray, hematologic studies, coagulation profile, sedimentation rate, electrolytes, and serum chemistries. Noninvasive vascular studies such as carotid Doppler/ultrasound or MR angiography and cardiac echocardiogram should be obtained, and in some cases intra-arterial angiography may be necessary. Systemic medical conditions that could worsen the cerebral ischemia, such as fluctuations in arterial blood pressure, cardiac dysrhythmias, hypoxia, hypoglycemia, or hyperglycemia, should be treated aggressively. Neurologic complications of acute brain ischemia include cerebral edema, hemorrhagic transformation of brain infarction, hydrocephalus, evidence of increased intracranial pressure, and epileptic seizures.

Patients with symptomatic internal carotid artery stenosis who have not proceeded to infarction should be considered for carotid endarterectomy. Consideration of this surgical procedure after brain infarction depends on the size of the stroke, extent of the neurologic deficit, and the general medical condition. Patients with established brain infarction and a stenotic carotid lesion are generally not treated with endarterectomy until approximately 8 weeks after infarction because of the risk of hemorrhagic conversion of the initial infarction. Patients with TIAs who are awaiting endarterectomy are typically anticoagulated with warfarin or receive antiplatelet agents. Risk factors for stroke should be treated or modified as much as possible.

The present patient initially suffered from recurrent TIAs in the vascular territory of the left internal carotid artery but unfortunately developed a completed ischemic stroke in the left cerebral hemisphere. Shortly after admission he had an episode of left amaurosis fugax and was promptly treated with intravenous heparin. Warfarin therapy was continued during 8 weeks of rehabilitation, and his symptoms and neurologic signs were minimal when left carotid endarterectomy was performed 9 weeks after the initial brain infarction. He has continued to do well on aspirin therapy, with aggressive control of hypertension, elevated cholesterol, and smoking cessation.

Clinical Pearls

1. TIAs should be regarded as warning signs of impending cerebral infarction and should be aggressively and rapidly evaluated to reduce stroke-related morbidity and mortality.

2. The risk of ischemic stroke is highest within the first several months following an initial TIA.

3. Acute stroke is a medical emergency that requires identification of the location of the lesion, determination of the underlying etiology, and initiation of appropriate therapy.

4. Most patients with symptomatic internal carotid stenosis should be considered for carotid endarterectomy.

REFERENCES

1. Adams HP Jr, Brott TG, Crowell RM, et al: Guidelines for the management of patients with acute ischemic stroke: A statement for healthcare professionals from a special writing group of the Stroke Council, American Heart Association. Stroke 1994; 25:1901–1914.
2. Feinberg WM, Albers GW, Barnett HJM, et al: Guidelines for the management of transient ischemic attacks: From the Ad Hoc Committee on Guidelines for the Management of Transient Ischemic Attacks of the Stroke Council of the American Heart Association. Circulation 1994; 89:2950–2965.
3. Levine RL: Cerebrovascular disease: Occlusive stroke and transient ischemic attacks. In Lechtenberg R, Schutta HS (eds): Neurology Practice Guidelines. New York, Marcel Dekker, 1998, pp 117–158.
4. Leys D, Mounier-Vehier F, Lavenu I, et al: Anterior choroidal artery territory infarcts. Study of presumed mechanisms. Stroke 1994; 25:837–842.
5. Moore WS, Barnett HJM, Beebe HG, et al: Guidelines for carotid endarterectomy: A multidisciplinary consensus statement from the Ad Hoc Committee, American Heart Association. Stroke 1995; 26:188–201.

INDEX

Page numbers in **boldface type** indicate complete cases.